T0260157

A Doctor among the Oglala Sioux Tribe

A **Doctor** among the Oglala Sioux Tribe

The Letters of Robert H. Ruby, 1953–1954

Robert H. Ruby | *Edited and with an introduction*
by Cary C. Collins *and* Charles V. Mutschler

University of Nebraska Press | Lincoln & London

Publication of this volume was assisted by
The Virginia Faulkner Fund, established in
memory of Virginia Faulkner, editor in chief
of the University of Nebraska Press.

Library of Congress Cataloging-in-
Publication Data

Ruby, Robert H.
Doctor among the Oglala Sioux Tribe: the
letters of Robert H. Ruby, 1953–1954 / Robert
H. Ruby; edited and with an introduction
by Cary C. Collins and Charles V. Mutschler.
p. cm.
Includes bibliographical references and
index.
ISBN 978-0-8032-2625-8 (cloth : alk. paper)
1. Oglala Sioux Tribe of the Pine Ridge
Reservation, South Dakota—History—
20th century. 2. Oglala Indians—South
Dakota—Pine Ridge Indian Reservation—
Social life and customs—20th century.
3. Community life—South Dakota—Pine
Ridge Indian Reservation—History—20th
century. 4. Oglala Indians—Medical
care—South Dakota—Pine Ridge Indian
Reservation—History—20th century.
5. Ruby, Robert H.—Correspondence.
6. Physicians—Nebraska—Pine Ridge
Indian Reservation—Correspondence.
7. Whites—Nebraska—Pine Ridge Indian
Reservation—Correspondence. 8. Pine
Ridge Indian Hospital (S.D.)—History—
20th century. I. Collins, Cary C.
II. Mutschler, Chas. V. (Charles Vincent),
1955– III. Title.
E99.O3R79 2010
978.004′975244—dc22
2009039102

Set in Minion by Kim Essman.

Contents

List of Illustrations . . . . *vi*

List of Maps. . . . . *vii*

List of Figures . . . . *viii*

Acknowledgments . . . . *ix*

Introduction:

The DeadliestWar . . . . *xi*

Timeline of Selected Events in the

Life of Robert H. Ruby, MD . . . . *lxv*

Editors' Comment on Editorial

Methodology. . . . . *lxix*

1. August 1953. . . . .*1*

2. September 1953 . . . .*22*

3. October 1953. . . . .*35*

4. November 1953. 49

5. December 1953. 67

6. January 1954. 78

7. February 1954. . . . .*100*

8. March 1954. . . . .*132*

9. April 1954 . . . .*154*

10. May 1954. . . . .*174*

11. June 1954. 204

12. July 1954 . . . .*220*

13. August 1954 . . . .*243*

14. September 1954 . . . .*274*

15. October 1954 300

16. November 1954 . . . .*313*

17. December 1954. . . . .*320*

Editors' Postscript. *324*

Appendix. *327*

Notes *329*

Bibliography *345*

Index *351*

Illustrations

following p. 112

Street scene, Pine Ridge, South Dakota, ca. 1940s

Street scene, Pine Ridge, South Dakota, ca. 1940s

Pine Ridge Hospital

Dr. Ruby's house, September 1953

Dr. Ruby in his U.S. Navy uniform, with Captain, July 1954

Dr. Ruby and daughter, Edna, 1954

Dr. Ruby in front of the new Pine Ridge Hospital, June 23, 2006

Charlie Yellow Boy, Edna Ruby, and Jeanne Ruby, Pine Ridge, 1954

Dr. Ruby on the front steps of Pine Ridge Indian Hospital, 1954

Lillian and Lawrence Mickelson with Edna Ruby, Pine Ridge, 1954

Typical reservation housing, near Manderson, South Dakota, 1954

White Coyote with team and wagon, 1953

Dr. Ruby outside their home in Pine Ridge, South Dakota, July 1954

Maps

1. Robert Ruby's Northwest . . . . *lxxi*
2. Washington State . . . . *lxxii*
3. South Dakota . . . . *lxxiii*
4. Indian Reservations in southwestern South Dakota . . . . . . *lxxiv*
5. Pine Ridge Indian Reservation
   and Environs . . . . *lxxiv*

Figures

1. Native American Church meeting altar arrangement..........*184*
2. Lacing pattern for drum used in "peyote service" *187*
3. Native American Church meeting altar arrangement..........*233*
4. Message to Great Spirit at Yuwipi service............. *268*

Acknowledgments

First and foremost, thank you to Dr. Robert H. Ruby for his willingness to allow us to publish his letters, which had been stored away for decades in the bottom of a cabinet in his home in Moses Lake, Washington. For several years we had been working with Dr. Ruby on historical projects related to his life, his writing career with his long-time coauthor John A. Brown, and Pacific Northwest Indian and white relations generally. In the course of our collaborations, Dr. Ruby frequently mentioned that he had been the head of the hospital on the Pine Ridge reservation and that he had written extensively about his service there. What he had composed were letters addressed to his sister, but when he spoke of his correspondence he often referred to what he called his "Pine Ridge diary." Like curious historians are inclined to do, we began asking him about the nature of his documentation. Initially Dr. Ruby shrugged off the importance of the letters, and our conversations with him really did not go very far. But we were persistent, and eventually he agreed to locate and share the letters with us.

The fact is that so much time had elapsed since Dr. Ruby had last looked at the letters (nearly a half century), he retained only a vague recollection of what was specifically contained in them, and, like us, he was startled to discover their elaborate and detailed descriptions of the functioning of the hospital and the overall state of affairs on the Pine Ridge reservation in the middle 1950s. The letters also revealed the story of Dr. Ruby and his late wife's experiences and the at once tragic and inspiring circumstances of the Oglala Sioux Tribe. Over time we came to believe that the letters were far too valuable to be stuffed back into that cabinet where they were likely to remain until someone at some point (and unthinkably to us historians) simply disposed of them. So the decision was made to edit them for publication. In guiding that process through to completion, we are grateful to the editors of the University of Nebraska Press for their receptive response and their immediate and sustained enthusiasm. We are also deeply indebted to the expert assistance and unflagging good cheer extended by Rose Krause, archivist extraordinaire at the Northwest Museum of Arts and Culture in Spokane, where Dr. Ruby's extensive collection of personal papers is housed. We thank Benjamin Reifel's daughter, Loyce Reifel Anderson, for her generous assistance in providing information about her father. At Pine Ridge we were assisted by Cheryl Hemingway, who shared with us rare family photographs of Pine Ridge, and Lisa Schrader-Dillon of the Oglala Sioux Tribe, who gave us an extensive tour of the still-standing old hospital building. Joe Svara grew up on the Pine Ridge reservation and from 1948 to 1957 owned and operated Joe's Market in Pine Ridge. Joe now lives in Sturgis, South Dakota, but met us in Rapid City to share his memories. Father Peter Klink, sj, president of Red Cloud Indian School (formerly Holy Rosary Mission), spent an afternoon filling us in on current conditions on the reservation. After all these years still a resident of McCall, Idaho, Dr. Ruby's sister (and the recipient of his letters), Marion Johnson, was always helpful and a delightful traveling companion (along with Dr. Ruby, she accompanied us to Pine Ridge), while closer to home we thank our families for their love, perseverance, and understanding: Cary's wife, Tina, and sons, James and Nick Collins, and Charlie's mother, Denise Mutschler.

Introduction

They drove throughout the day and into the evening, their unlikely destination Pine Ridge, South Dakota. It could be said "unlikely" because they had been married for only a couple weeks and to this point in their relatively young lives could claim absolutely no affiliation with either the Pine Ridge Indian Reservation or the members of the Oglala Sioux Tribe who lived there. It was August 1953, and Robert Ruby was a thirty-two-year-old U.S. Public Health Service surgeon assigned to Pine Ridge Indian Hospital. His bride, Jeanne (pronounced "Jean"), was three years younger than him and already a seasoned teacher of home economics. She had taught in several rural school districts in eastern Washington State. Together Robert and Jeanne had stuffed their belongings into their late-model olive green Pontiac coupe, scooped up their rascally black-and-white collie puppy, Captain, and pulled out of the driveway of Jeanne's mother's house in Chelan on the upper Columbia River. Although they could not have known it, they were setting off on a journey that in many ways would pave the way for the remainder of their lives.[1]

Even their first hours on the road were highly symbolic. On a hill, at a historic spot just above where the two-lane asphalt began to bend down into the majestic steep incline of White Bird Canyon on the River of No Return in west central Idaho, the Rubys edged over onto the shoulder of Highway 95. On this hallowed ground, near the site of the first major military engagement of the Nez Perce Indian War of 1877, they pitched camp. Robert and Jeanne prepared and ate a simple picnic dinner, rolled out sleeping bags, and passed a peaceful night with one sky above them. From White Bird Canyon, the Rubys resumed their flight into the future. For a couple days they delayed in McCall, Idaho, visiting with Robert's sister, Marion, her husband, and their children. Then, four days later, Robert and Jeanne were in Aberdeen, South Dakota. Robert had been directed to report to the Area Office of the Bureau of Indian Affairs (BIA) for an orientation meeting. Once that tedious chore was out of the way, Robert and Jeanne headed out again. Pointing their Pontiac in a southwesterly direction, they were within a day of catching their initial glimpses of their new home, their first home together.[2]

For the next year and a half the Rubys lived, labored, and learned on the Pine Ridge Indian Reservation. From the outset—and for the duration of their residency there—little seemed to go as planned. Robert had assumed he would be holding a staff position, but to his utter astonishment he was immediately named the hospital's medical officer in charge, a powerful administrative post that encompassed an extensive range of supervisory and bureaucratic responsibilities. Circumstance unfolded unexpectedly for Jeanne as well. She had thought her duties would be confined to concerns of home and family, but when a vacancy opened up in the government boarding school on the reservation, she reluctantly accepted the position of classroom teacher. It was in these ways then, within the orbit of their professional obligations and relationships, that the Rubys came to be looked at as important, recognizable public figures on the Pine Ridge reservation. On almost a daily basis they engaged in significant, meaningful interactions with the American Indian population, holding jobs, rendering services, and making decisions that directly impacted the Oglala Lakota people they were there to serve.[3]

The eighteen months spent by the Rubys in Pine Ridge, however, are noteworthy for another reason that could scarcely have been imagined in 1953 by anyone other than possibly Robert Ruby. From the very first days after he and Jeanne arrived on the reservation, he entered into an extensive, uninterrupted correspondence with his sister back in McCall. Diarylike, comprehensive, and candid, the letters that Robert wrote wove a profoundly revealing, personal accounting of reservation life at midcentury and, when assembled and presented as a cohesive document as they are here, deliver a memoirist's treatment of Ruby's experiences: what he saw and how he felt and reacted. Sweeping, frank, and insightful and crafted with the intimacy and sophistication that only a BIA insider could have, Ruby's letters described the massive, diverse, and complicated role that the government bureaucracy was continuing to play in the lives of the Oglala Lakota people into the 1950s and, perhaps more significantly, the ways in which the Native population was in turn negotiating and, as best as they were able, using the federal establishment to satisfy their own individual and collective needs and objectives.

Ruby's writings are informative from many perspectives. First, they provide a rare, first-person narrative of Indian health care, a critical and largely unexplored aspect of Indian and white relations in the twentieth century. The position Ruby held as medical officer in charge propelled him to the forefront of the most visible federal presence on the reservation. Pine Ridge Hospital functioned as a hub of community life where the most modern expressions of American society frequently intersected, and sometimes clashed, with those considered the most traditional and ancient. But in whatever guise, the hospital was more than anything a healing place where in Ruby's hands rested, both literally and figuratively, the physical well-being of the Oglala Lakota people.

As medical officer in charge, Ruby also assumed control over a sweep of programs and services that required his constant attention and supervision. Collectively these commanded appropriations that annually swelled into hundreds of thousands of dollars and employed a workforce that numbered among the largest on the reservation. It is not exaggeration that, other than the two positions of agency superintendent and superintendent of schools, the office that Ruby occupied was the most important and far reaching at Pine Ridge. The office, bringing him repeatedly into contact with the superintendent of the agency as well as with each of the other fifteen department heads that comprised the BIA administrative team, was the basis of collegial associations and interactions that privileged him with information and knowledge to which few others had access.

Second, Ruby proved an astute observer of people and cultures. Oglala Lakota history, traditions, and ceremonies intrigued and even mesmerized him, and he expended considerable time and energy documenting, often in exquisite detail, what he heard and saw. He traveled over the reservation and the region endeavoring to gain a sense of the place. In doing so, he sought out and befriended numerous members of the Oglala Lakota community, many of whom he interviewed, recorded, and photographed. In this regard Ruby initially found the Oglalas reticent and withdrawn in their interactions with him and, for that matter, with non-Indians generally. He made it a point, however, to try to set them at ease. Notably, he and Jeanne became the first agency employees to have Indians in their home socially, an act of uncommon hospitality and kindness that in addition to Jeanne's teaching and Robert's health care, helped win their confidence. It also drew the Rubys closely into association with many of the most prominent members of the tribe, those, for example, of the Red Cloud, Black Elk, and Standing Bear families—the children and grandchildren of those Oglala Lakota luminaries of the same name.

Third, Ruby's observations open a window onto the harsh socioeconomic conditions against which the Oglalas were constantly battling. For many tribal members, survival, even at a most meager level, posed a precarious proposition. Pine Ridge projected dolorous images of grinding poverty. The annual per capita income of the Oglalas ranked among the very lowest in the nation, and a vast majority of the reservation's inhabitants were eking out nothing more than bare existence. A large number were living in crudely constructed log shacks, and some only in tents—a deplorable state of affairs that was affording them almost no protection from the extreme climate, which could range from blistering summer heat to arctic winter cold. In addition, crime and alcoholism were rampant. Although federal law prohibited the selling of intoxicants on the reservation, several taverns located just two miles south across the Nebraska state line in Whiteclay, operated without restriction. Finally, the reservation appeared astonishingly out of step with modern industrial society. Few Oglalas owned cars and, exactly at the moment when the interstate highway system was beginning to fan out across the nation, horses and horse-drawn wagons remained visible sights at Pine Ridge. In sum, the reservation was different from anything Ruby had encountered, an always testing, always exacting foreign environment that demanded the best—and considerably more—than he or any public official could have been expected to give.[4]

A fourth reason the Ruby letters are valuable is the historical era that they seek to illuminate. The early 1950s represents a pivotal though understudied period of American Indian and white relations, a transition between two key phases of federal Indian policy: the Indian New Deal and termination. The former policy (dating from 1933 to 1945), despite its nod to cultural pluralism, tolerance, and revitalization, elicited criticism for tightening the grip of national controls over Indians and reservations. The latter policy (dating from 1945 to 1961) fell from favor for its attempts to scale back federal trust responsibilities. Ruby addressed the debate over these contrasting national prescriptions and what he foresaw as the potential ramifications of each for the Pine Ridge reservation and the Oglala Lakota people. An unintended but inescapable consequence of the Indian New Deal, he came to believe, was the gradual, ever-increasing dependence of the Oglalas upon government programs and services. For Ruby, it was a debilitating, unacceptable erosion of self-sufficiency that compelled him to embrace aspects of the policy of termination.[5]

Fifth, Pine Ridge was then, and it remains so today, among the most recognizable and important Indian reservations in the United States. Having served as a witness to numerous remarkable and tragic events in history, what has transpired there has often been considered the harbinger of a deeper story bearing national implications. Ruby recognized the special niche of this place in the collective American psyche, and he sought to reconcile what had happened in the past with what he was experiencing in the present with what he thought might play out in the future. In part, his motivation for writing stemmed from the forward-looking assumption that his observations, if preserved, might someday be of value. He was acting on a conviction that he was capturing snapshots of moments in time that were in jeopardy of being lost and could not otherwise be salvaged or much less reproduced, save through his admittedly imperfect although always tenacious attempts to get them down on paper, tape, and film.

Finally, the published memoirs of bia officials, particularly those documenting this historical era and subject, number relatively few. By making publicly accessible the writings of Robert Ruby, a contemporaneous voice is added to a historical account that has often had to rely on and has been dominated by government documents and reports. Similarly, they also provide a useful corollary to the plethora of American Indian memoirs, reminiscences, and biographies that have appeared in recent years, offering details, opinions, and interpretations that would have been inappropriate to include in official correspondence. By introducing into the mix the nonofficial writings of federal personnel such as Robert Ruby, a more textured and layered understanding of public policies and programs is made possible as is the construction of richer and more nuanced histories. The result is a better-informed readership.

Robert Holmes Ruby was born on April 23, 1921, in Mabton, Washington. He grew up there on a forty-five-acre farm that bordered the Yakama Indian Reservation. His father raised potatoes and also kept a garden, and when Ruby was a boy it was not an unusual occurrence for Indian people to stop by the family home seeking food. It was in his hometown, slogging as a journalist for his high school and local city newspapers, that Ruby got his start as a writer. What he wrote could boast scant historical content, but the satisfaction that he took away from the process of preparing his essays caused him to flirt with the notion of one day becoming a professional newspaperman. However, after graduating from Mabton High School in 1939 and enrolling in Whitworth College in Spokane, it was premed that he chose as his major. Yet his pen remained active. Again Ruby enlisted his services as a reporter, this time for his college newspaper. He had the good fortune of interviewing and writing on such notable public figures as Paul Robeson, Marian Anderson, and Lily Pons.[6]

In three years Ruby's coursework at Whitworth was finished, and he then continued his education by entering the Washington University School of Medicine in St. Louis. The years he spent in the Midwest, preparing for a career in health care, Ruby has noted, were one of only two times in his life that he lived apart from Indians.[7]

Following his graduation from medical school in 1945, the pace of Ruby's life quickened. He wrapped up a nine-month internship in Detroit and was inducted into the U.S. Army Air Corps. For twenty months he served in Denver, Los Angeles, and finally with American occupation forces in Japan. After his discharge in December 1947, he began training as a surgeon. Ruby took a fellowship at the Sugarbaker Cancer Clinic in Jefferson City, Missouri, and completed a year of postgraduate study at Washington University. He then spent four years in pathology and general surgery at a hospital in St. Louis.[8]

But the track that he was on soon veered in another direction. At the outbreak of the Korean War, Ruby was conscripted back into the military. Fortuitously, a clause contained in the Doctor-Dentist Draft Law of 1950 granted physicians their preference of service, and Ruby opted to join the Public Health Service, the government agency charged with supplying doctors to the U.S. Coast Guard, the American diplomatic corps, and the U.S. Indian Service. Visions of hobnobbing in some exotic foreign embassy briefly flashed through Ruby's mind, but when he received his assignment, it turned out to be with the Indian Service. He was given administrative supervision over the Indian hospital on the Pine Ridge reservation. Make no mistake. Pine Ridge was a world apart from the likes of a Cairo or Tokyo, but waiting was a life-altering experience.[9]

In 1953 Pine Ridge was a way-out-of-the-way frontier town of some 1,250 inhabitants, the great majority of whom were American Indian. The village lay on the southern edge of the two-million-acre (an expanse the size of several small states) Pine Ridge Indian Reservation, which sat on the extreme southernmost border of South Dakota. In Ruby's memory, Pine Ridge looked "just like an old western town with beaten-down frame buildings, mostly dirt streets, no sidewalks, and a few streetlights," a stark image that prompted him to remark, "It wasn't pretty." There was one main street, one school, one post office, one tribal agency, two service stations (Hemingway Texaco and Gerbers), two grocery stores (Hagels and Joe's Market), one bank, one variety store (the Pejuta Tepee), one hotel (Gerbers), one barbershop (Salaway's), many churches (for example, Catholic, Episcopalian, Presbyterian, and Church of Jesus Christ of Latter-Day Saints faiths), one state welfare office, and one hospital. There was no tavern, no restaurant, no theater (on weekends movies were shown at Holy Rosary Mission but only for students attending the school), no clothing, hardware, or department stores, no police department (other than the agency tribal police), no fire department, no funeral home (a mortician from the Chamberlain Funeral Home in Rushville, Nebraska, removed bodies, prepared them for burial, and then returned them to the reservation), no Laundromat, no car dealership, no pharmacy (medicines were issued directly to patients by hospital staff), no radio or television stations, no newspaper, no telephone service after 5:00 in the evening (that was when the operator went home), and no public library, swimming pool, or park. The nearest major city was Rapid City, 110 miles to the northwest. The much smaller, though more convenient Chadron, Nebraska, was half that distance to the southwest. In order to procure goods and services unavailable in Pine Ridge, agency employees also frequented other population centers such as Hot Springs, South Dakota, and Gordon and Rushville, Nebraska.[10]

Pine Ridge was located on the Great Plains and not in the American South, but elements of de facto segregation governed social relations in the town in a manner similar to that dominant in other sections of the country. In his masterful *Blood Struggle: The Rise of Modern Indian Nations*, the attorney and historian Charles Wilkinson has described the settlement—the largest on the reservation—as it appeared when Ruby lived there. Pine Ridge was separated into two halves, neither of which seemed to have anything in common with the other. "Highway 18 laid down a line of demarcation," Wilkinson asserted. "The west side was the white side, with the BIA office building, the jail, the BIA boarding school, and housing for federal employees." It was here where the Rubys and most of the hospital staff lived. Meanwhile, the other side of the road presented a different picture. "To the east," Wilkinson continued, "lay a shantytown, home to Indian people, a place devoid of the plumbing and electricity that served the community across the highway." In Wilkinson's assessment, neither the reservation nor its Native inhabitants exhibited much of the influence of non-Oglala society. "Many old men in Pine Ridge wore their hair in long braids, Lakota style, but the outlying villages—Porcupine, Wanblee, Yellow Bear, Kyle, Allen, and others—were even more resolutely traditional. Out in the backcountry, families sheltered in tipis, tents, and log cabins lived much as the Lakota had for centuries."[11]

Casting a long shadow over everything was the BIA. Characterized by Wilkinson as "'The Company' in a company town," there was virtually no aspect of reservation life that escaped the sticky reach of this federal agency. "The bureau dominated the economy as employer, purchaser, and consumer. It handed down the laws and ran the police and courts. It controlled the tribe's only economic asset, the fair-to-middling rangelands" and, "far from promoting Lakota interests," leased "vast expanses of grazing land to large non-Indian cattle companies at rates well below market value." Each district on the reservation was assigned a subagent who controlled almost every move. The permission of these functionaries, known as boss farmers, was necessary for an Oglala farmer to as much as sell a cow. Even more restricting was the fact that all lease payments had to be sent directly to the BIA, which in turn paid Oglala property holders not in cash but in vouchers, a procedure that in essence required the Indians to justify how they were spending their own money.[12]

Equally powerful were cultural and social repressions. In schools, both those operated by the BIA and ones under church supervision, children were immersed in the precepts of Christianity, but at the neglect of their traditional Oglala beliefs. And that was only one area of socialization. Students were prohibited from speaking their Lakota language, their braids were cut, and all Native life ways were denigrated as "pagan and savage." When something as seemingly benign as the sound of drumming wafted through the reservation, school instructors informed their impressionable charges that what they were hearing was "devil worship." Another example was the suppression of Sun Dance. The most important and enduring Oglala Lakota ceremony, having been banned since 1881 and driven underground by the BIA, Sun Dance was finally restored and allowed to be practiced publicly in the early 1950s. But as Wilkinson pointed out, it was only "under tightly controlled circumstances." Piercing, he related, was not permitted until the late 1950s, and even then strictly "upon certification from the BIA in Washington."[13]

Through all this, however, the Pine Ridge reservation remained the embodiment and keeper of the Oglala Lakota's most cherished possession. The vigilant guardian of their traditions, culture, and past and the basis and bedrock of their tribal sovereignty, it was as valuable as life, a bulwark that had enabled the Oglala Lakota to withstand the strongest assimilationist assault thrust against them. This vital sustainer of all things, timeless and with no beginning and no end and the very marrow of their existence, was their land. Ruby's letters reveal and lend weight to Wilkinson's apt assertion: That this place was so much more than the barren wasteland that often met the gaze of the traveler just passing through. For the Oglala Lakota the reservation, in all its manifestations, was simply the familiar they knew as home. As Wilkinson poignantly wrote, "To the Sioux, the reservation was the setting for the tribe's long history, the tragic and the uplifting and the ordinary, the place where all the ancestors had been buried in ceremony, the locale for all of Grandfather's stories. The land was a broad, ever-present charter—writ in sky and flowing grass, in low hills and cottonwood hollows and piney ridges—of freedom from the difficulties of daily life. Even the Badlands of the northern part of the reservation, a rough, choppy, eroded-out terrain of gullies and buttes, carried Lakota memories and were home to scattered families on plots far from any road."[14]

It was against this backdrop that Robert Ruby accepted administrative responsibility over the Pine Ridge Hospital. At the time he embarked upon his duties, he knew very little or absolutely nothing of the issues and problems articulated by Wilkinson, of the Oglala Lakotas and their history and culture, of the terrible trials that simultaneously burdened and challenged their survival. All this had to be learned, and to Ruby's credit, he did learn. With enthusiasm and energy, he immersed himself in the reservation and its people. As he elevated them as his foremost interest and priority, he seized on almost every encounter as an opportunity to increase his knowledge and understanding. Part of what Ruby came to realize was that at Pine Ridge he had been appointed to, and assigned administrative control over, a hospital and a health care system that were the products of complex and substantial histories, ones that had been a full seventy-five years in the making and were an integral component of the even longer and more complicated relationship that existed between the Oglala Lakota and the United States government.[15]

Morning for Indian health care in America emerged out of a most virulent night. The first formal attempt of the federal government to provide services dates to 1832. That year Congress appropriated moneys to purchase and administer smallpox vaccine. Missionaries active in Indian country also attended the sick, a few doctors were hired and assigned to agencies, and army personnel were employed. In the main, however, those pioneering efforts proved insufficient, irregular, and poorly coordinated, an ill-defined and incoherent pattern that, at least in the near term, persisted. In 1873 the BIA established a Medical and Education Division but then proceeded to dismantle the medical arm only four years later in 1877. Want of funds was offered as the reason for the reversal, and almost another half-century would pass before a similar administrative bureau was authorized to oversee the health needs of the American Indians.[16]

In a legal sense, federal obligation to furnish Indian people with health care was solemnized in treaties that, among other assumed benefits, promised medical assistance in exchange for cessions of land and land title. Over time the articles contained in treaties were sustained, extended, and bolstered through a succession of legislative acts, judicial decisions, settlements, and agreements. In the early reservation period and after the end of the Civil War the federal government began staffing Indian agencies with physicians who were required to supply their own medicines and attend to patients scattered over immense distances and living on widely separated reservations. In some instances, the accessibility of those doctors was so constricted—in 1874 only about half of the agencies had doctors—that some local agents felt compelled to learn the rudiments of medicine in order to be able to treat minor ailments and respond to emergencies. Perhaps not surprisingly, many reservation boarding schools, some entrusted with the well-being of scores of students, operated without the benefit of any medical supervision, and it is worth noting that in 1900 only eighty-three physicians were serving the entire American Indian population of the United States and its territories.[17]

Substantial federal support for developing a comprehensive and systematic system of Indian health care was marshaled in the activist term of Commissioner of Indian Affairs Thomas J. Morgan. Although Morgan has been the target of no small battery of criticism leveled by historians for what many contended were his heavy-handed tactics in carrying out federal policies of assimilation, he was an outspoken proponent of securing basic medical care for all Indians. In fact, their acceptance of modern treatment methods was perceived by Morgan as incontrovertible evidence of their acculturation. To him, those were the parts of a piece, the one a verifiable measure of the other, a potent symbol of Indians' evolution out of so-called barbarism and into civilization. "The Indian 'medicine' men are ignorant, superstitious, sometimes cruel, and resort to the most grotesque practices," Morgan proclaimed. "The only rational medical treatment comes not from among themselves, but is that which is furnished by the Government physicians."[18]

Morgan was not the first commissioner of Indian affairs to have taken up the mantle of Indian health care. In fact, his two immediate predecessors "sought to develop criteria for a more professional medical corps." However, according to the historian Robert A. Trennert, who has written extensively of developments on the Navajo reservation, their initiatives and proposals for reform sounded better than they were in practice, whereas Morgan managed to achieve tangible, quantifiable results.[19]

In 1890 the commissioner spearheaded a lobbying campaign to create an office of medical supervisor. As he envisioned the major tenets of the position, management of the health of the American Indian population would reside with this official as would the duty of formulating a ledger of qualifiers and job descriptors for the employees of the Indian medical field service. When Morgan submitted his ideas, no such all-encompassing administrative post existed within the federal bureaucracy. "This very important branch of the service is without competent supervision," Morgan decried shortly after he assumed office. "There is no professional head. The supervisor of the medical service should require the entire time of a competent expert."[20]

Troubling to the commissioner was the lack of uniform, prescribed official requirements and carefully crafted best practices in force regulating the hiring and monitoring the performance of medical personnel. Rather than approved criteria and clearly enunciated departmental policies and guidelines guiding decisions, the quality and expertise of staff was mostly left to chance. On the positive side, Morgan felt certain that "Many of the men . . . serving as physicians" were "of high personal character, of good professional attainment and experience," and faithful in the "performance of their duties." Unfortunately, those were traits not shared by all. In other instances, for reasons as serious as "immorality, neglect of duty, incompetency, or unprofessional conduct," Morgan had found it necessary to dismiss doctors from the medical branch. He was quick to point out, however, that under his watch care had been taken to have their places filled with individuals considered "trustworthy and competent."[21]

In Morgan's eyes, the most glaring deficiency in the hiring practices of the BIA was the absence of a formal assessment to quantify the competency of applicants. The process in place, as he discovered when he took office, obligated doctors only "to produce a diploma from some reputable medical school and to submit testimonials as to moral character and correct habits." The degree stipulation had been in effect since 1878, but from Morgan's perspective, it constituted a slight advancement. "Their appointments," he asserted, were "not guarded with that care which the nature of the services required of them demands." Morgan believed that rigorous standards needed to be devised, adopted, and followed. "No one should be appointed except upon an examination as to his health, his professional attainments, and his moral qualifications," the commissioner declared. "In addition to his qualifications for general practice, his ability to give instruction on hygienic subjects to school pupils should be tested, and he should possess such scientific and practical knowledge as will prepare him to have an oversight of the entire sanitary conditions of a whole tribe. In short, he should be capable of being a health officer as well as a physician and surgeon."[22]

To amplify the challenges of the reservation physician, Morgan contrasted the duties and requisite compensation of Indian Service personnel with that of their counterparts serving in the army and navy. What he found was disturbing. Compared to the American soldier, the

American Indian was receiving substantially less in the way of federal support for health care. For example, in the army and navy in 1890, 352 surgeon-physicians—this was how they were labeled—were treating a combined military force of 36,694. The Indian Service, meanwhile, employed 82 surgeon-physicians caring for a national Indian population set at 180,184. As one might suppose, the patient load carried by medical personnel depended upon the branch of service to which one belonged. On average, the army surgeon-physician was treating 137 patients annually, the navy surgeon-physician 72 patients, and the Indian Service surgeon-physician a staggering 830 patients. Salaries told a similar story. Surgeon-physicians assigned to the army and navy earned an average yearly wage of about $2,700, compared to the Indian Service surgeon-physician's $1,028. In total, almost one million dollars was appropriated in 1890 to the army and navy for medical purposes whereas the Indian Service received a sum of $84,300. Those amounts equated to $21.91 spent on each army patient, $48.10 on each navy patient, and a paltry $1.25 on each Indian patient.[23]

To address some of these jarring inequities, Morgan submitted a blueprint that he hoped would "bring medical aid within the reach of all Indians." To delay or fail to act on his recommendations, the commissioner warned, was to leave "thousands of Indians at these agencies . . . utterly unable to have medical care when necessary." Morgan couched his efforts as an attempt to stem "a large degree of needless suffering" and prevent "hundreds of deaths." His plan called for a thorough examination of those candidates applying for government medical positions and the payment of competitive salaries to those meeting the qualifications for and accepting employment. His proposal aimed to eliminate political considerations as a factor in making appointments, substituting the operational principle of "for cause" as the only basis for retaining and terminating employees. In addition, Morgan wanted a hospital "connected with every boarding school" and "at every large agency a general hospital for the severe cases of illness that require treatment which can not be given at the homes." Finally, so they could begin working professionally among their own people and holding up Charles Eastman, Carlos Montezuma, and Susan La Flesche as three individuals who had graduated from medical school and then gone on to successful practice, Morgan urged training Indians as doctors and nurses.[24]

Those ameliorating steps notwithstanding, Morgan anticipated a tough road ahead, at least in the near term. Militating against quick returns was an overwhelming demand for services counterbalanced against a grudging level of support seeping out of the Indian Bureau in Washington DC. Medical personnel worked grueling hours under the most challenging circumstances for subpar pay. "The duties devolving upon the physician are very severe," Morgan attested. "He has the work of a surgeon and physician, with the sanitary oversight of people with whose language he is unfamiliar and who are ignorant, superstitious, and predisposed to a great variety of diseases. He must be his own apothecary; he usually has no hospital and no nurses, and his patients have few of the most ordinary comforts of home, and little, if any, intelligent care in the preparation of their food or the administering of prescribed medicine. He is alone and has to cope with accident and disease without consultation, with few books, and but few surgical instruments."[25]

As it turned out, Morgan's initiatives were slow to gain traction, a sluggish response that caused the commissioner to ramp up the decibels of his rhetoric. In 1892 he characterized the miserly level of health care being provided to the American Indians as a "national disgrace." In raising the issue with the secretary of the interior again, Morgan called attention to the impossible situation that existed on the Pine Ridge reservation. It was "simply absurd to attempt, with only one physician," he postulated, "to care for the wants of more than 5,000 Indians, scattered over a territory almost as large as Connecticut." Emblematic of the Spartan support simmered a galling reality. Not a single hospital, not at Pine Ridge and not anywhere else in the United States, had been built specifically for the relief of Indians. "There still exists among Indian tribes the same urgent and pitiful need for proper medical attendance and hospital service," Morgan agonized. "Indian reservations have no hospitals and no place to which persons suffering from acute diseases, severe accidents, contagious diseases, or any other physical malady can be taken, and in which they can receive the nursing and care and medical attendance which they sorely need, and which ought to be furnished them in the name of humanity." Lives rested in the balance, Morgan pleaded. "Left to themselves they suffer unnecessarily and miserably perish." The commissioner reminded his superior that "again and again" he had "urged this matter." Estimates for funds had been submitted "which might be used in the establishment of hospitals among Indians." But a tightfisted Congress had failed to approve the appropriations, thereby reducing his most strenuous exertions to nothing and leaving both him and the Indian Bureau "powerless to remedy a great evil."[26]

The vision of the commissioner extended beyond the purview of just hospitals. He pressed for the authorization of a series of "asylums," including "almshouses for the blind, deaf, insane, the incurables, and the aged and other helpless and destitute Indians." In Morgan's opinion, failure to act was tantamount to the United States neglecting to meet its solemn trust obligations to the American Indians. "There is nothing for them," he warned fatalistically, "but neglect, pain and exposure until death ends their sufferings."[27]

In large measure the temporizing hopes of Commissioner Morgan were to be realized in the educational realm of Indian affairs. With the emergence of the off-reservation boarding school movement in 1879, doctors began to be added to the rosters of school staffs, and as the federal Indian education system expanded, appropriations were allocated for the construction of clinics and hospitals. In the early 1890s, in no small part as a result of the concerted efforts of Commissioner Morgan, nurses appeared on the federal payroll for the first time, and a field nurse program was inaugurated on reservations. Furnishing Indian families with direct home instruction on the benefits of cleanliness, hygiene, and routine doctor's care, field nurses also imparted nutritional advice, homemaking skills, and prenatal care. By the turn of the century, a degree of health care was to be had for most students enrolled in off-reservation boarding schools, facilities such as Carlisle in Pennsylvania and Chemawa in Oregon. In fact, on some campuses separate infirmaries were constructed for the treatment of tuberculosis, a scourge to Indian people and a leading cause of their mortality. In 1909, in conjunction with the efforts underway in off-reservation boarding schools, an office of medical supervisor was added to the Educational Division of the BIA.[28]

On November 2, 1921, Congress approved legislation that was to profoundly impact the future of Indian health care in the United States. Public Law 67–85, popularly known as the Snyder Act, moved beyond anything previously done. Authorizing discretionary appropriations for "the relief of distress and conservation of health" of American Indians and Alaska Natives, funds were earmarked for the benefit, care, and assistance of this targeted group and, as the primary means by which physicians and other medical personnel were to be hired, offered tangible evidence of a more active, direct, comprehensive, and systematic involvement by the national government in this emerging sphere. Under the statutory authority vested in the Snyder Act, members of federally recognized tribes who resided on reservations were declared eligible to receive services and the commitment of the American government to administer the health care needs of Indians appeared beyond question.[29]

The principles articulated in the Snyder Act were augmented in 1924 by the creation of a separate Medical Division under the authority of the BIA and the Department of the Interior. Another change occurred in 1926. That year "physicians from the Commissioned Corps of the United States Public Health Service were first assigned to Indian health programs." This ostensibly remained the status quo until August 5, 1954—although Indian New Deal–era legislation allowed the secretary of the interior to contract with states and territories for equivalent-level services—when the Indian Health Service was formed as a separate agency operating under the Public Health Service and the newly organized Department of Health, Education and Welfare, today known as Health and Human Services. The transition, which created the only national health program in American history for civilians, became official on July 1, 1955, six months after Robert Ruby left Pine Ridge.[30]

The introduction of health care to the Oglala Lakota living on the Pine Ridge reservation suffered through the same fits and starts characteristic of the national scene. In 1878, shortly after Red Cloud Agency on the North Platte River in eastern Wyoming was removed to its present location on White Clay Creek in South Dakota and reconstituted there as Pine Ridge Agency, health care came to represent a gradual but ever-growing focus of the local federal bureaucracy. To varying degrees, and sometimes with considerable overlap, tribal members received services through one of two government entities: the agency physician and the physician assigned to the boarding school at Pine Ridge. Often the same person occupied both positions, and from almost the outset the level of need far outweighed the ability, or the willingness, of the national government to meet the health requirements of the Oglala Lakota people. For several decades after the relocation of the agency, and up until the time when Ruby served as medical officer in charge, agents, inspectors, and doctors kept up a relentless drumbeat for increased appropriations, additional personnel, and improved facilities.

In terms of medicine and care, the early 1890s—those formative years in which Commissioner Morgan sat in office—represented flush times in the development of the village of Pine Ridge. During that period physicians were hired, a hospital was constructed, methods were standardized, and services were expanded. But at least one government official expressed grave concerns about the location of the agency and the benefits it could offer for healthful living. Chas. G. Penney, the agent assigned to the reservation, advised the commissioner of Indian affairs of a series of factors that he believed could deleteriously impact the quality of life of the Oglala Lakota people. Foremost among those were diseases borne of water and sewerage. "The question of water supply and house drainage must also receive immediate attention, if the location of the agency is not changed," Penney wrote. "For many years people have lived here in numbers, making quite a good-sized village, and absolutely without any attention to the laws of health. The whole ground is honey combed with privy vaults and cess pools, abandoned and in use, and the earth is reeking with filth, covered and out of sight, but none the less certain to do its deadly work as soon as the wells shall be contaminated. A pestilence is sure to follow, sooner or later, [on account of] persistence in this violation of the common laws of sanitation."[31]

From a federal perspective, another threat to the health of the Oglala Lakota was the tenacity of traditional methods of healing among them. Shamans—symbols of "barbarism personified" in the words of Pine Ridge Indian agent V. T. McGillycuddy—were active both during and after the Ruby era, but in the late nineteenth century they posed a substantial obstacle, or at least that was the perception. In August 1884 agency physician J. Ashley Thompson attributed "the large ratio of mortality . . . among children . . . to exposure and the harsh practices of their relatives, a majority of whom have not the remotest idea of the indispensable [necessity of] nursing and ordinary hygiene; hence it is, [that] many reliable prescriptions fail to benefit and they [that is, the patients, ultimately] return to their medicine men."[32]

Thompson's sense was that the Oglala Lakota did not "enjoy immunity from sickness any more than other races." However, so "wedded to the pernicious influence of the medicine men" were they and so often were those "empirics" encountered in the course of Thompson's daily rounds that he was prompted to conjecture that a "brief sojourn" in Pine Ridge would "impress one with a belief that they were nearly all—men and women—of that vocation."[33]

Thompson, partly due to the presence of shamans but also because of a general paucity of medical knowledge prevalent among the Indians, considered his duties onerous. The Oglalas' maladies ranged from "simple constipation to 'misery all over,'" he reported. "Tubercular diseases, diseases of the digestive system, of the respiratory organs, of the eye, and of the skin (the latter in great variety), of more or less gravity," were presented to him daily for treatment. In one sense, Thompson felt gratified. In most instances it had been possible for "routine treatment" to be applied. But things did not always go so well. He bemoaned that the Oglalas, after receiving their medicines, were usually never heard from again "for months, if ever, so little" did they comprehend "the necessity of systematic treatment."[34]

To alleviate some of the burden of laboring as a single physician responsible for the welfare of potentially thousands of patients occupying a vast geographic area and many exhibiting a pronounced aversion to his services, Thompson requested that he be furnished with at least one of the following: "an apothecary, an assistant physician, or limited hospital accommodations—about 10 beds—for such of the sick or injured who come . . . to the agency for treatment, and have to return [home] forthwith without receiving material benefit in one visit, because at present there is no provision for shelter and sustenance of the sick."[35] Thompson's recommendations were not immediately acted upon, but definitive steps toward addressing some of them were not to be long in coming.

Much of what is known of the earliest days on the Pine Ridge reservation, particularly those issues related to the budding field of health care, derives from the writings of Charles Eastman. A mixed-blood Santee Sioux from Minnesota, Eastman played a pivotal role in treating survivors in the aftermath of the Wounded Knee Massacre. Educated in medicine at Boston University, he served from 1890 to 1892 as the government physician at Pine Ridge Agency and, in an autobiography entitled *From the Deep Woods to Civilization* (1916), described the spare, crude structures he encountered in his inaugural assignment as medical officer in charge and his experiences caring for the Oglala Lakota people. In comparing the observations of Eastman to those of Ruby, it seems that in some respects time stood still at Pine Ridge. Eastman, in phrases reminiscent of those that would be echoed six decades later by Ruby, soberly recalled his initial impressions of his new station: "Pine Ridge Indian agency was a bleak and desolate looking place in those days," he reminisced, "more especially in a November dust storm such as that in which I arrived from Boston to take charge of the medical work of the reservation."[36]

Eastman was one of the first American Indian doctors hired into the Indian Service and was the same age, thirty-two, as Ruby when he located to Pine Ridge. Self-described as "athletic and vigorous, and alive with energy and enthusiasm," Eastman found himself thrust into an environment that tested those qualities. After reporting to the Indian agent for duty, he was escorted to his quarters, which, he discovered, consisted of a bedroom, a sitting room, an office, and a dispensary all arranged in a single long barrack that adjoined the police quarters and the agent's offices. As remembered by Eastman, this was a "flimsy one-story affair built of warped cottonwood lumber" that allowed the "rude prairie winds" to whistle "musically through the cracks." The trappings were austere. "There was no carpet, no furniture save a plain desk and a couple of hard wooden chairs," Eastman wrote, "and everything was coated with a quarter of an inch or so of fine Dakota dust."[37]

Eastman stepped up to the challenges set before him. To help him "in cleaning and overhauling" the premises, he engaged the services of an Oglala woman. He then shifted his attention to the real work at hand. His first order of business was sealing a hole in the wall through which his predecessors had dispensed medicines. Previous doctors, rather than examining patients from inside the barracks, preferred doling out sundry "pills and potions to a crowd of patients standing in line." Eastman, in contrast, hung a sign outside the entranceway that in carefully printed bold letters invited the Oglalas to come inside.[38]

His busiest time, Eastman recounted, occurred during a remarkable reservation-wide event known as the "Big Issue," in which the usually staid village of Pine Ridge was transformed into a "veritable 'Wild West.'" For the Big Issue, thousands of Indians either walked or rode in from across the reservation in order to receive their bimonthly distribution of government annuities and rations. Eastman painted a colorful portrait of the chaotic scene that invariably played out on the streets and inside the enclosed structures of Pine Ridge. Scores of patients were seen, and medicines were handed out "as if from a lemonade stand at a fair." In the course of his first Big Issue, Eastman learned firsthand of the Oglalas' penchant for self-diagnosis and their proclivity for self-prescribing their own "particular drug or ointment," their favorite being "a mixture of cod liver oil and alcohol." Eastman recalled the surprise of the Oglalas when he insisted upon examining each patient before giving them medicine and their similar response upon realizing that he was able to converse with them "in plain Sioux—no interpreter needed!" Eastman "made a record of interesting cases," noting specifically where the Oglalas were encamped. He intended "to visit as many as possible in their teepees before they took again to the road."[39]

Eastman took an abiding interest in the health of the Oglala Lakota, and his unceasing labors on their behalf proved highly rewarding. Soon hundreds of patients were being examined, a daunting caseload that unfortunately sapped Eastman's energies to the point that he eventually deemed it necessary to appeal to the Indian agent for the services of a dispensary assistant and a trained nurse. Included in his petition was a team and buggy, a hospital for the most serious cases, and a house for him to live in. To his surprise, all his requests were granted, and once hired, the dispensary assistant assumed responsibility for putting up "the common salves and ointments, the cough syrups and other mixtures which were in most frequent demand." But, for the most part, Eastman had little to work with. At Pine Ridge there was "no conveyance for the doctor's professional use, and indeed no medical equipment worthy the name." At the agency the "doctor was thrown entirely upon his own resources, without the support of colleagues, and there was no serious attempt at sanitation or preventive work." Out of his own pocket, Eastman purchased many of the needed medical supplies and instruments.[40]

Two factors accounted for much of the success that Eastman believed was achieved during his short tenure: his ethnicity and his heartfelt empathy for the members of the Pine Ridge community. According to a contemporary, Eastman managed to forge a formidable reputation that quickly "traveled the length and breadth of the reservation." He imposed "a new order of things" in which equal treatment was received by all and his instructions, which ranged from plain spoken medical advice to complex explanations of "physiology and hygiene," were understood by all. "No Government doctor," it was alleged, had "ever gone freely" among the Oglala Lakota as Eastman did. "[A] good part" of his "days and not a few" of his "nights" were spent "in the saddle," attempting to reach "the most distant parts of the reservation."[41]

By the early 1890s and just over a decade after the creation of Pine Ridge Agency, two hospitals were in operation on the reservation. The first, an appendage of the Oglala boarding school, was available to all members of the reservation community, including students. The second, a field hospital, was set up for those patients who could not conveniently be transported to the hospital connected to the boarding school. The school hospital—interchangeably known as Pine Ridge Hospital and Oglala Boarding School Hospital—was a relatively large three-story structure that had been proposed for construction in November 1889 and began admitting patients almost three years to the day later in November 1892. Featured was a full basement with storerooms and a heating plant, two wards for patients, and an attractive exterior landscaped in lawns, flowers, trees, and cement walkways.

But from the moment of its inception, Pine Ridge Hospital was beset with an inordinate array of problems. For one, the building sat on an isolated, exposed parcel of land that allowed the "cold winter winds" to strike "from all quarters." In addition, the design of the hospital was said to be flawed. It was equipped with only one means of exit, through the front door, and the upper two floors, where the patient wards were housed, had no running water. In fact, all water in the hospital originated from a single source, a faucet attached over the kitchen sink. Even greater causes for consternation were a sewage system placed too near the building and a steam plant so inadequate that woodstoves had to be resorted to. Unfortunately, those turned out to be a poor alternative because the large stoves needed "to heat the rooms to a comfortable degree" could not be used without restricting the number of beds in each ward to only two. Finally, space had not been set aside for storing and dispensing medicines, and even the shape of the wards was described as "defective" and "ill adapted to hospital purposes."[42]

Such was the imperfect state of repair of this new modern hospital, and administrators struggled to attract and retain personnel. According to J. S. Pede, the first medical officer in charge, "Owing to the incomplete condition of the building, its isolated situation and the meager means for convenience and comfort, but few employes could be found who could be contented with the service in the hospital." Pede commented, "Without exception all the employes constantly complained that the work was too severe and onerous." The exhaustive "climbing up and down the stairs between three floors, the bustle and litter made by two wards full of patients—at one time 19 in number—who bring with them many of the habits of camp life, and who understand nothing of the methods of treating the sick to which they are subjected," he related, "cause the female employes to break down in a short time, with the result that soon their places have to be filled by others." To ease the stress felt by his staff, Pede lobbied for the installation of a dumbwaiter and speaking tubes.[43]

Despite the deficiencies that were plaguing the building, Pine Ridge had been made beneficiary of a mostly functional hospital, one of the first in the Indian Service. In the spring of 1893, when Dr. Z. T. Daniel arrived on the reservation to assume the duties of agency physician, he was able to convey his pleasant surprise at finding "a small hospital here with a full corps of employees." Daniel had worked at Blackfeet Agency in Montana and Green Bay Agency in Wisconsin, and in comparison to Pine Ridge, he judged both of those stations lacking. At Pine Ridge he enumerated a hospital staff that consisted of a steward, a matron, a nurse, an assistant nurse, a cook, and a janitor. Two field matrons were assigned to outlying districts, and a field hospital had been established to accommodate those cases that could not be treated in the regular hospital.[44]

But infrastructure was only a single strand in a complex dynamic. Pine Ridge Hospital suffered in other areas as well. Most immediately, the restrictiveness of an institutionalized environment conflicted with the natural rhythms of the Oglalas while the very nature of a hospital setting, especially in terms of symbolism, was not always compatible with Indian customs, values, and beliefs. Daniel, in his annual report for 1894, flagged some of these social and cultural collisions. "Notwithstanding we have an excellent hospital here," he wrote to the commissioner of Indian affairs, "it is difficult to get the Indians into it for treatment." In earlier times the Oglalas "destroyed all buildings and tepees in which a death occurred," Daniel explained, and they held "an aversion to being sick in a house where a corpse has lain." He described the Indians as "intensely social," a characteristic that made them feel imprisoned when cloistered inside the walled rooms and narrow corridors of the hospital ward, where "their visitors are not so numerous, nor are the patient and visitors allowed to gormandize, as is their custom in the camp." Exacerbating Oglala suspicions was their equating of hospital diet to starvation and the ubiquitous rules that tended to govern all human activity: no drumming, no incantations, no singing of songs, no presents received from "sympathizing friends," "no vociferous proclamation of the sickness from tent to tent," and "no wailing by old crooning women which is so sweet to the Indian ear." The hospital, in sum, was "too quiet, too still, too mysterious . . . another world." The Indians disliked everything about it, Daniel concluded, with their minds obsessively and unbendingly consumed "on the deaths and failures." Even Oglalas employed at the agency refused to as much as step foot in the building, having affixed to it the eerie moniker of "the dead house."[45]

The design of the hospital and its other attendant problems proved untenable and required fixing. Therefore the upper floor was completely reconstructed in 1897 and the lower-floor rooms were replastered. With those improvements in place, government inspector James McLaughlin was able to describe the layout of the building that year as "conveniently arranged and neatly kept," relating that the "sick of the reservation, who desire to avail themselves of the privilege, are brought to the hospital for treatment, where every attention possible is given them." However, over the course of his inspection McLaughlin encountered only two employees—the agency physician and his interpreter—a skeleton staff that was impeding the effectiveness of the facility and depriving care from many of those needing it. The inspector recommended hiring three additional employees: another physician, a nurse, and a cook, thereby raising to three the number of doctors on the reservation. In addition to the agency physician working out of the village of Pine Ridge, a doctor at Kyle was assigned to the day schools. The secretary of the interior approved the nurse and cook positions but, citing the prohibitive expense of salaries, declined staffing a third physician.[46]

As one problem inevitably played upon another, the Pine Ridge reservation seemed to operate on the principle of two steps forward and one step backward. Emblematic of that competing inertia was the total destruction of the Oglala boarding school on February 8, 1894, by fire. Mercifully, there was no loss of life, and the hospital building was spared. In fact, patients continued to be admitted—although not children of school age—but in numbers so reduced that in November an inspecting official advised eliminating two of the nurse positions. Apparently the holders of those jobs had "nothing to do but draw their salaries every quarter."[47]

Even so, the medical resources of the reservation were constantly stretched to the limit. In 1894, 825 cases of sickness were diagnosed, treated, or prescribed for. The number of births slightly outnumbered deaths that year: 298 compared to 285. As reported by Dr. Daniel, tuberculosis and the complications associated with it constituted the primary cause of mortality. Asserting that it was practically the only disease contributing to the large death rate, he speculated that the Oglalas might very well in its absence "multiply and overrun the country." To illustrate the lethal nature of tuberculosis, Daniel related the heartrending experience of five Oglalas trained as Episcopal clergymen. After receiving substantial educations to prepare them for a lifetime of ministry service, two of the group had succumbed to tuberculosis. As Daniel described them, "neither were old men"; rather, they were young men "cut off in their prime." Daniel made the rather innocuous assessment that "were it not for tuberculosis," which wrought "such havoc with Indian youth . . . the results of their education would be more far-reaching." Regrettably, "in light of this dreaded scourge," he concluded, "no other than a modified pessimistic view" could be "entertained of it."[48]

Increasing the susceptibility of Oglala teenagers to tuberculosis was the popularity of cigarette smoking among them. "Any pathologist," Daniel informed the commissioner of Indian affairs, "will tell you of the disastrous effects of tobacco smoke on a pair of lungs predisposed to tuberculosis." To inhale the smoke of cigarettes was "to disseminate the nicotine through the lung tissue," Daniel explained, "which, in combination with the gaseous carbon from the wrapper, produces a depressing, irritating, and biting effect on the delicate organs." It was a "well known" fact, he lectured, "that carbon has a great affinity for oxygen, at high temperatures especially, and the union of carbon from the wrapping of a cigarette with the oxygen in the air cells produces a most poisonous body, known as carbonic acid gas, which will not support animal life." Referencing a practice nearly as pervasive with the children as with the adults, Daniel wanted it made a punishable offense for the Pine Ridge traders to sell tobacco to minors.[49]

In addition to smoking, Daniel linked the prevalence of tuberculosis to two other factors: a ration system that promoted idleness, poor diet, and other undesirable habits and the pervasiveness of intratribal marriage among the Oglalas. "No person can be healthy who does not work, eat well-cooked nutritious food, dress properly and bathe,"

Daniel asserted. It was his observation that "as a rule" the Indians did "none of these things," and therefore they were "sickly," simple as that. To validate his views on what he maintained were the pernicious consequences of marriage between members of the Oglala people, Daniel cited attendance in off-reservation boarding schools and the high incidence of tuberculosis prevalent in those institutions. For Daniel, if children fell prey to disease under ideal conditions—and to him off-reservation boarding schools were the epitome of such an environment—then there had to be another explanation for the disproportionate rates of tubercular infection. As he saw it, "Indian children are taken from the high and dry climates of the West, in apparently perfect health, and sent to Carlisle, Hampton, and other Eastern schools, and while there, under the most salubrious surroundings, develop tuberculosis and return to their homes to die, and they do die; they die here, they die in the mountains of Pennsylvania, on the Atlantic coast, in the hills of Alabama, and they will continue to die everywhere they go, of tuberculosis, until the race is so thoroughly crossed by "foreign blood" that it will stamp out the tubercle bacillus, and when that is done the Indian race in its original purity will be no more."[50]

Daniel favored keeping Oglala children on the reservation to spiriting them away to distant boarding schools where they frequently died or, at the very least, fell victim to some serious physical malady. He hypothesized that "It would be a very interesting study to take all the Sioux children who have been sent to all boarding schools, compute all the money spent on their education, the number who have died, the number who have lapsed into barbarism, or vagabondism, and the number who have really and substantially profited by their learning to the extent of being some service to themselves and to their fellow-men." Injecting his own analysis into what he believed such a study might reveal, Daniel asserted: "Here and there it is granted that some do well, but many would do well anyhow. Some men and women rise to usefulness and eminence in spite of all obstacles, and so will a few Indians, but they will be very few."[51]

In the face of his concerns, Daniel rated the overall health of the Oglalas and the medical offerings available to them as "good." Similar to what Ruby would report in the 1950s, he equated the level and quality of services to that which might be "found in the average town." Justifying his assessment, Daniel commented that "while some articles may not be first class, the important drugs are reliable. Within the last three years the medical and surgical supply list has been greatly enlarged and improved." Whereas the quality of water at the agency had been a source of anxiety, Daniel apprised the Indian commissioner that two new tanks had been erected, and because the water that filled them was generated by windmills, it was considered wholesome and safe for human consumption. Oglalas living outside the village of Pine Ridge obtained their water "from brooks and streams, with here and there a well," sources also deemed "healthy, with the exception of containing infusoria," or intestinal parasites. Finally, typhoid bacteria had not been detected, that welcome measure of good fortune a product of the sparse population of the region.[52]

Tuberculosis posed far and away the greatest threat to Oglala health. Figures compiled by James R. Walker, for eighteen years (from July 1896 to May 1914) the government physician at Pine Ridge, exposed a horrifying, unthinkable reality. In the ten-year period that elapsed between 1896 and 1906, 903 full-blood-degree Oglalas and 70 mixed-bloods out of a total reservation population of 5,000 had died of the disease. Based on Walker's statistics, nearly one-fifth of the tribe had lost their lives, an arresting—and relative to the American population as a whole—considerably elevated incidence of mortality. Whereas the rate of tuberculosis deaths among the general population of the United States numbered less than two per thousand individuals, the average on the Pine Ridge reservation was eighteen per thousand.[53]

In 1896, Walker's first year in Pine Ridge, W. B. Dew, the day school inspector assigned to the reservation, offered an indication of what the agency physician was up against. "There are many children on this reservation so afflicted with scrofula—having open sores constantly discharging—as would render them a source of danger to any that come in contact with them," he wrote. Because "the exhalations from these sores soon contaminate the air of the schoolroom," Dew added that it was necessary to have affected students "excluded from school."[54]

W. H. Clapp, the acting Indian agent at Pine Ridge, underscored the virulence of the disease. In his annual report for 1899, he attributed to tuberculosis almost all absenteeism experienced in reservation schools. Bemoaning that it was "alarmingly prevalent and in almost every instance quickly fatal," Clapp recounted the tragic fate of several pupils who had passed their physicals the previous September and then had been admitted to the boarding school. Each had since either died or lapsed into "the last stages of this dread disease." Fully one-half of the Oglala tribe, Clapp estimated, was infected. The highest rates were found among the children, and the crisis was growing progressively worse.[55]

Partially responsible were the horrendous living conditions ubiquitous at Pine Ridge. As late as 1910 the reservation continued to struggle with the same issue of sanitation that had been raised by agent Penney some thirty-five years earlier. That year Superintendent James Brennan informed the Indian Office that most Oglalas erected their log houses along watercourses, the same streams and rivers in which they watered their stock, discharged their human excrement, and disposed of their household garbage, but from which they also obtained their drinking water. The consequent level of contaminant prompted Superintendent Brennan to declare that it was "fortunate that these people live in tents much of the time and move about from place to place." He detected a fundamental relationship between the level of environmental pollution and the health of the Oglala people. "Beginning about the first of May in each year and ending in October there is comparatively little sickness among these people," he pointed out, a reality "easily accounted for when we study the Indian life and manner of living. He practically abandons his home during this period and lives an outdoor life. This manner of existing takes him away from [the] filth that is bound to accumulate when large families are housed in a single unventilated room during the other months of the year. As soon as their open air life ends and they return to their homes for the winter diseases incident to filth and bad air begin to develop."[56]

The first notable response against tuberculosis at Pine Ridge was mounted by James Walker. In 1896 Walker was forty-seven years old and an eighteen-year veteran of the Indian Service. Having served as a member of the U.S. Sanitary Commission during the Civil War, he was an 1873 graduate of the Northwestern University School of Medicine in Chicago. He had entered into successful private practice in his hometown of Richview, Illinois, but his own health frailties—he suffered from chronic dysentery—dictated him relocating to northern Minnesota, where he subsequently fell victim to hard economic times. In order to provide for his wife and children, he accepted a position with the Indian Service in December 1878. First assigned to the Leech Lake reservation in Minnesota and then to the Puyallup reservation in Washington State, eventually he worked at Carlisle Indian School in Pennsylvania, and from Carlisle he came to the Pine Ridge reservation. Walker remained at Pine Ridge for the duration of his career, until reaching the mandatory retirement age of sixty-five in 1914.[57]

As medical officer in charge, Walker dedicated himself to counteracting a disease that was threatening the very existence of the Oglala people. Deeply aroused by this humanitarian impulse, in 1897 Walker petitioned the Indian Service for the services of an assistant physician. This was necessary, he advised, so he could concentrate his energies on treating the reservation's exorbitant number of tubercular cases, which extended to approximately one-half of the Oglala tribe.[58]

Reporting a sufficient case load to justify employing six or seven doctors—not just the two allowed—Walker seized upon a rather unconventional approach to confronting the disease: he courted "the cooperation of the local medicine men" at Pine Ridge. But Walker's tactic was apparently not as open-minded as it seemed. While he did want to elicit the support and assistance of Oglala shamans, and even adopted and utilized some of their psychological methodology—particularly their powers of suggestion—his real objective had been to undermine their influence. According to Don Southerton, who has chronicled Walker's activities, the doctor "reported building friendships with the elders by 'praising the good they did, supplying them with simple remedies and instructing them in their uses . . . privately . . . [he] charged them with their trickery and persuaded them to abandon such methods.'" Although his purpose may have been to undercut the authority of Oglala healers, when the nature of his actions became known, missionaries on the Pine Ridge reservation complained to the secretary of the interior, alleging violation of the federal Indian policy of assimilation. An investigation eventually absolved Walker of wrongdoing, but in the opinion of Southerton, the doctor's capacity to combat tuberculosis was diminished.[59]

Walker, no different than Indian Service personnel from across the country confronted with the insidiousness of tuberculosis, determined that drastic steps needed to be taken if lives were to be saved. One like-minded official was Edwin L. Chalcraft, the superintendent of Chemawa Indian School in Salem, Oregon, at the same time that Walker was serving at Pine Ridge. Mirroring the situation at Pine Ridge and conditions elsewhere, infection rates at Chemawa were exploding off the charts, a harrowing state of affairs that spurred Chalcraft to action. In response, he devised an open-air treatment for consumptives that began as a tent colony in the spring of 1907 and quickly evolved into permanent wards made up of sixteen wood-frame cottages, eight each for girls and for boys. As Chalcraft described them, these structures were sixteen feet square "with polished floors 2 feet from the ground; hip-roofs with a large glass skylight on the south slope; and enclosed with walls all around to within 3 feet of the roof, canvass that could be rolled up enclosed the space between the siding and lower edge of the roof. The buildings were heated by steam and lighted with electricity." Of those students who underwent his method of treatment, Chalcraft boasted, not a single one died.[60]

As Chalcraft was busy on the Pacific Coast, Walker was active at Pine Ridge. To provide comprehensive care and check the spread of the disease, Walker, like Chalcraft, proposed the construction of a tuberculosis sanitarium. His plan called for a tent camp—not unlike that of Chalcraft's initial invention—laid out over four sections. Walker believed that this would enable him to begin to get a handle on the 539 diagnosed cases of tuberculosis on the reservation. He suggested starting in an economical manner, apportioning one tent for every two patients, while requisitioning funds for a kitchen and a dining room, a laundry, a warehouse, a barn, outhouses, employee housing, and fencing. The tents, measuring twelve by fourteen feet, would be furnished with a single bed, a chair, a drinking cup, a washbasin, a cuspidor, and a chamber pot for each occupant as well as a camp stove, a water bucket, a pitcher, a slop pail, a washstand, and a lantern.[61]

Walker requested a staffing allowance of a physician in charge, a cook, a laborer, a laundress, a nurse, and a matron, with the laborer being accorded police powers. Fresh food, a necessity in treating the ill, would be supplied from beef cattle, milk cows, and chickens. A farmer equipped with a work team, harness, wagon, agricultural implements, and seed would provide for the cultivation of the fields. Walker estimated the overall cost "at between three thousand and thirty thousand dollars 'depending on the quality and completeness of the plant.'"[62]

In the summer of 1908, Walker forwarded to Francis E. Leupp, the commissioner of Indian affairs, a draft of his proposal, but he was to be disappointed in the reaction it received. Leupp had visited Chemawa Indian School, observed the wooden buildings raised by Chalcraft, and endorsed the school superintendent's approach. Thus, when the commissioner reviewed Walker's documents, he responded only by furnishing the Pine Ridge physician with a set of the blueprints drawn up by Chalcraft in Oregon. Walker's dissent was apparently grounded in the frigid South Dakota winters and the havoc they could—and were likely—to wreak on tent life.[63]

Failure to authorize a tuberculosis sanitarium was emblematic of the national government's piecemeal response to meeting the essential health care needs of the Oglala people. For a span of nearly two decades following the retirement of James Walker, the level of services and the quality of facilities dropped relative to the number of tribal members positively disposed toward receiving treatment. Increasingly, the Oglalas found themselves in closer and more frequent contact with non-Indians and further alienated from traditional methods and life ways, intensifying the potential for health problems and disease while heightening the stresses placed upon available medical supports. But as the number of Lakota seeking assistance soared, the ability of the reservation's medical staff to satisfy that demand at best remained static and at worst declined. The result was a threshold of suffering and morbidity that exceeded anything experienced previously.

A landmark event in the evolution of health care at Pine Ridge occurred in 1912. Automobiles that year were acquired by the agency for the first time—one for each of the two physicians on the reservation. According to Superintendent Brennan, the cars constituted a boom, greatly enhancing the efficiency of the doctors by making it possible for them "to cover a great deal more ground than" before. With that benefit in view, Brennan pressed the Indian Office for the funds to purchase an additional vehicle to be reserved for a third staff physician. "These machines," when "supplemented by horses for very bad weather and times when the machines are out of commission," he purported, significantly "extend the field of the physicians and give much better returns in service for the money expended."[64]

However, as always seemed to be the case at Pine Ridge, gains could be fleeting. Four years later, Superintendent Brennan apprised the commissioner of Indian affairs that there was only a single automobile at his disposal for medical purposes. He requested two more, one less than an inspecting officer who lobbied for a third additional vehicle. According to Brennan, the physician at Kyle was driving his own car, "an imposition," and he reiterated his earlier assessment of the efficiency of motorized transportation: it "more than doubled the capacity of the physicians to make calls, in this country of great distances." By 1921, the agency had been equipped with a fleet of three Ford touring cars, modern assets that were enabling the reservation's three physicians "to do much more effective work than heretofore."[65]

And that was followed by an even greater breakthrough. Of incalculable importance and another milestone in the history of the Pine Ridge reservation was the opening of a new hospital at the boarding school in 1914, replacing a structure that had been continuously in operation for twenty-two years. Unfortunately, this hospital—of all brick construction and supporting twenty-one beds—remained the only medical facility on the reservation, a deficiency that required the one physician on staff to fulfill, as best he was able, the health care requirements of the entire Oglala population. An unsatisfactory if altogether impossible situation, it inspired Brennan to launch a spirited, although in the short term ineffectual, campaign to have a general hospital built. "It is reported that a new hospital is to be constructed on this reservation in the near future," he wrote encouragingly to the Indian commissioner in 1914, "and I earnestly hope that this dream will come true, as such an institution is badly needed." He reminded his superior that there had been agitation from him and from others for a number of years, and a site for either a hospital or a sanitarium had been "selected and set aside nearly ten years ago for this purpose."[66]

Unquestionably there was ample justification for going forward with a general hospital on the reservation. As one indicator of the rising interest in services, a tent colony was set up on the boarding school grounds in the summer of 1914. Several Oglala families took this unprecedented step in order to avail themselves to "the benefit of constant treatment" from the school hospital. In response, Superintendent Brennan mulled over the prospect of establishing "a permanent camping place for such purposes near the agency." As he saw it, the only drawback was the potential for abuse if "not closely watched." The Oglalas, he cautioned, "would like nothing better than an excuse to camp near the agency, leaving their allotment and gardens."[67]

While the Oglala Lakotas were proactively taking matters into their own hands, Brennan offered the perceptive comment that the principal threat to health on the reservation was not epidemics but too few physicians to treat "the ordinary run of sickness." Although a staff of three doctors was budgeted for the reservation, typically only one or two of those positions were filled at any one time, and sometimes there was not even that level of support. Significant blame for that situation rested with Pine Ridge. For Indian Service personnel it was simply not a coveted appointment. In his 1914 annual report, for example, Brennan lamented that the physician's position had sat vacant for "practically the entire year." The office was "very hard to fill and keep filled," he explained, because "whenever an appointee reports for the position, he is no sooner on the ground and started than he is offered a position at increased salary at some other agency and, naturally, he accepts and moves on," leaving "the entire district on the reservation without proper medical attendance."[68]

A related issue was the competency and experience of Indian Service physicians. The constantly revolving door of personnel caused some tribal members to come to the understandable conclusion that the reservation was simply a testing ground for the young and a haven for the incompetent. Without doubt the quality of staff posed an ongoing concern, for both the Oglalas and the federal government, and even a brief survey of staff assigned to Pine Ridge lends credence to some of the Indians' suspicions. Take, for instance, the year 1916, when there were three physicians on the reservation. The first, located in the village of Pine Ridge, was thirty-two years old. He had been in the Indian Service for several years, possessed a reputation as being "energetic," "willing," "interested in his work," and for "never refusing calls." His specialization was internal medicine, and he also performed surgeries. "Well liked by the Superintendent, employees and the Indians," he had been slated to assume charge of the general hospital had it been built while he was there. The second doctor was twenty-five years old and a recent graduate of a medical school in Philadelphia. His background encompassed seven months of private practice and one year of hospital service. He was said to be "well prepared . . . active . . . and doing good work" at his duty post in Manderson. Finally, the last physician was "considerably over" fifty years of age. A longtime employee of the Indian Service, he did "not pretend to be thoroughly up to date in medicine," but his superiors believed he was trying his best to meet the needs of his patients. According to Indian Service records, he was "well liked by the Indians and whites in the community" of Kyle. Considered collectively, then, and at this single snapshot in time, all three physicians were seemingly popular on the reservation, but one possessed very limited experience and another was not current on the latest medical practices.[69]

In every way possible, Superintendent Brennan applied pressure on the Indian Office to beef up the level of staffing, particularly in the area of doctors. In 1910 he reported that "it is impossible for four physicians to cover the entire reservation—comprising four counties"; in 1912 he said: "The reservation is so large and the population so scattered that the number of physicians is entirely inadequate to give the proper attention to the cases arising which call for practice on their part. There are practically seven thousand people scattered over an area ninety miles long and sixty miles wide"; in 1914 he expressed relief that "there have been no epidemics during the past year, merely the ordinary run of sickness. Our principle trouble has been the lack of physicians to handle the routine business." And so it went. But the national government, in failing to develop sufficiently the medical infrastructure at Pine Ridge, was flirting with disaster in the advent of an emergency.[70]

The staffing issue reached a flash point in the fall of 1918. That year the worldwide influenza epidemic raged across the reservation, unleashing in its wake unprecedented sickness and death. Undoubtedly there would have been some loss of life no matter what preparations had been made, but at Pine Ridge the medical corps was wholly ill-equipped to respond to the health crisis that ensued. In 1918 there was no agency physician employed on the reservation, only one doctor assigned to the boarding school and another stationed at Kyle. The school physician had responsibility for 250 boarding students, a like number of students enrolled in Holy Rosary Mission four miles north of the village of Pine Ridge, and approximately one-half the remainder of the general reservation population. The doctor at Kyle maintained oversight over all day school students and the other half of the reservation's adult population.[71]

Partly due to the deficit in medical personnel, circumstances deteriorated rapidly in the days after the scourge hit. The physician at Kyle— and his entire family—were "among the first to contract Influenza," an initial strike that debilitated him to an extent that he was able to provide no more than minimal assistance "during the worst part of the epidemic." Meanwhile, the physician in charge of the boarding and mission schools thought to take the extraordinarily farsighted step of quarantining each of his campuses, a directive that was kept in effect throughout the ordeal. At the height of the outbreak some 3,500 Oglalas were stricken, and by the time it had finally run its course, an estimated 350 to 400 had died. It is noteworthy, however, that no fatalities were reported among boarding and mission school students, and in the aftermath of the tragedy, the agency superintendent felt compelled to issue the telling statement that while it was a fact that "the deaths . . . could not" have been "prevented," it was also true that "the one physician could not cope with the situation."[72]

In the spring of 1922 a less virulent strain of influenza passed through the reservation. There were no fatalities, but the 168 cases diagnosed in the boarding and mission schools underscored the essential need for increasing the number of medical doctors on staff. Similar to the composition of the field staff in 1918, only a single physician was servicing the village of Pine Ridge, and with the care of students monopolizing all of his time, no time was left "for reservation practice," the most glaring neglect occurring in obstetrical cases, virtually all of which were going "unattended by physician." Influenza struck again the following spring, causing several deaths, and in 1927 outbreaks of whooping cough and red measles proved "serious and far reaching," producing "a great many deaths among the infants and children under three years of age."[73]

And there were lingering threats. In 1919 the agency superintendent reported that the purity of the water had not improved, triggering a few mild cases of typhoid fever among boarding school students. Without swift and substantial intervention undertaken by the Indian Office, the agency physician worried that a "disastrous" epidemic might occur. The decades-old problem persisted that the water that supplied both the agency and the boarding school fed directly from White Clay Creek to the standpipes and from those to the consumers without filtering. The superintendent conjectured that "since the creek is not a very large one" and was "used as an outlet for refuse, as well as watering stock," it was only a matter of time before it became polluted "to such an extent as to be injurious" to the health of children and agency employees. In order to supply potable water to Pine Ridge, the superintendent recommended drilling several deep wells "at an early date." In this instance the national government reacted swiftly. Pipe was sunk the next year.[74]

But the health of the Oglalas was trending downward. In 1922 the agency superintendent offered an unusually candid, pessimistic assessment. "There are, without doubt," he feared, "considerable numbers of cases of tuberculosis and other diseases which are wholly without treatment, save such aid as the Indians themselves may provide." In terms of tuberculosis, so little was being done that most of the infected were receiving no medical assistance whatsoever. Fault lay not fully with the national government; the Oglalas often declined treatment. But more often than not, there were no services to turn down. According to the superintendent, the only effective method of treatment was sanatoria hospice, and patients had been referred to facilities located in Iowa and Idaho, but that option was not always feasible. "The distance of these institutions from the Reservation, coupled with the reluctance of the Indian people to leave their homes during illness, and the shortage of funds for such purposes," the superintendent reported, had limited the number of patients he had been able "to send away." Lauding the remarkable results attainable through sanatoria care, the superintendent pleaded with the Indian Office for the construction of such a resource on the Pine Ridge reservation. It was their sole hope, in his view, for arresting the disease and saving lives.[75]

In 1923 the agency superintendent reported that proposals for both a general hospital and a tuberculosis sanatorium had been submitted. It had been suggested that the sanatorium be located "somewhere in the Black Hills," described as "a sort of Mecca for all Sioux." The sanatorium initiative failed to garner BIA approval, however, and an application for a general hospital was substituted in its place. But that request did not go without opposition. "There are many objections to a local hospital," the agency superintendent explained. "The expenditure of money would be considerable, and it appears that more real service could be given the Indians if a similar sum were expended in increasing the number of physicians on the reservation. Such a plan would limit the territory of each physician, thus giving him time to actually cover his district." He urged that whichever arrangement was finally adopted be put "into practice as early as possible, since the health conditions on this reservation are not at a desirable standard." Several years later, another superintendent went further, recommending approval of a general hospital consisting of 200 to 250 beds.[76]

The problem was two-fold. More students required sanatoria care, and across the reservation more Oglalas required hospital services, than could be accommodated. In both instances, funding and facilities were inadequate to meet need. And even when there were open beds in the school hospital—which was actually often the case—government officials were wary of filling them with nonstudent patients for fear space would be unavailable in the advent of an epidemic. Due to the highly communicable nature of tuberculosis, placing tubercular patients in the school hospital was not an option either. The longstanding solution of local officials was the construction of either a sanatorium or a general hospital open to all members of the reservation community, whether infants, very young children, adults, or students.

By any standard the reservation was wracked with disease, which was at once partially a result of and made worse by another hard truth: a widespread prevalence of malnutrition. In the first decades of the twentieth century the Oglalas continued to subsist largely on government rations, provisions that afforded an unbalanced diet heavy in meat (mostly beef) and starchy dried goods but that was light in fresh fruit, vegetables, and dairy products. Besides the lack of variety contained in the food, the distributions to families were insufficient. In tandem, the dual factors of quality and quantity contributed to an ongoing health crisis among the Oglalas.

Hunger posed a gut-wrenching reality. A survey of reservation conditions conducted in 1925 revealed "beyond a doubt that many Indian families" went "for days at a time with the scantiest food supply." According to this study, "many homes were found where the only article of diet was beans; others were found where horse meat and cattle meat in a questionable state, was the dependence until the next ration day. Many families were found who had been without flour for several days. Other instances were encountered where bread and coffee appeared to be the sole diet." The agency superintendent admitted that "a detailed account of just what the Indians lived on last winter, would not be appetizing. There were probably no cases of actual starvation, but the numerous conditions arising from lack of sufficient food, were clearly in evidence." There could be "but little doubt," he asserted, "that the high infant mortality"—statistics indicated that nearly 25 percent of Oglala babies died before reaching the age of three—was "due to deficient nutrition."[77]

According to almost every commentator on the subject, the precarious state of health on the reservation was directly attributable "to the economic condition of the Indians." In the first decades of the twentieth century, disease and sickness were visible everywhere. Some 30 percent of the Oglala population was infected with tuberculosis, and the death rate resulting from the contagion hovered at four times the national average. Another 13 percent suffered from trachoma. A large number of children evinced evidence of "diseased" tonsils, adenoids, and noses that required surgical attention, and "practically every Indian on the Reservation" was "under nourished" and without other necessities such as soap and clean water. Only "one family in twenty" owned "a milk cow" and not more than one percent of families had milk to drink on a regular basis. The average Oglala family comprised ten members living in a one-room log house that was ten by sixteen feet in size, dirt floored and dirt roofed, and poorly lighted and ventilated. Many Oglalas ate and slept on the bare floor, hauled their cooking water in barrels, and were without bathroom, bathing, or clothes-washing facilities. So alarming grew the reports of deprivation and want that a delegation of the American Red Cross was dispatched to investigate.[78]

Documentation of the extreme socioeconomic conditions, together with the lethargic response of the Indian Office to do much of anything about it, and in tandem with the publication of the Meriam Report in 1928, which spotlighted public attention on the appalling conditions that existed at Pine Ridge and throughout Indian country, resulted in positive intervention finally being undertaken to alleviate suffering and improve the health of the Oglala people. In the late 1920s the national government reinstituted the field nurse program that long had been inactive on the reservation. One nurse was assigned to each of the four outlying districts of Oglala, Allen, Manderson, and Porcupine. In addition, a women's auxiliary was organized to gather, study, and disseminate information related to home and family, and the allowance of physicians on the reservation was increased to five. Other measures were also introduced, including a home construction program, a schedule for administering routine vaccinations, and a comprehensive system for testing the agency's water supply. As a result, agency officials were able to profess, and with a degree of sincerity, that the health of the Oglalas, while far from optimal, was improving.[79]

Much of that positive momentum revolved around the realization of a coveted and long-held objective. On January 25, 1931, fully seventeen years after Superintendent Brennan had first raised the issue with the BIA, the following telegram arrived at the desk of the commissioner of Indian affairs: "TWO FLOORS OF NEW HOSPITAL IN OPERATION TWENTY NINE PATIENTS ONE NEW BABY ONE MAJOR OPERATION." The forty-seven bed general hospital was a three-story yellow brick structure built on a hill about a quarter of a mile north of the agency buildings on a location that, ironically, was the former site of an Oglala burial ground. Human remains were unearthed there during the excavation for the basement of the building. The hill on which the hospital sat held other historical ties as well. It was said to have been the scene of one of the last military engagements to take place between the Oglala Lakota and federal troops. Lakota warriors reportedly had used it as a staging area from which they attacked a group of Pine Ridge agency scouts in 1890. Seven years later, in 1938, another health highpoint occurred when Sioux Sanatorium opened on the former campus of Rapid City Indian School. Although located a considerable distance north of Pine Ridge, it would serve as the primary critical care center for many of the reservation's tuberculosis cases, a function it still performs today.[80]

Despite the obvious advantages attained through the construction of a new general hospital and the opening of a tuberculosis sanatorium, the Great Depression years proved especially challenging for the Oglala Lakota. So extreme grew the hardships and suffering that many children, simply in order to receive the provision of food, clothing, and shelter, were enrolled in the thirty-one day schools and one boarding school in operation on the reservation. Insight into this distressing period can be gleaned from the Depression-era diaries of Marion Billbrough Dreamer, who was an elementary school teacher on the Pine Ridge reservation from 1932 to 1942. During that span she taught at Day School Number Five (also known as Lone Man Day School) near Oglala and at Grass Creek Day School near Manderson. A recent graduate of Washington State College (now Washington State University), Dreamer applied for and received an appointment at Pine Ridge, stayed for ten years, married an Oglala Lakota man, and ultimately left deeply disillusioned. Underlying her dissatisfaction was what she believed was an overtly controlling BIA (apparently in its relations with both Indians and agency employees) and frustrations that arose from having to deal with an impenetrable "reservation bureaucracy." The depth of her unhappiness eventually compelled her to terminate her relationship with the Indian Service.[81]

Dreamer's primary responsibility was teaching, but long distances, bad roads, and limited transportation caused her to expend considerable time and energy tending to the health needs of her young charges and their families. According to Laura Woodworth-Ney, who has published excerpts of Dreamer's diaries, Dreamer "accepted her unofficial role as a nurse, observing the health of her students carefully and intervening when she deemed it necessary." At times the obstacles she confronted, which extended beyond simply those related to a depression economy, appeared overpowering. As Woodworth-Ney has documented, "General poverty, undernourishment, and wretched sanitary conditions contributed to a high incidence of infant mortality [on the reservation] and an alarming frequency of communicable disease," including trachoma and tuberculosis.[82]

Because Dreamer was often the only official on hand capable of rendering medical assistance, she had to be prepared to meet almost any exigency. Among the more routine were requests for her to transport adult tribal members to a medical doctor or a medical facility. As a day-school instructor having access to an automobile, she was able—and with the generous and substantial assistance of her husband—to accommodate most of those seeking aid. For example, when one Oglala man complained that his wife had been suffering with her teeth for two weeks, George Dreamer agreed to drive her to a dentist in Chadron. Similar trips were undertaken into the village of Pine Ridge. Sometimes it was for purposes related to health care, at other times to pick up groceries and supplies, and on occasion to conduct pressing business.[83]

In a majority of instances, however, Dreamer was on her own to ad-

minister treatment. From nursing earaches to furnishing baby powder and salves to dispensing medical advice, Dreamer was involved, directly and often profoundly, in delivering health care to those around
her. Woodworth-Ney related a situation that occurred in April 1937.
A student of Dreamer's fell ill, giving "out by noon" each day for several days in succession. The teacher responded by sending the student
and her sister home before school was out for the day. Outwardly concerned, Marion and George Dreamer, in an attempt to urge the mother
to take the sick child to the hospital, drove out to the house where the
girls lived. The advice given operated to good effect, and the Dreamers accompanied the family into Pine Ridge, but when they got to the
hospital a doctor could not be roused, and to her great dismay, Marion Dreamer observed the other sister (who had been in the hospital
the previous week) "running around with out any shoes." In the end,
all the efforts of Dreamer and the afflicted girl's parents had no effect, as the condition of the sisters continued to deteriorate. In her diary, Dreamer lamented the family's "desperate circumstances." There
were "two beds for nine of them with hardly any bedding," and "Today Irene is just as tired out as Mary Rose. She has sit around the school
house all day."[84]

That same month another student's health teetered so precariously
on the brink that the Dreamers felt they had no choice but to take deci-
sive steps to ensure that prompt attention was given. Marion Dreamer
described the situation in her diary. "All the children except Katherine Kindle are in school again," she wrote. "Her sister told me yesterday that she was sick and did not seem to get any better. She has been
sick for three weeks. George took her to the hospital to-day and the
doctor kept her there."[85]

Sickness and disease exacted a toll on school attendance, and the
number of children sitting in class on any given day served as a fair barometer of the state of the health of the student body. Trachoma, a serious infection of the eye that without proper treatment could lead to
blindness, was a common ailment. Woodworth-Ney explained, "Doc-

tors periodically conducted examinations at school, usually sending those who needed further treatment to the hospital." But that was not always possible, and Dreamer never forgot one especially horrific scene in which a visiting physician "laid the children on a table, held the eyelids back and scraped them with a sharp knife."[86]

Death posed another inescapable reality. Statistics are hard to come by, but average lifespan of the Oglalas was in all likelihood considerably below the national average, while rates of infant and child mortality were in turn substantially elevated. Dreamer documented one four-day period in 1937 during which three deaths occurred. Two were of infants, and the Dreamers were involved in the funeral preparations made for them. Marion Dreamer wrote in her diary: "Mrs. He Dog died, Geo took Willie to Pine Ridge to get things for the feast. The Little Brings Him Back baby died too. Geo began digging the He Dog grave." A few days later, Dreamer added that "Geo went to McKinley Slow Bears to take his little baby to the cemetery. It is about a month old and died last night. It was buried in the Catholic Cemetery at Oglala. They took it in the back of the car."[87]

Sometimes illness and death struck with such dual ferocity that parents had to make the unfathomable choice between attending the funeral of a child or expending their energies trying to procure treatment for the living. This was the heartbreaking dilemma that confronted the Slow Bear family. Dreamer recorded that she had had to excuse two of the Slow Bear daughters from school so that they could "take care of their younger brother while their father was at the cemetery." According to Dreamer, "Mrs. Slow Bear did not witness the burial of her baby . . . because 'she had to take another sick child (Rose Mary) into the hospital." Of course, the most trying for Dreamer were those times when one of her own students passed away. One instance of this occurred when an entire family of school-age children had to be kept home because of tuberculosis. Dreamer subsequently learned from a relative that one of the girls had succumbed to the disease.[88]

As revealed in the experiences of Dreamer, Pine Ridge presented a brutally demanding environment that seemed little changed since the creation of the reservation. In 1950 the federal government conducted a survey of health and living conditions, and the findings duplicated decades of federal agency reports, providing a stark indication of what Robert Ruby was to confront in his duties as medical officer in charge. At midcentury, 60 percent of families continued to live in log houses. Tuberculosis, malnutrition, pneumonia, dental caries, measles, conjunctivitis, and scabies remained the primary risks to health. Potatoes, rice, macaroni, and other foods high in carbohydrates and low in protein were the principal diet. There were only four physicians on the reservation in addition to one director and one assistant director of nurses supervising a staff of seven nurses. Perhaps more telling, of a reservation population that had grown to nearly eleven thousand, only thirteen tribal members were college graduates, and almost 20 percent of children between the ages of six and eighteen were not enrolled in school. Average annual family income was placed at $1,290, less than a quarter of the national average of $4,237 and a figure rendered even more troubling when it is factored in that average family size was at least double at Pine Ridge to that of the national average of three per household.[89]

If gains had been made anywhere, they were in infrastructure. By 1953, when Ruby located to Pine Ridge, a complex system of hospitals and other health care facilities was under operation of the BIA. Across the continental United States and Alaska, there were sixty-two hospitals and three tuberculosis sanatoria. The largest of these, having a capacity of between 150 and 425 beds, were classified as "medical centers." The others were termed "general" hospitals. Most were relatively small, servicing on average fewer than 50 patients per day. During Ruby's tenure, Pine Ridge functioned as a modern, comprehensive, medical-surgical general hospital with a bed capacity of 46, one of the largest of ten medical units under Aberdeen Area jurisdiction. It supported a clinic, an emergency room, an ambulance corps, and a pharmacy, and it also maintained dental, optical, and pediatric departments. In fact, such was the diversity and range of services available at Pine Ridge, other BIA hospitals in North and South Dakota were under direction to transfer their elective surgeries there. In Ruby's estimation, the care patients received was probably "equitable to that of most of the small town hospitals of the time." He believed that they "didn't lack for much," as Pine Ridge possessed "most of the apparatus that was just beginning to come available to keep people alive."[90]

While Ruby was there, Pine Ridge Hospital teemed with activity. Some 1,400 patients were admitted annually, on average just under 4 per day. In a given year the hospital experienced 210 births and 30 deaths. The surgical unit performed about 20 operations per month. Five doctors were on staff, or at least that was the number budgeted for. In addition to Ruby, who simultaneously held the positions of medical officer in charge, orthopedist, and surgeon, there were four others: an ophthalmologist, an obstetrician and gynecologist (who was also the anesthesiologist), a pediatrician, and an internist. Rounding out the hospital's personnel were one dentist, nine registered nurses, three practical nurses, eleven blue girls or housekeepers, one X-ray technician (who in addition performed all lab work), two medical clerks, and four janitors.[91]

But these positive developments masked serious, fundamental problems churning just below the surface that were verging on bringing about a complete re-organization and re-alignment of Indian health care. A great value of the Ruby letters is their on-the-ground documentation of a national Indian health care system in crisis, a system that had atrophied and was languishing in its final throes. The year and a half that Ruby was at Pine Ridge coincided with the transfer of Indian health care from the BIA to the Public Health Service, a transition that took effect on June 1, 1955. In part, the shift emerged out of a termination-era ethos that sought to assimilate Indians into the mainstream and lessen federal involvement in Indian affairs. A larger point, however, was the unavoidable fact that under BIA supervision Indian health care had been inadequate if not an abysmal failure, the germs of which were dramatically in evidence at Pine Ridge and contributed to the frustration and cynicism that came to jade so much of Ruby's outlook. The BIA lagged far behind the armed services, the Veterans Administration, and the Public Health Service in recruiting and retaining physicians. Bluntly put, the BIA health service suffered from a chronic case of the "unders": It was underfunded, understaffed, and under-equipped. According to James R. Shaw, the first director of the Indian Health Service, under the BIA, "The pay was terrible, the doctors were isolated, they had bad facilities, no continuing medical education, and worst of all, they were subordinate to the local BIA superintendent."[92]

In comments suggestive that Ruby's was not an isolated experience, Emery Johnson, another Indian Health Service director, described the brief time that he spent working as a physician for the BIA:

After finishing my one year rotating internship, I started at White Earth, Minnesota on June 30 1955, the last day before the transfer. I found that a new stove that had been ordered for the medical officer's residence had been "requisitioned" by the BIA Superintendent, the official "boss" of the reservation. For most of my time at White Earth I was the only physician; we had to go 25 miles to make a long distance telephone call. When I got there I was immediately inundated with patients with eclampsia, motor vehicle and gunshot trauma, diarrheal dehydration, appendicitis, and pneumonia. The stove was not all that was missing from my quarters. There was no laboratory equipment, even for hemoglobin determinations. Most of my surgery was performed with local nerve blocks, but I also used spinals, or drop ether.[93]

The most immediate cause of the transfer, however, was the incontestable reality that the BIA had fallen devastatingly short in its charge to raise the standard of Indian health to a level commensurate with that of the rest of the American population. Statistics compiled on Indian health speak for themselves. During the period that Ruby administered Pine Ridge Hospital, life expectancy for Indians floundered nine years lower than the national average. Infant death rates—among health professionals "a seminal indicator of health status"—"were nearly three times higher than among other races, and a quarter of all deaths occurred among infants under one year of age." In addition, "maternal deaths associated with childbirth were also three times higher than among whites," while the rates of death "from diarrhea and dehydration were 300 percent higher among Indians." Impossible to ignore was the fact that 10 to 25 percent of the Indian population remained infected with tuberculosis, an alarming figure which in the years during and immediately after World War II formed the basis of a national scandal and served as a potent symbol of the shortcomings of the BIA as a purveyor of health care. According to one study, the health of the American Indians lagged "approximately three generations behind the rest of the country, due primarily to culture, language, and attitudinal problems, as well as economics, isolation, *and above all, lack of service*" (editors' emphasis).[94]

It was in this context that Robert Ruby toiled on the Pine Ridge Indian Reservation and constructed the contents of his memoir. Originally written in the form of a series of letters addressed to his sister, they present a first-person account of many subjects condensed into a single volume. Ruby's observations of government practices, medical care, and physical survival convey a sense of how the BIA functioned in the mid-twentieth century while offering glimpses into the rigors and hardships of daily life in Indian country. The book is also a narrative of one man's experiences as a new member of the medical profession, and it is a chronicle of his coming to the threshold of a deeper understanding of cultures and circumstances not his own.

As is usual for a memoir, this is a report of observations, perceptions, and experiences more than a critical assessment. Memoirs are written from the perspective of an interested party, leaving the analysis to others, and for the analytic scholar Dr. Ruby's writings contain a cache of documentation. As a participant in the daily operations of the Pine Ridge reservation, he recorded the lives of his patients and the agency staff. Of both, he formed opinions that he willingly shared in unvarnished prose often recorded in the heat of the moment and just minutes or perhaps an hour or two after an event took place. Doubtless the views and attitudes of a young surgeon from a white, middle-class background differed substantially from those that might be obtained from an Oglala Sioux living at Pine Ridge in the 1950s. Historians know all too well that sources are complicated, often incomplete, may address only certain aspects of a complex situation, and can express themselves in a manner considered insensitive or even callous when evaluated against modern sensibilities. Dr. Ruby's memoir offers the perceptive reader several complementary views of his time at Pine Ridge, distilling a detailed look at life there and many of the issues that confronted the Oglala Sioux, the BIA, and the management of Indian health care. But it must always be kept in the forefront that it remains the work of a white physician. The hope of the editors is that the publication of this memoir will stimulate others to add to the scope of our understanding of Indian health care and especially those deriving of multiple perspectives, including the Pine Ridge Lakotas.

A casual reader might infer that Pine Ridge reflected a passing phase of Dr. Ruby's life, one that he filed away in a back drawer along with his copies of the letters that he wrote. (In fact, his correspondence sat hidden and untouched for a half century, until Ruby and the editors met to write a brief retrospective of the works of Ruby and his longtime writing collaborator, John A. Brown, for an article that was subsequently published.) Certainly in its final pages the tone of the memoir suggests as much, projecting an impression of impending finality, that Ruby was prepared to walk away and never return. Ruby began writing with an exaggerated sense of cheerful good humor and perhaps naïveté, an attitude that permeates his opening passages: his recounting of his trip to South Dakota and his descriptions of setting up housekeeping in the village of Pine Ridge. By the close of the year, however, the feeling is markedly different: the mood is more somber, the comments are more pointed and biased, and in the end, cynicism and disillusionment pervade. Today, Ruby recognizes in his letters his "sometimes intolerance of those Indians there in the early 50s ... [his] frustration for seeing why one could not snap his fingers with an admonishment and expect results ... [his] impatience with slow or in some case[s] no response of change in their ways of living then." But it would be wrong to presume that in December 1954 Robert Ruby had seen the last of Indian reservations or that he had abandoned his interest in Indian people.[95]

In 1955, after having entered into private surgical practice in Moses Lake, Washington, Dr. Ruby maintained a close association with the American Indians, and he gradually developed a second career as a writer of their histories and lives. His first book, which was composed while he was still in Pine Ridge, was self-published, and his labors as a historian evolved from there. Some works were Ruby's alone; others were prepared jointly with John Brown. Except for a book on Columbia River ferryboats and one on prohibition-era bootleggers, the Ruby and Brown scholarship concentrated solely on American Indian history. If the prolific nature of their relationship can be used as a barometer—in forty years Ruby and Brown published twelve books—it would appear that the fatigue Ruby felt at Pine Ridge was only fleeting, and that with the passage of time and with the advantage of distance and the progressive attitudes toward Indians that emerged in later decades, Ruby's opinions moderated as well. His medical career and his life-long involvement with Indians extend beyond the scope of this volume, but his eighteen months in Pine Ridge were not the culmination of a young man's fascination with the West and its people; they were the beginning of a lifetime of historical exploration, scholarship, and service to others. In the same sense that a healer seeks to achieve the wellness of the whole being rather than strictly the attainment of physical health, Ruby was embarking on a pathway at Pine Ridge steeped in people, medicine, and words that has continued to the present.[96]

Timeline of Selected Events in the Life of Robert H. Ruby, MD

1921   Born in Mabton, Washington.

1939   Graduates from Mabton High School and enters Whitworth College in Spokane, Washington, enrolling in pre-med.

1940   Returns to Whitworth College for second year.

1941   Returns to Whitworth College for third year.

1942   Shortly after U.S. entry into the Second World War, drafted into the U.S. Air Corps as a private. University and college students are conscripted into the military, but pre-med majors and those enrolled in some of the sciences are allowed to finish their degrees. In the fall enters the Washington University Medical School in St. Louis, Missouri.

1943   Medical student, Washington University Medical School, St. Louis, Missouri. Graduates in June from Whitworth College based on three years of credits earned at that institution and one year of credits earned at Washington University.

1944   Medical student, Washington University Medical School, St. Louis, Missouri.

1945   Graduates from Washington University Medical School. In July begins required nine-month medical internship in Detroit, Michigan.

1946   Completes internship in Detroit in April. Two weeks later, reports to Fort George Wright near Spokane. Promoted to officer's rank based on medical training. On June 30 assigned to the air base at San

Bernardino, California, and on October 15 transferred to San Antonio, Texas, for basic training.

1947 On June 5 assigned to Lowry Field outside Denver, Colorado. On July 12 boards the USAT *General C. G. Morton* to serve in the U.S. Army of Occupation in Japan. Arrives in Seattle on December 16 aboard the USS *Mayo* and is discharged.

1948 In January travels to Fort Lawton in Seattle to study basic science before taking exams for medical license. In March begins six-month surgical residency at the Sugarbaker Cancer Clinic in Jefferson City, Missouri. In October begins year-long postgraduate course in St. Louis for doctors returning from military service.

1949 Completes postgraduate course in June; then begins a surgical residency in the St. Louis County Hospital in Clayton and the Barnes Hospital in St. Louis.

1950 Korean War begins, and national government calls up physicians who have not met the twenty-month service requirement during and after the Second World War. Ruby falls into this category by a few weeks, but draft law allows physicians-in-training to finish their schooling, enabling Ruby to complete his third and fourth years of surgical residency.

1951–52 Continues surgical residency, St. Louis County Hospital in Clayton and Barnes Hospital in St. Louis.

1953 Completes surgical residency on June 30. Returns to Washington State and marries Jeanne Henderson in Spokane in July. Leaves for Pine Ridge, South Dakota, in August as an officer in uniform in the U.S. Public Health Service.

1953–54 Medical officer in charge, Pine Ridge Hospital, Pine Ridge Indian Reservation, Pine Ridge, South Dakota.

1954 Edna Phyllis Ruby born in Pine Ridge Indian Hospital; Ruby believes she is the first non-Indian birth in the Pine Ridge hospital. Also, publication of his first book, *The Oglala Sioux: Warriors in Transition.*

1955–91 Surgeon, private practice, Moses Lake, Washington.

1965 Publication of *Half-Sun on the Columbia: A Biography of Chief Moses*, Ruby's first collaboration with John A. Brown.

2001 Publication of *Esther Ross: Stillaguamish Champion*, his last collaboration with John A. Brown.

2004 John A. Brown dies.

2009 Robert H. Ruby continues writing historical articles from his home in Moses Lake, Washington.

Editors' Comment on Editorial Methodology

The original material consisted of a series of letters from Dr. Robert H. Ruby to his sister, Marion Johnson, using a typewriter and keeping carbon copies for himself, which he preserved. As he began transferring many of his papers to the Northwest Museum of Arts and Cultures in Spokane, Washington, Ruby retained the rights to this correspondence, with the idea that he might want to edit the letters as an account of his experience in South Dakota. The editors met Ruby while writing an article on the historical work of Ruby and his colleague and co-author, John A. Brown. Following the publication of the article, Ruby invited us to edit his memoir of the time he spent on the Pine Ridge Indian Reservation.

Our methodology has been to edit for clarity and readability, but to retain Dr. Ruby's voice. As written, each letter was self-contained, sometimes with reference made to previous events. The editors removed repetitive sections and sometimes modified wording for clarity. In some instances minor corrections to dates and spelling were made. Editorial comments were intentionally kept separate from Dr. Ruby's narrative, to avoid breaking into it. The historical analysis of the memoir has been confined to the introduction and a brief conclusion written by the editors. Explanatory material about the contents of the memoir has been added in the form of endnotes, again to avoid disrupting the flow of Ruby's narrative.

Dr. Ruby regularly wrote about the persons with whom he worked as well as his patients, freely using their names in his letters. While this is not remarkable in private correspondence, identifying people can be problematic and even unacceptable in a book. Most of those mentioned in Dr. Ruby's letters were not elected officials with official lives that they expected to be bared and opened to public scrutiny. The editors decided that it was important to allow private citizens to maintain their anonymity, particularly in those cases where it was deemed reasonable to believe that embarrassment might follow through the disclosure of their identities. Ruby encountered a wide range of persons possessing a great variety of personal and social problems, including substance abuse (mainly alcohol), child neglect, abject poverty, joblessness, demoralization, and out-of-wedlock sexual activity, and his tendency was to record everything that he either witnessed himself or heard about through others. For the sake of privacy, the editors have excised from the text the names of persons who might feel embarrassment, and vague descriptions have been inserted in place of the names. In a very few instances, pseudonyms have been used. The social issues encountered by Dr. Ruby remain serious challenges and ones that the Oglala Sioux Tribe is working diligently to overcome.

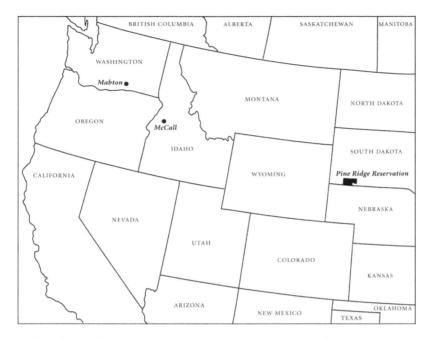

1. Robert Ruby's Northwest. The spatial relationship between Dr. Ruby's childhood home in Mabton, Washington, his sister's home in McCall, Idaho, and the Pine Ridge Indian Reservation in South Dakota. The newly married Rubys drove from Washington State to McCall and then to South Dakota to start their married life and Dr. Ruby's career as a physician and surgeon.

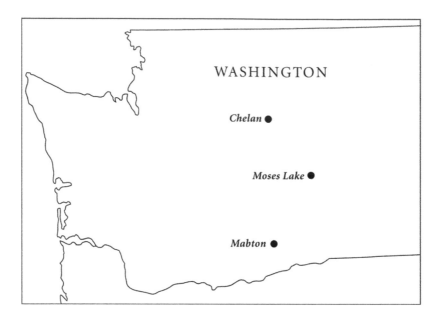

WASHINGTON

Chelan ●

Moses Lake ●

Mabton ●

2. The three Washington communities most important to Dr. Robert H. Ruby: Mabton, where he was born and raised; Chelan, his wife Jeanne's hometown; and Moses Lake, where he established himself in private practice in 1955 following their return from Pine Ridge.

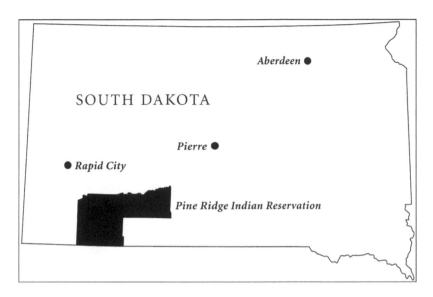

3. The locations in South Dakota most relevant to Dr. Robert H. Ruby: Aberdeen, where his superiors in the Bureau of Indian Affairs were headquartered; Pierre, the state capital; Rapid City, the nearest major commercial center off the reservation, and the Pine Ridge Indian Reservation, where Dr. Ruby worked.

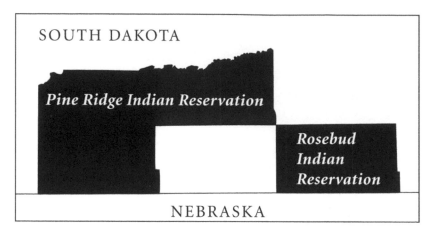

4. Indian Reservations in southwestern South Dakota. The Pine Ridge Indian Reservation and Rosebud Indian Reservation. Dr. Robert H. Ruby was based on the Pine Ridge Reservation, but he and his colleagues worked across reservation boundaries on some occasions.

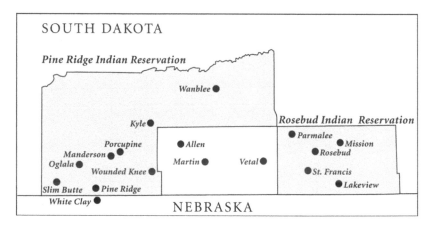

5. Pine Ridge Indian Reservation and Environs. The communities on the Pine Ridge and neighboring Rosebud Indian reservations. Dr. Robert H. Ruby became familiar with the small communities on the two adjoining Indian reservations and neighboring towns during his tenure at Pine Ridge.

One. August 1953

I am still not accustomed to the work attitude of government personnel. SLOWNESS is the best word I can use to describe it. In meetings officials talk about quantity and quality. But words fly faster than results. There is protocol for official methods, manners, channels, procedures, and so on. But unofficially I've been told not to worry my head about it. In the government service it would appear on the surface that to make errors is a grave sin. But you soon learn that if you do not enrich or profit by mistakes personally, you are not held accountable.

Sunday, August 9, 1953

I received my commission in May as a senior assistant surgeon in the United States Public Health Service. As soon as I received the papers, it was only a few days later that a letter arrived from Pine Ridge, South Dakota, from the Bureau of Indian Affairs, with the glad tidings that a "mansion" was being reserved for me. Pine Ridge was to be my station, since I had been allocated to the Department of the Interior.

This promised mansion was to have three bedrooms. It would be completely furnished, except for dishes and linens. It would be only a stone's throw from the hospital so that I could walk from my promised estate to the hospital without getting my nose cold in the cold wintry air.

Our trip to South Dakota was uneventful. We had no car trouble, just a smooth journey. The first night after leaving McCall we stayed in Pocatello, Idaho.[1] I did not know what was customary concerning dogs in motels so I didn't ask anyone. I just sneaked Captain in.[2] And

I did so each succeeding night, until I learned that dogs are permitted in most motels, at least those that are not carpeted. The second day we drove through Yellowstone National Park. We saw lots of wildlife. Captain was especially interested in the bears. There was one mother bear with two of the cutest little cubs. But more beautiful than the drive through the park was the drive from the northeast entrance up over the mountains, above the timber line, and then a sudden drop down into Red Lodge, Montana, where we stayed the second night in a log cabin motel.[3] That drive was out of this world. So many lakes that can be seen up there so high. The distance is only fifty miles but it takes a good two hours going along as fast as you dare. This particular highway was built in 1938. It is fairly new as you can see. It is only open four months out of the year.

Such a contrast to the next day out, our third. The drive from Red Lodge across southern Montana was so flat. We made our greatest distance in that day, ending up in Hettinger, North Dakota.[4] Ran into rain this day. The next day we arrived in Aberdeen, where we stayed for four nights.[5]

We had time in Aberdeen to do little chores. Our new staff orientation conference started on Thursday at the Bureau of Indian Affairs Area Office. That evening we had a banquet, and I'm not exaggerating. I had a steak that was a good two inches thick. For once I had all the steak I could eat at a sitting. The next day at noon another doctor just coming into Pine Ridge and myself sneaked out of the meeting and after picking up Jeanne and the dog we were off to Pine Ridge.[6] Dr. Joseph Walters rode down with us. It is a good trip, 380 miles from Aberdeen.

But let me tell you about the swank place, THE place of Martin, where we had dinner and spent the night. Atmosphere! And How! After sitting at the tables covered with linoleum, chipped about the edges, and the chipped paint of the legs in the place that looked to be furnished about the era of the flapper age, twenty-five years or better back. I asked the girl where the washroom was. She said, "Over there." It wasn't a room, only a slight depression in the side of the wall. Therein was a crude shelf. On it was a bucket of cold water, dipper, and beside it an old wash basin decorated with a pattern of sand around it. A mirror, which had been well splashed, was on the wall. Underneath was a larger bucket into which the used water was tossed.

Joyously riding into Pine Ridge the next morning, we were yet ten miles out and still the metropolis couldn't be spotted, when a young Indian removed his hat and greeted us with vigorous motion of his upper extremities. "They must know we are coming." I did feel royally welcome. It wasn't long until "clunk" and then "thud." We had hit some sort of bird, after already having three very narrow misses with other flying foul. I checked the speedometer, seventy-five miles per hour. It could be that the foul aren't used to people flying low. So I quit playing footsie with the gas feed and slowed to a creep, sixty miles an hour. Result, no further traumatization of flying foul.

We didn't drive within miles of any pine trees, but soon in the distance there was a ridge, by stretching the imagination. And sure enough, there were pine trees on it. Then I knew we were near the metropolis of Pine Ridge. Soon we went over a little knoll, and down in a hole on the other side was the town of Pine Ridge.

The joint was teeming, teeming with shacks, referred to as houses. The majority are used to house Indians, being the town is on reservation land. Main Street! It was surfaced with gravel, and well run over to make nice big holes and wash boards. There was a service station, three grocery stores, a post office, and that is about all, outside of churches galore. There is every denomination of church here, including the Church of Latter Day Saints, the Adventists, the Christian Scientist, and so forth and so on. EXCEPTING one, and that is a Methodist church. But some local yokel told me that at one time the Methodists did have a church here. It is the first town I've seen that did not have as many bars as churches. There were none. But being a reservation, no drinking is allowed.

In the distance I could see one building. It was a large brick structure, a nice-looking building, high on a hill. Our mansion, no doubt. But goodness, were they giving us three stories? I thought it was three bedrooms. We drove up. It was the hospital. On the grounds was another brick structure, the nurses' quarters, and two wooden homes, one large and already occupied, the other small, that was to be Dr. Walter's home. There were no other buildings, excepting utility buildings. Was it that our promised mansion was so large it had to be out a ways?

Being that it was only 8:00 a.m., an early hour, no one was stirring. We therefore had to go looking for the administrator of the Bureau of Indian Affairs. After getting him up out of bed, he gave us a key and directions to our new home.

"Oh, there it is." Our home, a small wooden structure. I later learned that the building was hauled on a truck all the way from Montana from a previous government reservation that was recently closed. Our house was obviously new. The new paint kept the windows, doors, and other movable parts from closing or opening with ease. Not all the window locks were on. The light fixtures were not in.

Our promised mansion. Well, because of its rather limited size, I told Jeanne she could store "junk" in the basement. But there was no basement. As luck would have it, a rather large garage had been provided, with more room than is necessary for our car. We could store in there. It wasn't long until the maintenance men were there. They had to figure out how to get the antiquated electric stove in since some enterprising individual had STOLEN the new gas range provided. Another maintenance man spent all morning getting our automatic water heater in gear. At last, hot water. Now we could start on the enormous job of washing everything up. Our completely furnished house had not one stick of furniture in it excepting a bed. And that had been put in the preceding day after the superintendent called from Aberdeen the preceding day telling the officials at Pine Ridge we'd be in and had to have something to sleep on. But the bed was in pieces. It took only a brief pause to set it up so that it could become a catchall for junk until we got situated.

The adequate corner windows were without not only curtains but also shades, making it necessary to run around from bath to bedroom without lights at night. My wife quickly went to work. She laid out our dirty clothes from three weeks of travel on the dirty highways. But there was no washing machine. Then came our first kindness. The wife of the superintendent came to pay a visit, brief of course. She came in just after all of our shipped things had been laid smack in the middle of every inch of available floor space, after we had gotten our work underway and looked like it, too. She offered us the use of her washing machine until we got one, saying she had lots of the notoriously hard water around these parts. I thought it was a swell idea. I told my wife she could go over daily with her clothes until she became such a bother that the mistress would be sure to remind her husband more frequently as it got unbearable that the Rubys were without a washing machine. Perhaps we'd soon be given one.

Perhaps my wife has intuition. Or it could be that she was holding some information from me. She took several items of furniture and more than, far more than, what should be considered adequate knickknacks and what have you, to decorate this little place. We quickly went to work unpacking box after box of things. Soon what limited shelf and closet space there was seemed to be bulging at the cornices. The remaining items were left packed. Soon we went around scooping up piles of dirt, and quantities of dead insects of all sorts. I then decided to haul the boxes and some items to be stored across our beautiful yard to the garage. First I had to make a path through the weeds that reached to my head. Such tall, succulent weeds made it hard to get the garage doors open also. I learned my first bit about the Indians. All labor around here is done by Indians. Huge mounds of dirt had been hauled in and dumped three for four feet apart all around the house. But Joe Horn Cloud and Dixon Little Bear promised that this would be leveled soon.

But in order to make our house completely livable it was necessary to "borrow" furniture from other government houses. This was no great task, especially since Dr. Walter had brought furniture enough for a complete setup. This provided me with a complete afternoon of wiping down beds, bureaus, dressers, chairs, and so forth.

The next day I had a breathing spell and decided to examine the surrounding neighborhood. To the east where I can look from my desk as I write is an old government house that has been burned. Such an intriguing sight. To the west from the dining room I can see an inhabited Indian home. It is only a stone's throw from our yard. The outside privy is well in evidence. The drive leading to this abode takes off from our own drive. In the time I was looking over our new home, I noticed that many Indian children were appraising our setup. Their cat was curious enough to take a trip over. Their dog and puppy also took note of the Rubys.

We do have to eat, so the Rubys went shopping. The day before our arrival saw the end to a three-day Indian festival, so the stores' excuse for being out of stock was that the Indians had bought them out. We had to make a visit to two grocery stores in order to get a fair semblance of what would do us for a few days. Being out of money was, we thought, our worst fix, especially since there is no bank in this city. But identifying ourselves made it easy to cash checks. In one store we were introduced to a shopper as the new doctor and his wife. "Oh, which one, Dr. Walter or Dr. Ruby?" asked the man. I told him. But I was curious to know how he might have known our name, since it hadn't been mentioned to him. He answered, "I'm the postmaster, and you've been getting mail for a month." That seemed to help my spirits.

Dry Cleaners. No. Drivers from neighboring towns, twenty-five and fifty miles away, make trips in and collect dry cleaning. The water here is so hard that it leaves a well-healed scar around any basin after a wash. The grocery stores are stocked with lots of water softener and the basic items. One of each. If you want a can of peas you have the grand total of one brand to pick from. And the same with any other item. There is no hardware store in town, but I felt exceptionally fortunate to find at one of the grocery stores a padlock for our garage, since none had been provided. It was an Indian, one of the Bear family, one of the Feathers, who warned me that it was unwise to leave an auto sitting out. It could well be minus fixtures the next morning if that were done.

Really we are more than delighted with our cute little house. I honestly can't wait until you all get to see it. Joe Horn Cloud said it was under three hundred miles to Cheyenne. If you people should come by train instead of auto we'd be delighted to drive and get you. I haven't talked that over with Jeanne yet, but I know she would because we are really isolated from any real places to shop and that would be a good outlet for her. The first thing we are going to do is to get a catalogue to do some of our ordering. We need curtain rods and then Jeanne is going to make curtains.

I was so sore yesterday after moving furniture, hauling furniture, et cetera, that I could scarcely move. Jeanne washed every item of glassware, pots, and pans we have. I helped some on that, but I wiped down all the furniture. Jeanne brought quite a bit of furniture, otherwise I don't know what we'd have done. They brought us a dining room table. A beautiful piece of furniture. Today we hung some pictures. You'd die to see where I hung that Siegfried Reinhardt sketch of me.[7] In the guest room, your bedroom when you visit. To keep the rats out, I guess. There was a bed here for us, but I wanted one for you people in your room. We got one. It is nice. Only I think a little too soft perhaps. Then we have Jeanne's davenport, which is a Hide-a-way for the kiddies. I found an ash wood bureau for you. Only it's got things in it now. Your room, which I am in, now, has this desk of Jeanne's that I use for my den. Jeanne uses this room then in the days for sewing, ironing, and other tasks.

Send everything that comes for me simply to me, Pine Ridge, South Dakota. Guess after my name you better write simply Indian Hospital. Leave off the excess Pine Ridge in front of the hospital and leave off the usph. Be sure to send my bank statements.

We were discussing furniture last night with Dr. Walters, who came over amid the litter for chicken dinner since his wife isn't coming for several months yet. We sure do like our first little house since being married, and we are anxious for you to see it.

Honestly Kid, this town makes me feel at home—Reminds me of Mabton in *so* many ways.[8] Jeanne thinks so, too.

August 17, 1953

Hello from Pine Ridge: Setting up housekeeping in our house was not without its moments. It was without a phone. My work is one in which there are repeated and constant phone calls, 70 percent of which are unnecessary and superfluous.

The telephone exchange in Pine Ridge is a small office. The operator knows everyone and everyone's business. Her board is not large. To get the operator, an individual leaves the phone on the hook as he rings an antiquated crank. The operator on answering plugs the caller into his party. The entire town is on a party line. So obviously there can be no more than one conversation going at one time. And what's more, when the operator rings a party, every phone in town rings. The phone office is open five days a week, Monday thru Friday, 8:00 to 5:00. On nights and weekends there is no phoning excepting to the hospital. The operator can hook up her board so that in some way anyone in town can ring the hospital. If there is an emergency, the hospital can summon the police by turning on a red light on the top of the hospital building, which is on the hill above the town. The tribal police below, seeing the red light, answer by phone or respond by going up to the hospital.[9]

My first day of making phone calls kept my arm sore from cranking. My first day at the hospital I could not get used to the phone ringing and not having to answer it. When someone calls the hospital, the office girl answers. The call cannot be plugged into different offices or floors. Rather the office girl gets on a loud speaker and announces that someone is wanted on the phone. So the nearest phone available on the floors and offices is picked up and used. When the office girl hears your voice, she knows you've answered and hangs up her own phone.

That first night in our home we invited Dr. Walters in spite of the floor being a conglomeration of packing boxes and general confusions. My wife agreed that it would be all right to have a doctor in for dinner, one of the doctors who had come into town with us. We soon found that in spite of all the materials we had brought with us, we would have to order various items. One of the household books of necessity is the Sears Roebuck Catalogue. Our first letter was one to the Sears Roebuck Company asking for a catalogue.

I think my first day at work could be best called one of confusion. There was the blur of new names, new faces, new rooms, new routines. It seemed to me that every time one turned around each move had to be initiated with forms of red tape. The government wants six copies of every order. Before an order can be placed, however, the money has to be obligated with six copies of the obligation, and so forth and so on.

Mr. O. R. Sande, who is the superintendent of the Pine Ridge Indian Reservation, called a meeting to throw more confusion in the way for the new doctors.

I was so impressed with the necessity for knowing so much routine in ordering, making reports, and so on, that after the meeting Mr. Sande told me not to be concerned. Things will take care of themselves. I must have shown my great worry for trying to comprehend some of the routine.

Mr. Sande went at great length to ask that the Indians be respected and cared for as individuals. They must have that personal touch and be respected as a free person. But they must not be thought of as having their medicine provided free, because it was not that. The taxpayers were paying for their care. The doctors must render the care provided a fee-paying patient.

I did some figuring as Mr. Sande talked. After having looked the hospital over and taken a fair squint at the lack of equipment, it seemed to me that by the time I have obligated necessary money for needed equipment to do surgery and orthopedics, by the time the orders were placed and other forms, red tape, and so forth was waded through, that

9

there would be much of it not getting there until my tour of duty of two years would be up.

There I sat in the dining room eating cookies, drinking coffee, and taking in all Mr. Sande had to say, and I was the only one in a suit. No one in the Indian Bureau wears suits. It is sports shirts and slacks.

It so happened that this, my first day on duty Mr. Sande called a meeting of the heads of his different staffs. I was asked to come to represent Health. The acting medical officer was ill in the hospital. I had understood Mr. Sande to say I'd be the assistant acting medical officer. Therefore I figured I was there for that reason. Again, the meeting seemed to me one of importance, so much so that I should wear a suit. Everyone else at that meeting that night looked to me as if they had stopped in on their way from a picnic.

The next day Mr. Sande clarified my position for me. He had been on the phone with the Area Office in Aberdeen. I had been elected, chosen to be the medical officer in charge.

The first thing Mr. Sande asked me to do besides care for inpatients, care for outpatients, ordering equipment and drugs, be custodian of the hospital, its equipment, personnel, and grounds, and take care of the health of nearly eleven thousand Sioux Indians, and do their surgery and surgery on patients referred from other reservations, was to read volume 6, part 3, of the Indian Bureau manual, about three hundred pages, and make suggestions on all of its content as to how it might be reworded to read more clearly.

Chowder, return the first two pages of this letter for my notes.[10]

We are now a two-car family. As the medical officer in charge I have a government car. I'm the only one in the bureau or on the entire reservation that can have a car twenty-four hours a day. So that leaves Jeanne with our car for her use. It is very convenient.

If only you could have been with us Saturday. We drove fifty miles to Chadron, Nebraska, to do our shopping.[11] Our biggest spree was in the meat market. We bought ham, sausage, hamburger, steaks, veal chops, cheese, roast, spare ribs, brains, and so on and so on. We had the brains scrambled with eggs Sunday for breakfast. We bought gobs of groceries, three big boxes full. I bought Jeanne some gladiolas for her table. Had the car serviced. Went to Penney's for curtains, rods, and so on and so on. We had a good time.

Marion, find out who has an amateur radio sending station there in McCall. Get their call number. Tell me their name and call numbers and then I'll make a definite date and call you on the radio set that Dr. Walter here has and talk to you. Do this soon.

The craziest thing yet is that on my nights on I take the deliveries. I delivered twins the other day. And to top it off, the first one came breech. I am doing a gall bladder this week. Last night (Sunday) an Indian got his leg cut off, rather mangled, when a train ran over it. So I did an amputation last night.

I'll sure be glad when you see our house. We have it pretty much in shape now. And is Jeanne ever cooking. Baking rolls, cakes, and so on. Chowder, why don't you and Skinny take the train?[12] You kids could get on at Boise at 5:00 in the morning. You would arrive at Cheyenne, Wyoming, at 5:00 in the evening. We'll pick you up there. That will be only one day on the train.

August 23, 1953

I would say that our three main scourges are dust, bugs, and weeds. It would be necessary to take off a thick layer of dirt daily from the furniture if it were to look halfway clean. Weeds make a border to our dirt yard. They rise to the height of the clothes line. I had to get out the other day and chop out a few of the larger ones so we could wend our way beneath the clothes line and to that we could hang a few of the smaller items on the clothes line without them being brushed by the weeds. There are every shape, description, phylum, and gender of bugs around here. At night the place is swarming with the creatures. Crickets make highways across the floors. I find the mosquitoes particularly distasteful.

Shopping is our big problem. We travel fifty miles to Chadron in

11

Nebraska to buy up stocks to last a month. It makes a nice Saturday afternoon drive. And brings us back to civilization.

Believe I've already told you that the Indians have many horses. They run loose. It is nothing daily to have horses pass across the yard. The Indians are flattered when white people ask to ride their horses. The horses are quite spirited. Though they are not fed, merely left to scrape for themselves, they are well fed, fat, and look to be in fine shape.

Right now as I write there are Indians galore on foot, horseback, and car headed for the rodeo that is less than two miles from our house. This weekend will see lots of casualties. Broken bones. Alcohol and wild animals don't mix too well. The folks here justify it by believing that there are fewer casualties than in football.

My first night on duty at the hospital was not without difficulty. There being no phone in our house, the attendant or relatives of some ill person had to come for the doctor. We were living "in the new house behind the burned-out house."

One of the people to come after me the first night, because we had no phone service, was Joseph Big Thunder. When I got to the hospital I found it was an OB case. The patient had a breech delivery. I quickly recalled what the books and my professors years ago had told me about delivering babies. The mother and I had no trouble.

It was only four nights later that I delivered twins. As if that wasn't enough, the first of the two came breech. After I'd been there a week I delivered my third bottom-first baby.

Indian mothers deliver easily. Breech babies and twins are more frequent than for white mothers. The first stage of labor from beginning of pains until they are fully dilated averages in time as white women. But the second stage of labor from full dilatation to delivery is practically no time. The usual rectal examination to determine the degree of dilatation is of no value because the Indian woman dilates fast and delivers immediately. She will go from a centimeter of dilatation to full dilatation in a minute or two.

For the white woman the average length of time for the third stage of labor, from delivery of infant to delivery of the placenta, is twenty minutes. For the Indian women it is three to five minutes.

I've not delivered a woman yet that needed anesthesia or an episiotomy. I do appreciate this help from these mothers. They are a great help in getting them delivered.

Clinics for the eleven thousand Sioux Indians on our reservation are held each afternoon Monday thru Friday. Indian children quite often come to clinics unaccompanied by an adult. The majority of Indians understand English. Those who do not generally are the very aged. There are only a few of the very young who do not understand Indian.One of the first Indian expressions I learned was the equivalent to "Where does it hurt?" This to me had the phonetic sound of "Doko de nee aa za?" I worked it to death the first week.

The Indians are notorious for removing their own casts from fractured extremities at their own initiative and by themselves before fractures are fully healed. I was simply horrified when one man, thirty-seven years of age, fractured the bones of one of his legs. A long cast had been applied elsewhere, since the injury had been sustained off reservation. In less than a month the man had removed the cast from below the knee and the thigh and from just above the ankle and foot. He was left with a cylinder on his leg. The leg bones are major weight-bearing bones and often need immobilization for six months after a fracture. Immobilization is by cast, which extends beyond the bone broken, across the joints above and below the fractured bone; to maintain immobilization.

Indian men keep their hats on in buildings. But the most impressive compliment I can pay the Indians is that they show appreciation for things that are done for them at the hospital. Indians know and use the word "Thank you."

The Indians, both sexes and all ages, are notorious for marking their bodies with indelible ink of some sort for tattooing. This takes the form of names, initials, and designs such as the swastika-like figure.

The Indians use slang as frequently as the white men. "Oh-kedoke" is frequent. One of the most difficult things to become used to, I believe, is a broad "a" when they speak. These Sioux sound fresh out of Boston at times, and again some of them sound exactly like the Katherine Hepburn voice.

When the order came through "nominating" me as the medical officer in charge, it became necessary to attend agency meetings as a department head. There are some fifteen departments in the Bureau of Indian Affairs. I had to practice the new attitude. No longer must the Indian be isolated and protected. He must be made one of our society and integrated with our society. The Indian must be made to assert himself and show his independence.

I was shocked when I saw in print that the Indians must be continuously "graduated," relocated, and resettled in the years to come. Here is a quote from a report that may startle even the uninitiated in Indian affairs as it did me. "Much space in your program is rightfully devoted to the problem of how to modify those Sioux attitudes and traits which retard the Sioux' progress in their modern economic environment. It is regrettable that selfless magnanimity, generosity, broad charity, fearlessness, tolerance and a highly developed sense of personal dignity should be characteristics which impede the integration of the individual possessing them with a society professing to be Christian, but it is a fact that these Indian traits handicap the possessor almost as much as the Indian habit of intermittent instead of continuous effort. As you imply repeatedly, we must first inculcate in the Sioux the desire for material things, indoctrinate them with our own attitude toward possessions before the transition from the life of a nomadic hunter to that of a settled cattle rancher can be completed successfully. But we must be careful that in this transition the finer values of Indian character are not irretrievably submerged."

This is from a report of preparations made in 1944, when William O. Roberts was superintendent of the Pine Ridge Agency, for a long-range program to bring Indians to self-sufficiency at a standard of living enjoyed by others.[13] The Bureau of Indian Affairs was to provide public services in the fields of education, health, social welfare, relief, law enforcement, roads, and probate, which services are not rendered to Indians on reservations by local authorities since the treaties give the Indians land tax exemptions and the state and counties are unwilling to supply these services.

The above is not so shocking when one learns the Indian race is two-thirds or more white infusion. I think from those I see in the clinic, greater than two-thirds are obviously mixed blood. Buffalo days are gone. The Indian must be implanted with practical virtues that anyone on his own steam must possess. The Sioux must be aroused to become ambitious. The immediate need is developing the Indian to act on thinking. "Selfless magnanimity," "generosity," and "broad charity" take such forms as collectively and individually to make the Indian "dead broke." There are Indians who practice reckless disposition of property. There is one I know who uses all his money for liquor after selling land.

The luxury of Indian ways is moving about, absenteeism of the children from agency schools, the tendency to spend money and dispose of property regardless of amount, extravagant use of time for social affairs, and inertia or resistance.

I should offer this. The exact program is not to promote Indian ways that are the same as white ways but rather to stress the willingness and desire to do whatever is at hand that will contribute to better living and greater health standards.

The agency health program operates not just the hospital, medical clinic, and dental care. There are clinics out on the reservation staffed with a nurse for medical and dental care. There is an active program to examine all school children in the fall at the start of the reservation's school. It will not be long until the Indian children return to school. The districts in the reservation are Wounded Knee, Porcupine, White Clay, Medicine Root, Eagle Nest, Wakpamni, and Pass Creek.

I spend much of my day going over official communications from the Bureau office and Area office. One of the most amusing things to me is the slang injected into official communications, such as "covering with a fine tooth comb," "as sad as a barrel of spoiled apples," and so on.

The Sioux still harbor a certain amount of resentment for whites because of earlier historic violent confrontations. They also resent such things as the way too much of the money set aside from them in the Bureau budget goes for the homes and living expenses for white BIA employees.

I am still not accustomed to the work attitude of government personnel. SLOWNESS is the best word I can use to describe it. In meetings officials talk about quantity and quality. But words fly faster than results. There is protocol for official methods, manners, channels, procedures, and so on. But unofficially I've been told not to worry my head about it. In the government service it would appear on the surface that to make errors is a grave sin. But you soon learn that if you do not enrich or profit by mistakes personally, you are not held accountable.

Had lots of surgery this past week. I did a gall bladder that was one of the worst infected messes I've seen. I closed a perforated peptic ulcer.

I've found a few moments this week to read some Indian history. Marion, I'm intensely absorbed in Indian history. I'm also reading "Edwin Booth, Prince of Players." An interesting book. Mrs. Johnson sent me the copy of the *Christian Herald* which I wanted to read and which I forgot.[14] I was very happy she did. I wrote her a letter yesterday.

Jeanne has her curtains up. That seems to be the last major item of work to be done in our house. Excepting that I have to get some DDT to spray this big hoard of insects that plagues us each evening. And now we have a mouse.

We had a nice Sunday. Got up late. Went to church. I washed the car, washed the dog, and cleaned those weeds from under the clothes line. Then we had a steak dinner on our dining room table. Then I laid down a while and went to sleep before starting writing letters. Last night we went for a drive. There were so many Indians in town, congregated for the rodeo.

The moon is so big, round, and full. Think I'll see if Jeanne wants to take a walk.

[no date]

I am having my troubles as the medical officer in charge of this hospital. Each person has their grievances. They come to me with their problems. In most of the cases it helps for the individual to talk out their difficulties. Psychotherapy. One of the nurses, Miss Pratt, is "sore" at Margaret M. McGill, the acting director of nurses, because Miss McGill does not rotate her. She keeps Miss Pratt on night duty and has since May. Being on night duty now the night outside light is shut off at the nurses' home so Miss Pratt has to go home in the dark. Miss Pratt kept her car in the garage, she said. Birds roosted over the top and got it dirty. When she gave up the garage, Miss McGill had the birds cleaned out. Someone else has the garage and Miss McGill will not give it back to her. Miss Pratt suggested buying a present for one of the nurses when she left. Miss McGill, as director, would have nothing to do with it. But she went out and bought a present and solicited money from others for a present, excepting from those she did not favor, and then gave the present to the departing nurse without their names on the gift card and after she, Miss Pratt, had suggested it. And so on and so on.

The hospital is three stories: a basement for the cafeteria, maintenance shops, X-ray, and laboratory. The floor above is administrative offices and a few beds for overflow of patients. At the far-east end is my office. It has a phone for outside calls. There is an X-ray viewing box and a fine library as well as a private "john." The third floor is all for patients, the operating room, and delivery room. The cast room is in the basement floor at the far-west end under the clinic building.

We can handle fifty patients and are now running a census of forty-six patients. We are understaffed, and I've been writing memorandums to the Bureau office for a week trying to get some action from them. If action is taken, it will not make any major changes for a year.

When I first came into the hospital I learned that there had been a fire in the elevator shaft. So the elevator was not working. I learned also that this hospital has no fire escape. I was here nearly a month before the elevator was put into working order. It was impossible to carry bedfast patients from the upper floors down to X-ray. Patients suffered for lack of X-rays. When critically ill patients came to the hospital, they had to be carried up the narrow stairs by whoever we could round up to help.

We were out of 5 percent glucose and water for intravenous injection. We ran out of the large size of X-ray film that is used for chests. Here with the Indians, where so many chest X-rays are taken as tuberculosis has been rampant, it was a serious lack of supplies. Our X-ray technician loaned a few he had until we could get more. I have found only one flashlight in the whole hospital. At one time the typewriter in the doctor's office and the front offices were both on the blink.

And with the lack of personnel and equipment, they want to make this a referring center for other reservations to send patients here. This includes quite a number of reservations. I have heard that they are planning on shutting down all other reservation hospitals in the area and making this the only hospital to take referrals. I don't see how that can happen, since we have hardly the personnel to care for our own patients. This reservation is one hundred square miles. Already we have had referrals from other reservations for surgery. But with our lack of help, we can do surgery only three days a week, Tuesday, Wednesday, and Thursday, excepting emergencies, which are done at any time. In the time I've been here already I've utilized most of those days. Excepting that at first I balled things up not knowing that these were surgery days. I scheduled surgery other days and caused the overworked staff to come back for extra duty.

In the clinic approximately a third of the patients are pediatric problems, and we have no pediatrician. Children come in occasionally with new or clean clothes, not ironed. The older Indian women wear braids, and shawls, and some wear the deerskin moccasins. Most all Indian women wear earrings thru pierced ears. Very few of the old Indian men wear braids.

I occasionally take pictures of the patients coming out of the seven districts for clinic care. They never mind but usually want me to be sure and send them a print. Now that fall has arrived, some Indian women tell me about preserving winter's supply of fruits and berries, all wild. The wild plums are smashed up with the use of old-time hand stone grinders.

An Indian came to the hospital not long ago peddling the wild plums, and the wild grapes from which Jeanne made jelly. We have used wild crab apples. The jellies and jams from wild fruits and berries (including elderberries) are a delicacy not to be missed.

Saturday we went fishing at Denby Dam and the White Clay Dam on the reservation. We got bass, perch, and bullheads. We got frogs and ate the legs. What a delicacy. The frogs were thick at Denby. There the water is shallow, and the weeds and moss thick. They hop out quickly and get lost easily.[15]

One of our best "finds" was a place to buy vegetables. Five miles out of town is a Catholic Mission.[16] And there Brother Schlinger is the gardener. He came from Switzerland twenty years ago. His primary work is to raise vegetables to feed six hundred children attending school at the mission. He was busy making sauerkraut when we first went out. He has every vegetable imaginable. Since he does not raise them to sell, he lets the hospital personnel have them very inexpensively. It is the excess that he sells. I thought I was smart buying a fifty-pound sack of potatoes from a peddler at the hospital one day. They were a pound less in the stores at Chadron where we do most of our shopping.

It is a thrill to go home these evenings and see the kitchen lined with the day's canning of vegetables and preserves that Jeanne has made for winter use. The aroma is delightful.

At first we were afraid we were going to have some help from a small mouse, some help getting rid of our winter's stores. In Chadron we got a mouse trap and were rid of him inside of two hours after the trap was baited with cheese and set.

Occasionally our collie dog Captain comes in handy. He hauls in trash from all the neighbors and piles it in our front yard. But the other day he hauled in a red bucket, which came in handy for planting a wild plant we got the other day while fishing.

One morning all department heads were called in and told Senator Mundt of South Dakota would be in Pine Ridge the next day, and we were to prepare a list of certain things for the senator to let him know about our respective departments.[17] The meeting was to be in Superintendent Sande's office. I was there bright and early. No senator. After some amenities, Mr. Sande got a call that the senator would be late. He had not gotten to bed before 1:00 a.m. I waited around and talked about stamp collecting with Mr. Stanley Walker, head of the Highway Department on the reservation. I decided an hour was all I could waste. I just got up to leave when I saw Mr. Sande talking to some gentlemen in the hall. As I started out I told Mr. Sande I had surgery. He introduced me to a very distinguished looking man. It wasn't the senator, though. Next he introduced me to another man. Surely he was the senator. No. Finally at the end of the line I was introduced to a short, fat, tubby, undistinguished looking man. That was the senator. After introductions and an effusive gush, politician style, he asked, "Oh, are you in charge of the hospital? That building high on the hill we saw all lighted up last night?" I replied that I was and excused myself to go back to work.

The other night our clerk came to do some work. She had to get into a storeroom in the attic and to dig out an old patient chart. The switch that turned on the attic lights also turned on the outside red light. The police were up in no time.

Our drive yesterday through the Black Hills was very nice. But after being used to the Rockies there is certainly no comparison when it comes to height and grandeur of the Rockies. The Black Hills seem tame. They are beautiful in a more restful sort of way. We saw the summer White House used by President Coolidge. Then we saw the lodge where President Eisenhower stayed for four days this June.

The Black Hills are a favorite for tourists. A new monument has been started to honor Crazy Horse, the chief who led the battle against Custer. And then Mount Rushmore. What an inspiring sight. The monument was carved from a sheer wall of granite. The faces of Washington, Jefferson, T. Roosevelt, and Lincoln were started around 1930 by the sculptor Gutzon Borglum. He died in 1941 before the monument was completed. His son, Lincoln Borglum, finished the remaining touches on the faces. When I got to the monument I stood gazing at it for some time, spellbound. I was fascinated at that structure. A museum on the grounds explains the construction. I think no other manmade monument equals it.

We proceeded on up to Spearfish, where the Black Hills Passion Play is held three nights weekly during July and August each year.[18] There were cars there from all over the United States. We saw the last performance for the season.

The stage is equal to three city blocks in length. There is no changing of scenery. There is the temple, the garden of Gethsemene, the cemetery. The Roman courthouse where Pilot holds forth. The courtyard, other structures, and a central building with a curtain where several scenes were performed, such as the Last Supper. It was next to the Crucifixion the most beautiful and stirring scene. Live horses, burros or asses, and even camels are used in the play. There was the walk to Golgatha, the hill where the Crucifixion occurred, off in the distance and high up a mountain where Christ marches with the cross. What a sight. A luminous light shines on him. A weird noise heard as the heavens opens made goose bumps.

The play is done to perfection. There was not a flaw in the performance. Joseph Meier as Christ did not portray a very radiant character. He didn't charm or command all the attention as a dynamic person might. It was, however, a sight to behold. The amphitheater is large and holds a vast crowd. For a very few minutes a heavy rain came down. Very few people got up and left. We were drenched.

After the performance we drove three hundred miles to home base. I was on duty bright and early the next morning after three and a half hours sleep.

Two. September 1953

On August 26 the Indians had a knock-down-and-drag-out celebration for Eugene Rowland, a returned Korean prisoner of war. The crowd was respectful of the occasion and broke up by late evening. Nothing like that the Saturday before when at the dance during the rodeo days it was necessary to use tear gas to break up the noisy drunken crowds after they overturned a police car.

[no date]

Up north on the Pine Ridge reservation and just above the reservation are three large plateaus of land. One is Red Shirt Table, where many of the Indians live, Cooley Table, where some live, and Blindman Table, where only one family lives. These areas surround the very rugged Badlands. A patient in the hospital now with tuberculosis of the peritoneum is Nettie Blindman, a sister-in-law of the Blindmans, who have lived for years alone in this wilderness.

It is no trouble to contact anyone on the reservation. We have a method here that is better than smoke signals, better than the wireless, or mail. And that is word of mouth. News spreads throughout the reservation like wildfire. Mr. Lawrence T. Mickelson, the school principal, wanted to get news to a girl way out by Wounded Knee that he wanted her to cook at the school in the place of another woman who fell and fractured her leg. So Mr. Mickelson merely announced at the football game last Sunday afternoon that he wanted Mrs. So and So to come see him. She was there the next morning. When we want someone to come to the clinic, we merely let out the news, and from the four corners they are here.

Funerals: Death in a family is great cause for wakes and other means of "commemoration." The family has to have money to bury a family member. Mr. Sande tells me they come for money for burial purposes and bury people in good suits of clothes. Something far better than they wear during life. It is customary for the family to give away everything of the deceased right after he dies. What usually happens is that the family is so much in grief, the near-family and close-family, that when the distant relatives come they are not taken up so much in grief and get away with all of the deceased's belongings.

Mr. Sande allots money to them for emergencies. The Indians come in at the slightest provocation and with any excuse for money. One of my patients sold some of his land. Mr. Sande keeps the money and proportions it out to him a little at a time because the man would spend it all in a week if he had his hands on it. He is a big drinker. He developed a ruptured ulcer and came to the clinic after I'd been here only a week before. This man was so moribund, he couldn't sign his own operating permit. So I got Mr. Sande to sign it. Superintendent Sande, with two concerns, came uninvited to the hospital and went into the operating room to observe the surgery. Since the patient was under the influence of alcohol and thus could not sign a surgery permit, it was up to Mr. Sande to do so for him. Secondly, he was concerned for the safety of the people he was charged with. So, not being sure of the new surgeon's skills, he decided to check me out. After a successful operation for which he had signed the permit, he was relieved and commented on the foul odor that occurs from a peritonitis from a ruptured bowel. Mr. Sande's assessment was, "It smelled like a manure pile in a barn yard."[1]

The three of us here at the hospital went to the Oglala Community School to do physicals on the students. That is the boarding school here in Pine Ridge. We got through the upper six grades. All the children were dressed nice. And with three exceptions, the 250 students we ex-

amined were all clean. The girls are more noisy than the boys, I do believe. The girls fooled with the light switch, turning it off and on and
such things. There are so many Indian children with high blood pressure and with aortic and mitral murmurs as evidence of old valvular
disease from rheumatic fever.

Well, the story of the year is that they wanted Jeanne to teach chemistry.[2] She told them she would teach for a couple of months until they
could find someone, but she didn't want to sign a contract for all year.
They didn't take her up on her two-month teaching. But the other day
they came to her and asked her to teach sewing classes. She signed a
contract for one month. The previous teacher left because her husband
who worked here was transferred. Jeanne has a class of sophomores
and juniors in the morning and a class of seniors in the afternoons. She
was warned the children were disciplinary problems. But she has found
them quite the opposite. Good children, attentive, and already after only
three days of teaching they are confiding in her with such problems as
"How old should a girl be before she gets married?" Of the girls in her
class, most have four siblings. Four out of five of the homes have sewing machines. In the class of twenty seniors all but one is Catholic. And
they talk rather disparaging of the Catholic Mission five miles from
here, saying that the nuns are sure hard on the children.

Indians do not use sign language anymore. For practical purposes,
they don't. But a few do know a few of the signs. Deaf Indians use the
old sign language. And Indians separated a distance use it so they won't
have to shout. It was used in earlier days for talking between tribes since
each had its own spoken language.

The Sioux today are polite but not appreciative. In the days of the
buffalo and free plains, the Sioux roamed about in large bands. These
groups lived together. Men walked about without making eye contact
with women. Promiscuity was scarce. Today it is frequent. Even prostitution occurs on the reservation. In the late summer months there are
numerous rodeos. Nine months later the hospitals see an increase of
illegitimate births. In the old days law and order was strict when deal-

ing with criminal behavior. Sioux people remind white employees of their bitterness for the violence at the battle of Wounded Knee. The elders pass the hate to their youngsters. The Sioux are slower to acculturate to white ways than most Indians. One worker asked one time, "What is the Indian Bureau?" Answer from a bureau worker: "Just another agency to make the Indian more dependent."

Friday, September 11, 1953

The people here do not rely on food sources from the wild as much as I expected. They are not the hunters, fishermen, or berry pickers as one would expect after reading about them. Though they still shoot deer and use the hides to make leather goods (moccasins particularly, decorated with small beads that are made in Czechoslovakia), they prefer to get food from tin cans.

Recently Congress passed a bill and the president signed it to allow the Indians to buy liquor and bring it onto the reservation. The bill was unnecessary. People have been bringing liquor onto the reservation for some time. There are beer cans and whiskey bottles galore over the reservation. Many Indians who looked non-Indian had no trouble buying beer any place off reservation. The biggest outlet was bootleggers who smuggled in beer in and sold it all over the reservation.[3]

The Indians love celebrations. Lillian Mickelson, wife of Lawrence Mickelson, the school principal, told us one of her husband's greatest problems was keeping students in school for the entire school year. On August 26 the Indians had a knock-down-and-drag-out celebration for Eugene Rowland, a returned Korean prisoner of war.[4] The crowd was respectful of the occasion and broke up by late evening. Nothing like that the Saturday before when at the dance during the rodeo days it was necessary to use tear gas to break up the noisy drunken crowds after they overturned a police car.

The week before on Saturday night the jail keeper brought his one and only prisoner to the hospital when he volunteered to donate blood.

Old George Iron Cloud, the jailor, said it was the first time in seventeen years the jail census had been that low.

We have no blood bank at the hospital. When a transfusion is needed or anticipated the prospective recipient is tested for blood type. A file of donors on the reservation is consulted. A driver is then rounded up to go fetch the donors. Prisoners, glad to leave prison for a short while, sign up to donate blood.

Indian justice is controlled by tribal police, courts, and lawyers. All of this is under scrutiny of the Department of the Interior. The federal government moves in when federal laws are violated.

There are no longer Indian chiefs with authority who rule the tribe. The title Indian chief today is more an honorary position of respect but usually no influence. The tribal government operates by a tribal council, elected every two years. The officers are a president, a vice president, a secretary, and councilmen. Charles Under Baggage, the current president, is temporarily out of his office. He was in Washington DC on business for the tribe not long ago and disgraced himself and dishonored his position by getting drunk. The vice president, Samuel Stands, carries on.

We made our way to the Presbyterian church, a small grey stucco building with a bell tower at the front. The building fronts on the main street across from the largest grocery store. The two Indian ministers who alternate Sundays were out of town for a presbytery meeting. So Mrs. West, the wife of the head of the Agriculture Extension Agency, held forth. She gave a very interesting talk, using the parable of the growing corn as her subject. There are twelve church benches in the building. This first Sunday for Jeanne and me to attend church there were six couples. One was Superintendent Sande of the Pine Ridge reservation. Another was Lyman J. Carr, our lab technician at the hospital, and his wife.

Most Indians living on the reservation have horses. I came here from St. Louis, where I worked at a hospital with a large emergency service, where daily we treated numerous broken bones as a result of auto accidents. But here we are in an "uncivilized world." We have frequent patients with fractures, caused by horse accidents. We may see up to four such accidents a week. Years ago there used to be forty-four million horses in the United States. Today there are eleven million. Horses will soon be a thing of the past. But not yet, we still see Indians riding the roads here in old wagons.

We entertain occasionally. Mrs. Mickelson was over for dinner one night before school started. Her husband was in Aberdeen with Superintendent Sande for a visit to the Area Office. I kept her plied with questions as she tried to eat. She told me there are over five hundred students in the twelve grades here at the school, the Oglala Community High School and Grade School. Athletics are followed enthusiastically by the Indians. And even though school has not started, the football squad is already on campus for practice.

Mrs. Mickelson informed me that Sitting Bull should never be referred to as a chief, as is so often done. The stir caused by the removal of Sitting Bull's bones from Fort Yates on Standing Rock reservation in North Dakota to Mobridge, South Dakota, this spring is not over yet. The three granddaughters present at the removal are residents of the Pine Ridge reservation. They are Nancy Kicking Bear, Sarah Little Spotted Horse, and Angelique LaPointe. Their picture was in TIME magazine last spring. A nephew, Clarence Gray Eagle, lives off the Pine Ridge reservation.

The classes at school are so large that each class has two teachers. They are short of teachers this year. On the campus the buildings look fairly modern. The boarding school has large acres of grazing land for their fine herds of cows and horses. The tribe raises all the meat for the boarding school children. The reservation cows supply the milk. The tribe bakes and has laundry facilities to cover the school on the campus.

The Indian houses are all small. A complete house could be placed into an average white man's living room with room to spare. There is space to sit, stand, turn, and be in another part of the house without taking many steps. Half the houses are modern. Half that are not have privies. Most all houses in town have electricity and electric refrigerators or electric or gas stoves.

September 11, 1953

Today Angelique LaPointe came into the hospital. She brought one of her nieces for a chest X-ray prior to entering Day School Number 5 at Oglala. Angelique is freshly back from Mobridge, South Dakota, where the monument to Sitting Bull was dedicated on the first of September. Angelique had a clipping of the monument and of her sister and cousin and uncle who were there. Grey Eagle, her uncle, is merely an uncle by marriage and not a blood relative to Sitting Bull. Miss Little Spotted Horse is Angelique's sister and Nancy Kicking Bear is a cousin.

Angelique says that the newspapers said she and the others signed some papers to have Sitting Bull's bones moved to Mobridge. But she says she did not. She said Nancy Kicking Bear is the one who moved Sitting Bull and signed the papers to have that done. There is going to be a trial, she says, with North Dakota out to get the body back to Fort Yates on the Standing Rock reservation.

Angelique remembers that Sitting Bull had nine children. There were two sets of twins; all were boys. There were three girls and two other boys. Angelique was born in 1902 after her famous grandfather died. Angelique is the daughter of Sitting Bull's oldest daughter. Angelique's family name is Little Spotted Horse. She first married a man named just Spotted Horse. She divorced him and married LaPointe. Incidentally, there are many Indians here with French names.

Angelique has a gun and a belt that was Sitting Bull's. Her mother gave it to her. She had a piece of paper that was some sort of map that Sitting Bull had made, but some member of some historical society in North Dakota bought that from her recently. Angelique has long black hair she braids. Each braid has a broach set with numerous rhinestones clipped around the end of the braid. On each side of her head she wears a comb partly covered with beaded leather. She wears the usual kerchief around her neck, long dress, and store-made shoes. She looks younger than fifty years.

When I was at the Holy Rosary Mission tonight I saw Felix Walking. He was one of my patients. Felix was brought into the hospital on August 16 from near Rushville in Nebraska. His left foot was mangled years before when he was run over by a train. He now has a prosthesis. Everyone on the reservation knows Felix. He is quite a painter. He paints buildings and also paints pictures. He usually stays out at the mission. He makes paintings for the mission, which they sell to tourists.

Felix told me when he was in the hospital last month that he would make a couple of portraits for me. One of an Indian man and another of an Indian woman. Tonight I met Brother Keevan at Holy Rosary who showed me some of Felix's work. There was a beautiful painting of Chief Red Cloud that Felix had done from photographs for one of the fathers out there. It was such a wonderful portrait that I asked Felix to paint one for me.

[At approximately this time Jeanne Ruby became pregnant. When they confirmed her pregnancy, the Rubys contacted family by telephone with the news—Eds.]

September 18, 1953

Miss Walborg Wayne, the acting medical director of this area, and Mr. Michael Kessis, the administrative officer from the Area Office, were in Pine Ridge to make a visit to the hospital. They found problems galore. Everybody around here knows Mrs. Ethel Merrival. She calls herself a champion of Indians, and she is bucking the council, the Bureau Office, and whatnot. Though I've not seen her, I know about her. She tears down and criticizes everything. The minute there is trouble, she is there to enlarge on it. She writes our congressman frequently. Many people go to her when they have complaints. She is Indian.

A patient's family slapped one of our nurses because they thought the nurse had been mean to their sister. The facts are that the nurse had not been mean. This family didn't get the story from the sister at all but from other patients in the hospital. Then they came out and slapped the nurse. The nurse did nothing. But it was witnessed by one of the doctors, Dr. Joseph Walters. So since there has been an assault and battery against a government employee when she was doing her duty, it is a criminal offense. As such, the hospital is going to ask Mr. Sande to have the federal prosecutor step in.[5] Of course, the family went to Mr. Sande with their complaint in the first place. So they are investigating from that end too. Well, Mrs. Merrival has stepped into the picture and is promoting the situation since it spells trouble for the Indian Bureau. It doesn't really since the hospital is not at fault, but it does create dissension and stories about the hospital.

One family had a patient in a hospital in Rapid City.[6] They were up there. The patient needed some kind of operation. The doctor called up and didn't say the patient couldn't be moved. So we sent a car for the patient. The patient didn't come back with our driver. So I sent word that the family had to pay their own bill then since we were equipped to do surgery here now, and the family agreed to this. Since then the family now wants the treatment authorized to take place in Rapid City. So they called Mrs. Merrival in on the deal. I wrote Mr. Sande a letter that they were pulling a fast one and that I wouldn't pay for that surgery to be done in Rapid City with hospital funds.

When Mr. Kessis and Miss Wayne were down on September 16, they found the hospital was missing a typewriter and a new car. Before Dr. Shelby from the Area Office resigned, he had arrived at an agreement with the superintendent here to clear as surplus certain houses that were used previously by doctors. The furniture in these houses used by doctors was bought with hospital funds and was supposed to have been returned, but it is missing. So there is apparently some misappropriation of funds.

Miss Sara E. Holden, our new director of nurses, arrived September 15. She is supposed to be a crackerjack. The first evening we had a conference. Miss Holden was sent here with the purpose of making this hospital a smooth running organization. She was full of vim, vigor, and fire and thought she could get this hospital organized. The next day she sat in on conferences with the Area Office people and learned about many of the hospital problems. In spite of my warnings to her of our gigantic problems, she was much enthused. The next day she was discouraged.

The big federal program now is called *Withdrawal.* It is an attempt to withdraw the Indian Bureau all together.[7] Let the Indians become integrated with the other peoples. The biggest movement now is to get the Indians to leave the reservation, see the outside world, become educated, and make their own way. I believe it would be a good thing. Perhaps health services would have to be maintained for those off the reservation. Plans now are to have a separate Health Service. Those in the Bureau Office believe integration is rapidly approaching. Most steps are taken with Withdrawal in mind.

One patient is Jack Iron Boulder, an elderly man who used to be a council member at the Standing Rock reservation for most of his existence. He saw Chief Sitting Bull the day before he was shot near Fort Yates. He used to kid the followers of Sitting Bull and call them "Hostile Indians."

Everybody in the Bureau Office wants to sponge off of Health funds. Especially Mr. Albert T. Pyles, who heads Education. I hear he likes to spend others' funds instead of Education's. The Area Office said we are paying the salary of two laborers who are not at the hospital and whom I've not seen. So Miss Holden is going to be the snooper to see who is using them.

September 21, 1953

Apparently the visit of Area Office officials to Pine Ridge helped some. Today one of the Ford cars belonging to the hospital was returned. Miss Josephine Olinger, our field nurse at Kyle, was down at the garage, and they told her it was ready. She said it was mysterious as to where it came from. No one at the garage seemed to know. But the typewriter has not found its way back, nor the furniture bought by hospital funds.

We are understaffed. Things were so bad for awhile that we simply had to cut down on the number of people we admitted. When I came, clinic days were five days a week. We eliminated Wednesday. Now we are eliminating Thursday. Visiting hours were every afternoon and every evening. Now all evening hours are being eliminated since only one nurse is on duty. The only afternoon hours will be Wednesday, Thursday, Saturday, and Sunday. This eliminates people wandering in to see patients and then going to the clinic and vice versa.

I'm having trouble getting instruments and equipment soon enough for some of my patients who need operations. One of the secretaries in the front office needs vein ligation. When I told her we had no vein stripper she wired to Aloe's Surgical Company and got a reply immediately on what they had available, and then she sent in an order pronto. Ah, but that is government service.

September 25, 1953

I thought our troubles were over. But it seems the further we dig the more we find. Not only did Superintendent Sande have one of our cars that he was driving around, but another old car of ours is sitting in the "junkyard," a 1948 Pontiac, which had a brand-new 1953 motor put in it, paid for from Health funds, and now another department is driving it around, the Maintenance Department. Not only is their driver working for the Maintenance Department full-time, but he is supposed to be here at the hospital. And he buys gas on the hospital or Health fund account sheet. So the Bureau has taken one of our men, and though we are paying his salary, providing him a car and the gas, he is working elsewhere and we never see him.

September 29, 1953

The more I see of the work being done for the Indian the more I am sure that we are not helping the Indian but making it far worse for him by making him more dependent. There is no absolute free education in the United States except for the Indian. And for Indian children school is absolutely free. The children are boarded, fed, taught, prescribed glasses and medicine, and even their clothing and shoes are bought for them. And at the same time the Indian does not pay taxes. There are very few Indians who do pay taxes. Those few who pay taxes are those working for the government and have to pay withholding taxes.

There are church schools on the reservation. There are families who will send some kids to the Catholic school to get handouts from the Catholics and send other children in the family to Protestant schools to get handouts from the Protestants at the same time. I performed physicals on athletes from the Holy Rosary Mission five miles out this last week. They are a better behaved group of boys than those from the boarding school.

My trip yesterday to Kyle was nice though somewhat tiring. I started out from here at 8:30. I should have been in Kyle by 10:00. In Wounded Knee I went up to the hill where there is a narrow tall white church and the cemetery, the common grave for all those who fell at the Battle of Wounded Knee in 1890. Then I went on up to Porcupine. The Porcupine bluff is a small, isolated-looking high hill of dirt. From here I was only twenty miles from Kyle. But I got on the wrong road and came out at Batesland. But then Miss Olinger, our field nurse, had called down here, and they decided I must be lost. After having gone about twenty-three miles I saw a white church up on a hill and decided I must be coming back to Wounded Knee. I was wondering what to do when who should come looking for me but Miss Olinger. I was on the right road and had only seven miles to go to reach Kyle.

Once at Kyle I went to work. The school building is fairly new, a nice building serving eight grades, but terribly short of teachers. I examined all 50 children in the school. The enrollment is 150. One hundred were off with their families picking potatoes. Trucks come onto the reservation and get the families. The children go along and, of course, are not supposed to work. The families contract for so much a bushel or a row to pick potatoes. The families put the kids to work shaking vines and so on. Then they get a sum of money, which they blow before they get back to the reservation.

In the town was a public school with only twelve kids. I was told it is for those who are "too good to go to the Indian schools." Such a waste of building space and under-utilization of teachers. The Indian schools are federal, and the public schools are county.

The school principal at Kyle tells me they have a quantity of boots and shoes yet at the school. These used to be given to the Indians. The kids were supposed to work for them. The Indian enjoys all the rights of this country. They are citizens. They should be taught to assume some responsibility. I have found one thing that is so prevalent here in this agency: there are too many employees who do not want to lose their jobs. So they aren't helping the Withdrawal program one bit. They are stifling it, in fact. For instance, instead of investigating the family and seeing if a certain family can buy glasses or such for their child, they simply go ahead and buy the glasses for any kid. There are children in the boarding school who are there simply because they can sing or play the piano or play football and the particular teacher having that class or activity will get children in the school. Then there is the case of one girl going to a special school. She had a friend who wanted to go with her. So the teacher made a welfare case out of the second girl so she could join her friend. No welfare case existed, and it didn't make any difference that our welfare worker ruled that no problem existed in the second girl's home.

All this is bad for me, too. I could be spending my time here working in the clinic and doing surgery. But I would say that 50 percent of my time is spent doing administrative duties. Tonight, for instance, our chief nurse and I were climbing over cars in the garage looking for serial numbers. We spent a good hour looking for the serial numbers on typewriters. Such a waste of my time when I should be spending it with patients.

Three. October 1953

I realized then the water was too hot so I just turned on the hot water tap in the utility room to a trickle to take care of that steam. Thought I'd let it run all night. However, that tap only shortly afterward shut off. I guess it shut off, because in the morning Jeanne was awakened by a rumble, rumble. She woke me. It was the water in the hot water tank. It was boiling. So I immediately turned on the hot water faucet in the bathroom. We got nothing but steam. Our whole house was soon a hot house. We tried to flush the "john," and all we got was steam. So I turned on the cold water faucet at the bathroom sink, and all we got was steam and warm water. The hot water had backed up into the cold water faucet pipes. That did it. I was ready to resign, after nearly a week heating the water on the stove in small pans to do dishes and then to try and wash clothes. And that I had to do since Jeanne had a rash and couldn't get her hands in water. I was ready to execute my request for transfer.

October 1, 1953

Things may rapidly come to a head. Then again, they may not. Anyway, I wrote a memorandum to the garage that only certain people were authorized by me to get gas and car repairs on hospital cars.

My secretary, an Indian, refused to take a history on a patient, a white man. That is her job. But the man is head of Forestry and doles out the money to the Indians. He has a tough job, and his work is not appreciated. So they, the Indians, do not like him. Her personal feelings went above her work, whereas she should have been very impersonal. That was straightened out.

Mr. Sande tells me he thinks "WITHDRAWAL" is coming soon.[1] So he told us not to fix up too much here, just the necessary things we want done at the hospital. I told him that I thought Public Health would take over the hospital, so then there was no harm in fixing things up. He said that perhaps that wouldn't happen, though that has been my impression all along. The Indians do not want Public Health to take over the hospitals because then the hospitals wouldn't be "theirs." And surely the Indians regard them as "theirs" now. When they are displeased they can raise a complaint with Mr. Sande or go all the way to the secretary of the interior. The Indians feel they can run the hospital through the Bureau of Indian Affairs.

Yet it is here, and this is theirs to do with as they please. For instance, before I came here, one of the doctors told a mother to shave her son's hair because he had some infection in it. She promptly told him to do it himself. That started a useless row that went all the way to the Bureau Office in Washington DC. How much nonsense. And the surgeon that was here before me had a similar altercation. An Indian woman thought she needed an operation. Dr. Lam, the surgeon, told her she did not. She went to the tribal council, and that took a good part of their time. Well, of course, she didn't get an operation. But you see how the thing works. Mr. Sande said Dr. Lam cured her by putting her on the table, taking out a knife, and saying "OK, where do you want me to start?" That ended it. But Mr. Sande asked, "Why can't you just make a slight operation on such people anyway?" Well, I nearly collapsed. Consider the risk of death from unnecessary surgery. Sara Holden, our chief nurse, refers to him as "The Old Goat." I always know who she is talking about.

Another reason why I think WITHDRAWAL should come soon is that the Indian is a smart person. He has run opportunity and assistance into the ground. He appreciates it only in that he can get all he wants. Here in the Soil and Moisture Conservation Department they contracted with Indians to terrace their lands and build dams. The government bought the machinery, and the Indians would pay only labor. The individual Indian was to pay back for the labor necessary to fix up his land. One Indian who owns cattle and has now sold them won't pay his bill for $600. And though the Bureau Office gets the checks and has to give the funds to the Indians, they can't compel them to pay bills. The department head can't. Mr. Sande could, but he won't always back his department heads. Many Indians agreed to pay for killing ground hogs, which apparently ruin the land. That was done by the government, and now there are Indians whose land was helped, and they won't pay for that.

There are quite a few Indians who are leaving the reservation for relocation. Seems to be this Withdrawal business that is sending them out. All departments are being cut in funds. Part of the Withdrawal.

October 2, 1953

Do you know what peyote is? Peyote is a cactus that produces a bean. Eating the bean produces hallucinations. It is and should be illegal to use it. There is now a cult that uses it. The Indians call its use a religion. So for that reason some Indian agencies have been asked to go slow with arrests. There are a few of the peyote cultists here on this reservation.[2] One Indian girl was a psychoneurotic. The family knew the girl was not right in the head. So one day our social worker wanted to have her examined at one of the mental institutions. The family said, "Oh, no. She is cured." "Well how did you do that?" asked Mrs. Forshey. "We fed her fourteen peyote beans," was the answer. There are many of the Indians who have powwows when someone is sick, peyote and otherwise. Mrs. Forshey has trouble getting some of them to come to the hospital at times.

Friday, October 2, 1953

I'm on call tonight. The past week has been hell for me. I get tired haggling over such darn nonsense in government procedures. Such a waste of my time. I operate occasionally, too. This week I performed an open reduction of a forearm and plated a bone fracture, and also fixed a hernia and did a thyroid operation this week. Next week I'm doing a breast operation.

October 4, 1953

Today we went to the Badlands of South Dakota.

Mr. Frank Afraid of Horses and his family live on the very brink of the unknown. Their house teeters on the edge of the Badlands. Frank is a seventy-eight-year-old Sioux Indian. An amazing man who has made the trip down there many times, too. He is as agile and nimble as a small youngster.

Frank said he would show us a path to take. We started down the almost perpendicular slopes. Soon we came to a canyon that water follows when it rains. From here, the going was easy. The sensation of the Badlands from the bottom of the spires is that their surface is like heated, molten lead, minus the steam.

We found some skull bone of some long-forgotten animals. We found countless pieces of petrified wood. And I found one tiny agate. Frank gathered petrified wood. He stacked most of it. I presume he will haul it up later. At his home he has some prehistoric bones. Frank has his path marked by piles of rocks he has made. We went to the edge only of the first flat area. The basins are the areas where the agates are supposed to be found. It was late, and we had to start back.

Pine Ridge, South Dakota
Friday, October 9, 1953

We are having troubles at our house. Jeanne has a rash that is spreading over her arms and legs. She spent today in bed. Poor girl is so miserable. They had homecoming at school and no classes anyway, so she didn't have to teach. But if she is no better, I'm not going to let her go to school Monday.

October 11, 1953

I think the climax was last Thursday. We had just had our new dial phone installed. I was glad to see that antiquated phone that operates with a crank out of the house. But on Thursday the phone wires were crossed in some manner, and the thing wouldn't work. That day our oil furnace just wouldn't go on. Our water heater wouldn't work, for what seemed like the billionth time. The phone is working now but no water heater. We have been out of hot water for nearly a week now. And with Jeanne ill and with clothes to wash, baths and dishes to do, it has been heating small bits of water most all the time in small pans over the electric stove. I'm really sick and tired of waiting for maintenance men to come and fix our house.

Today Mr. Sande took one of our station wagons to haul some congressmen around. That is all right, but in all fairness or out of courtesy he should at least call me or inform me. The other station wagon was in the garage. We use them for ambulances. So that left us with nothing. Thank heavens it was back tonight.

I lost out on the glasses for school children deal. Mr. Eldon La-Course, the administrative officer for the Bureau, got Education and Health on the phone in Aberdeen, and we had a four-way conversation. The idea is to have every child who doesn't have 20/20 vision tested for glasses. That averages two out of five kids. But it does not mean that Health buys glasses only for kids at $6.75 each, but we have to pay for refraction at $5 per child. That is over $2000 for the more than five hundred pupils at the boarding school alone. There are twice that many children in day schools over the reservation maintained by the Bureau also.

Tuberculosis among the Indians is quite common. Within the past year the tribal council here has adopted a policy to work for the prevention and cure of diseases using the policy adopted by the South Dakota state Department of Health. That means that people with tuberculosis can be apprehended and held at some hospital for treatment if they refuse treatment. But that is not being done. I can't do that because I'm not in authority to do so. I say this because some people wonder why I don't apprehend certain diseased individuals. Doctors can't do this. Only the officials of the South Dakota Department of Health can do this.

But it seems to me that of the numerous people we send to the tuberculosis sanatorium in Sioux Falls, half of them sign themselves out after being there only a few days. But what can you do? In many ways the Indian is over-educated on disease prevention, having been taught so by the white man.

There is a lot of divorce among the Indians these days. In the olden days the Indians were more than "Victorian" in their habits on marriage. Now they equal the whites. The result—many broken homes with many children who pay for the circumstances with their upset lives. I shall never forget young Marvin Little Thunder. He fell and a piece of wood punctured his hand, thus resulting in a gross infection. His parents were divorced. So he stayed with his grandparents way out in the reservation. Before they brought him to the hospital his grandfather cut his hair. I'm sure he didn't use a bowl because it wasn't that even around.

Speaking of hair, Henry Little Goose is a fifty-year-old Indian male in the hospital with a cellulitis of his leg following an injury in which he hit his leg with an ax. He is the first Indian male patient we have had who has long braided hair. I've seen maybe two or three other males with long braided hair.

Felix Walking, the artist, did two nice paintings for me: one of Sitting Bull, the other of Chief Red Cloud. He had a big write-up of his injury in the local scandal sheet. Felix now stays at the Holy Rosary Mission. There he does paintings for the Catholic mission, and they sell them to tourists in the summertime. Felix is an untrained artist with a real talent. One of the first portraits he did was of Chief Red Cloud as he appeared to be at about the beginning of the war.

October 14, 1953

This is just to fill you in on events. Monday the maintenance men installed an electric element in our hot water tank. The hot water tank is a gas affair, but the gas unit has been torn out for a week now since it refused to work altogether. Well, they said now we should have some hot water. And hot water we had! That evening, Monday, the water was boiling hot. I practically scalded my hands. I realized then the water was too hot, so I just turned on the hot water tap in the utility room to a trickle to take care of that steam. Thought I'd let it run all night. However, that tap only shortly afterward shut off. I guess it shut off, because in the morning Jeanne was awakened by a rumble, rumble. She woke me. It was the water in the hot water tank. It was boiling. So I immediately turned on the hot water faucet in the bathroom. We got nothing but steam. Our whole house was soon a hot house. We tried to flush the "john," and all we got was steam. So I turned on the cold water faucet at the bathroom sink, and all we got was steam and warm water. The hot water had backed up into the cold water faucet pipes. That did it. I was ready to resign, after nearly a week of heating the water on the stove in small pans to do dishes and then to try and wash clothes. And that I had to do since Jeanne had a rash and couldn't get her hands in water. I was ready to execute my request for transfer. Miss Holden, our director of nurses, had a conference with the front office and brought up our troubles. They said they'd see that something was done. It was. But not until today [Wednesday].

October 19, 1953

I think the old adage "When the cat is away, the mice will play" applies here at this agency. The cat would be represented by the Area Office representatives, and the mice could be almost anyone in the Bureau here. When Mr. Kessis, administrative officer for Health for the Area Office, was here, he located one of our cars and asked whoever used it last to return it to the office. That was done. When the administrative visitors were gone, we had a station wagon come up missing. I've hunted for it for one week and finally found it. Mr. Sande has it over in his garage. The thing that makes me angry is they don't tell me where it is so I spend valuable time looking for cars when I could be seeing patients. Then, once the cars are borrowed without permission, they use Health funds for gas and maintenance of the car.

Dr. Robert Bragg, who is to be assigned here permanently, came in today.[3] He will be a great help to me. He will relieve me of some clinic duties so I can spend more time working in administration.

October 20, 1953

Miss Walborg Wayne, acting medical officer of the Aberdeen office, was here with a group of nurses from the Washington DC office. Her primary trip was to visit many hospitals and check on the nursing problems. So she could only devote one hour's time to a conference with me and Miss Holden to take up the problems that we have. But she couldn't give us much help, only moral support. The problems have to be worked out by the Area Office people. So she did tell me that Mr. Kessis would be here, and he was coming here for the one purpose of clearing up these items. He is the one who can deal with the Bureau people and get them to straighten up and fly right. I have just started a list of things to present to him, and it has many items already.

October 20, 1953

Do you know what Yuwipi is? It is pronounced "you-wee-pee," with the accent on the "wee." I can't give you a definition just yet. But I would put it this way. The medicine man practices Yuwipi or holds Yuwipi. It is a spiritual rite. For instance, when someone gets sick, Yuwipi is practiced or held. When a girl from near here in Nebraska was lost, the Indians held a Yuwipi.

When someone is sick a medicine man is summoned with a specially prepared summons token. It consists of a piece of cherry wood about eight inches long. Tied to one end is a small piece of cloth in which has been placed some tobacco, half the amount you could stuff into a thimble. The member of the family knocks on the door of the medicine man and places the tobacco and cherry stick down in front of the door. The medicine man sings a chant. Then he invites the family member in, who tells him about the family illness. The medicine man then goes and sees the patient. There he may use herbs and will go through some spiritual ceremony.

To become a medicine man requires first of all that a previous family member must have been a medicine man. The role is inherited. The young "pre-med student" gets his gift by going by himself to some high hill where he stays two weeks. During that time he communes with the spirits. In the old Indian spirit world everything was thought to have a spirit. There was not one spirit, one great spirit, such as the Christian God. But everything had a spirit. There the young medic would see all the animals there were. They would come up to him. He would talk to them.

Charlie Little Bear's grandfather was a medicine man. Though still living, he doesn't practice his "art" now. When he went to the high hill to become a medicine man he saw a huge snake several miles in length approach him. It came right up to him and looked him in the eye. The young "medic" couldn't even see the end of the snake whose body was as big around as a wash tub. This same medicine man cured his wife when she had a stroke. One side of her face drooped and she couldn't even talk. So he drew a picture of her in the dirt. While his wife kept pointing to indicate the place on her face where it hurt, the medicine man took a stick and kept hitting that same place on the dirt picture of his wife. At the same time he kept chanting a special song. Presently the pain left his wife's face. She could talk, and the droop came out of her face; only a little remained.

Another Indian man told me that his grandfather was a medicine man. Louis Mosseau said one day he was lifting a calf into a buggy, and a spring broke. He was leaning backward. His back hit the wagon, and he couldn't even straighten up. Someone came along and took him home. There his grandfather took a piece of wood and put it in Louis's mouth for him to bite on. Louis was lying on his side. Then his grandfather threw him over, and he hit really hard on his back. It snapped in place. After that he put some brewed herbs on Louis's back that he'd prepared. Louis could feel it draw like a real strong liniment, and he felt better, he said. Sometimes when a "patient" has a pain somewhere, the medicine men will suck on that area with their lips. They simply draw out the pain.

October 24, 1953

We had dinner guests on Thursday. For our little house, it was a gathering. We had Dr. Harvey S. Gassman and his wife, Yetta, and four children and Elizabeth Forshey, the social worker for the agency. She is formerly from St. Louis. Lawrence T. Mickelson and his wife, Lillian, were over as well, and Mr. Kessis, who is here doing some sleuthing for me. Miss Holden joined us, and the two of us made thirteen. And believe it or not, we are giving a dinner for about as many this coming Thursday.

October 25, 1953

Wednesday evening Mr. Kessis came down from the Area Office in Aberdeen. He spent all of Thursday and Friday sleuthing here at the Bureau for Miss Holden and myself. He got lots done and said he would stay over the weekend if I wanted, but there is nothing he could have done over the weekend, and besides he pretty much straightened things around for us.

Final decisions now are the following.

Hospital funds for glasses:

1. MOC [medical officer in charge] will set aside a specific amount of funds for glasses, an amount that he thinks he can spare from

his funds. Glasses may be purchased for school pupils until that amount is spent.

2. All applicants for glasses must be reviewed by social service to see if the family should pay or if federal funds should be spent.

Ambulance service:

1. The hospital is not to furnish ambulance service for the reservation or even off-reservation cases excepting to transport patients to and from one hospital to this one or vice versa.

Admission of patients:

1. The Indian hospitals may admit persons other than Indians on a fee-paying basis.

Hospital cars and gas funds:

1. The Pontiac four-door that Maintenance is using is to be transferred to another reservation.

2. The Plymouth, which Miss Olinger had and which Dr. Bragg is currently using, will be transferred to Maintenance.

3. Gasoline purchased from Health funds is only to be done so by those people authorized to do such by MOC.

4. Gasoline purchased by persons outside the Bureau, such as the TB mobile unit, are to be billed for gasoline taken.

Two people on hospital funds not showing up here for work:

1. Mr. Kessis found these people have been loaned to Administration. However, no provisions were made for Administration to pay Health. This will be taken up with the Washington DC office.

2. The truck driver will have to do some trucking for the hospital. Dr. Stanley L. Sheppard's house is to be given to Mr. Lyman Carr or saved for a new dentist coming in.[4] We may cancel existing contracts for milk and laundry and get new contracts for those services if we so desire. Certain things we need for the hospital are to be provided by Maintenance.

October 27, 1953

One of the Maintenance division men at the hospital is Joe Adams, who is in his sixties. His family is also related to Crazy Horse. Joe's father, now deceased, was Alex Adams. Alex's grandmother was Chief Red Cloud's daughter. Red Cloud had four boys and one girl. Anyway, Joe told me some of the stories that his father used to recite to him when he was a boy. The Sioux Indians roamed south as far as Oklahoma, Utah, even into California, and they were much in Colorado. In fact, the reason there is so much mixed ancestry is that the government troops were stationed in Colorado in the 1870s. The Sioux traveled much. They robbed other bands of Indians. They would always rob by night.

To become a warrior a boy was started on his bravery tests and lessons at the age of fourteen. He would be sent with a pail, perhaps three miles away, to get water after dark. Then as he grew up, he could go with the fighting forces as a flunky. He would tend camp, pack supplies, and so on.

Joe says that when Crazy Horse was killed he was carried from Crawford, Nebraska, in a wagon by his father and mother and two friends on horseback. The stories vary on some of these points. But he says the trail his folks took was similar to that given by others. The party went to Chadron, Nebraska, and then through what was then the main thoroughfare, the shortcut of today, the one Jeanne and I take always to Chadron when we go shopping.

The Indians still hold the Sun Dance here at Pine Ridge each summer. But the Sun Dance is not like the Sun Dance of years ago. Joe remembers his father telling him about the earlier Sun Dances. A young man in the tribe wishing to take part in the Sun Dance the next year would make the fact known. Then everyone in the camp or band would respect him. He had to live a good life, free of sins. He was looked up to all year and revered. Then when it came time for the Sun Dance, the chief of the band would pierce the skin of his left front chest with a stick, usually of ash. The stick was whittled down until it was very sharp. It was burned over hot coals. Then, with just the right amount of skin and subcutaneous tissue, the stick was used to pierce through approximately an inch width of skin, which was picked up with the fingers of the left hand by the one doing the piercing. With the stick through the skin a rawhide string was tied around the stick on each exposed end. This way the stick would not fall out. To the piece of rawhide a long piece of rawhide was tied to a large pole standing in the center of the Sun Dance grounds. With his eyes closed and praying, the man would take so many steps forward and so many steps backward until the rawhide was taught. This was the dance portion to it. Then he would jerk on the rawhide. All the time the man was praying to the spirits for all the things he wanted for the band of Indians to which he belonged. The person never ate during all the time it took him before tearing the skin to free himself, sometimes one day and sometimes two days.

You know the U.S. government used to give the Indians rations of flour, beans, bacon, baking soda, and other staples. At about the time of the Crazy Horse incident there was general unrest over the insufficiency of the rations. So one of the things the government did to subdue the Indians was to increase the rations. The Indians had ration cards. In Nebraska, I believe at Crawford, Jake Herman has been able to trace rations given to Crazy Horse's wife and the new husband she married after Crazy Horse was shot. It was her new husband who took the new name of Crazy Horse and was exhibited as "the real Crazy Horse" by Buffalo Bill Cody.

October 27, 1953

One of our patients here recently was Henry Standing Bear. Most of the Indians said he was a smart old man. He once, not long ago, gave a speech in Denver on Withdrawal. Henry was for it. His speech was printed in the *Denver Post*. He died here about two weeks ago. I signed the death certificate as cerebral vascular accident. I believe I've told you they are chiseling a monument to Crazy Horse outside of Custer, South Dakota. Well, Henry Standing Bear was in on that. Crazy Horse would never be photographed. Work could not proceed on the statue until Henry approved a photograph of some Indian, whose likeness was to be used for the Crazy Horse monument. Henry knew a man who remembered what Crazy Horse looked like. But Henry's elderly acquaintance died before they got him to pose as a reasonable facsimile of Crazy Horse. So Henry found a photograph of someone who looks like Crazy Horse for the sculptors to work from in making this new huge monument, which is not yet finished.

Joe Ashley Chips, from Wamblee, whose grandfather was a medicine man about the time of Crazy Horse, knew Crazy Horse. Joe says that he could contact the spirit of his deceased grandfather, who had been a medicine man, through Yuwipi, and that old Chips would tell them just where Crazy Horse was buried. But they couldn't tell anybody because Crazy Horse doesn't want anyone to know so that his bones will not be molested. Especially since the white man took the Indians' hunting grounds and their buffalo and herded the people onto plains or reservations. But Joe says they still have these spiritual meetings, called Yuwipi, and contact the spirits.

Four. November 1953

Did I tell you a saying common among the Indians? The Black Hills are a sore point among the Indians. The fact that the white men have the area, that is. They are also sore at Chief Red Cloud, who traded the Black Hills around 1877. In prolonged illness or for any illness that may bring them to the hospital and when referring to the immense cost to the government, they say, "Oh well, the Black Hills is paying for it."

November 1, 1953

We started out early yesterday morning, Jeanne, Lyman Carr, and I, with Jake Herman, one of the five members of the tribal council. We headed north from Pine Ridge, past where the hospital is located, and where the Indians shot at the Agency Office in 1890. The Indians had the belief that wearing a certain jacket of buckskin would protect them from the white man's bullets. We went over Cheyenne Creek. Jake pointed out where an Indian with TB lived before the beginning of the [twentieth] century. A friend took him to the doctor one day. The doctor told the friend the old man would die soon from his ailment, but he would send along some medicine anyway. The friend told the old man, who thought the doctor had put a curse on him. For that reason the old man went out seeking vengeance for his impending death and shot a school teacher as he rode his horse to school. When we came to the Holy Rosary Mission we turned east and went up over the reservation. Jake showed us where, in 1913, a movie was made. At the time Buffalo Bill Cody was there, and General Miles, General Moss, and Wells, an interpreter.

As we rode along, Jake, who is sixty-three, told us old Indian customs. When he was a youngster, his father told him if he ate a raw turtle he'd be a brave man. Of all the animals, the badger is the only one the Indians never killed to eat. The reason: the badger, they felt, ate human flesh, and where there was a badger hole there possibly was a grave. But they had a belief in which a badger was killed, laid on his back, and then slit down the stomach and the internals taken out. The blood that accumulated there was left to jell or coagulate. Then, when the sun was high, by looking into the jelled blood, an Indian could see the image of himself when he would die. Therefore, if a young Indian saw a real old image of an Indian, then he knew he'd live to be old. The jelled blood made a mirror.

Whenever an Indian saw a spider he would step on it and utter this saying: "See/a wauk ee/on neeck stie/pee." [This is a phonetic spelling.] The translation is: "Spider lightning will kill you dead." The Indian believed it would then protect the Indian from being struck by lightning.

Indians always believed the spirit of departed members of the family returned to earth. They, the children and adults, always prayed to the grandmother—never to the grandfather—to the spirit of the grandmother who was dead. Today with Indians, as with whites, it is the grandmother who never spanks the children but who loves them and cares for them. So the Indians believed the grandmother's spirit would help them. When they wanted to accomplish a particular thing or find something, they prayed to the grandmother's spirit to help them that day. If they looked hard enough, or worked hard enough, they would accomplish that particular thought. If they did not, it was their fault, not the spirit's.

Jake told other stories. In early morning or evening old men would go and sit on high places, maybe for two hours, and sing a mournful song that was their way of mourning for departed relatives. It was a sort of psychotherapy, for that way they got a lot out of their system.

Then he told me about law and order. When an Indian murdered another Indian, there was no trial. They all knew who the murderer was. The usual reason for murder was when some man stole another's wife. (Chief Spotted Tail, the chief of the Rosebud group, was shot and killed for stealing another man's wife.) The killer was forced out of the band for a year. Usually he'd go to a high hill to stay. He could return to his band in a year. The perpetrator would either kill himself or join another band before the year was up. We passed the old home of Kicking Bear, who was one of the leaders of the 1890 Ghost Dancers. As we drove along Jake would tell us the names of the younger generation who were currently living in the homes and to whom most of the homes originally belonged. The homes are one-story, two-room log cabins. They do not have electricity. They use kerosene, oil, and occasionally bottled gas to heat with. The yard has a privy and one to ten wrecked cars. Phone lines run along the roads, but they go only to the towns where there is one phone everyone uses.

We saw only one two-story house that stands today. It was an antiquated building built by Bat Pourier. Bat was a fairly wealthy Indian, an old scout and interpreter for the army back in the 1860s. After 1880 the army built some two-story houses on the reservation for the sub-chiefs. None of the two-story government houses are still standing.

We passed through the town of Manderson, named after one of the army colonels or generals. There are perhaps ten buildings in Manderson. It is up on Wounded Knee Creek about where White Horse Creek and Wounded Knee Creek come together. We angled from north to northwest and skirted the Badlands. Here we stopped and spent a great deal of our time in Cedar Creek between the Porcupine and Wounded Knee buttes.

Jake said when Buffalo Bill took his show to Europe, one of his men, Standing Bear, married a German girl. After they came back to the reservation this German girl's sister came over from Germany and also lived on the reservation. She came for her health. She adopted Indian customs and wore braids. She was liked by the Indians. About 1900 she died and was buried on a knoll on the reservation. The knoll is covered by weeds. A half-torn-down wire fence surrounds the grave. On the grave are some pretty rocks placed there by Indians. There is one other grave out there, of either old man Penican or Rocking Bear. Jake likes to believe it is Rocking Bear's grave. Rocking Bear was also called the "White Indian Soldier" because he was an early Indian scout and a good one.

Long ago the Sioux buried people in trees, and after the bones dropped to the ground they were buried. Then, before 1900, common trunks were used for burials. Now they use caskets or wooden boxes. The Indians decorate the graves with pretty rocks. Caskets are made by the Rehabilitation Department of the tribal council for the reservation. These are sold or given to them and then paid for by Welfare. All Indians get a casket for the dead.

Jake is proud of the Indian rehabilitation program. He spoke to me about the recent scandal of about three weeks ago where congressmen came to investigate the whereabouts of missing funds that couldn't be accounted for. He said the initial amount in question was $30,000, but this built up to $100,000 or more. A team is making a report for Congress that will show where the money should be. The funds were to have been used for loans to Indians to build homes or start businesses. The Badlands are on the reservation except for the portion set aside for the National Park. However, Jake told me the Indians have the privilege of living in the park and building a home there. Tribal members hunt deer on horseback. When they shoot one, they eviscerate it, hang it in a tree, and come back later in a car or pickup to take it home. Jake tells me no one runs off with a hanging deer if they come upon it before the hunter picks it up. The Indians today have traded beef for buffalo.

Jake told us he once ate six peyote seeds. It made him visualize one of his departed uncles. First he was blue, then various other colors. Soon he saw snakes and then animals. The following day, he felt very pleasant. There was no hangover. Then he said to himself, "I'd better not take this stuff again." And he hasn't.

November 7, 1953

I just returned from a trip to Aberdeen. The purpose was an Area Office medical and dental conference on November 5 and 6. The conference was held in the Capitol Café. About thirty officials were there, including a few superintendents. The biggest discussions concerned tubercular patients who signed out of the Sioux Sanitarium against medical advice, or AMA. These AMA patients are numerous and a menace to others in society. They come to our hospital. A diagnosis of tuberculosis is made, and then they are sent to the Sioux Sanitarium in Rapid City. They sign out in a few days time. What should be done about it? One agency, the Cheyenne agency at Cheyenne River, has been enforcing the contagious disease code of the state of South Dakota, which that agency tribal council has adopted. They have had a few trial cases, mostly as examples. When a member of an agency gets off the bus on return from the Sioux Sanitarium as AMA, they are picked up and taken to the jail. They are kept there until they are willing to go to the sanitarium voluntarily for treatment. No one, of course, can be forced to take any treatment, so they are given the choice between jail or the treatment. A local tribal council is helpful in rounding up such characters and jailing them.

Talk was thrown around of building special jails for people with communicable diseases who refuse to go to the sanitarium for treatment.

The Social Service Department talked to us, mainly about eyeglasses. Afterward, Mrs. Ruth K. Heinemann, the area social worker, said to me, "I spent eight years in Pine Ridge back several years ago. You can see I didn't do much of a job on Mr. Pyles." I had to agree with her. Mr. Pyles has been giving us fits here. He brought a huge list of peoples' names to Social Services to screen for indigents. Social Services was wrong in coming to me to see if I'd screen them first before Social Services did, thus saving them time. But I had written some pretty strong memorandums to various branches about the school trying to get parents to buy glasses first. It apparently helped quite a bit; others who had the same idea were afraid of saying just that because of politics.

The Relocation and Rehabilitation Department talked to us. It is a new department. Two years old. Their purpose is to take Indians off the reservation who are able to go out into white society and live and work with them and earn a living. This department pays the Indian's way to a city and gets them a job. Rehabilitation talked to us simply because all these people are to get physicals first. It was brought out by someone that many people return to the reservation, chiefly because they miss their communal living and get homesick. In a big city an Indian woman has lots of unknown neighbors, but she doesn't sit on the street corner and get all the local gossip and gossip about the government. It costs the government less for them to live in a city than it costs for all the welfare and other programs provided on the reservation. The government will get jobs for those returning should they want to leave again, but they do not pay their transportation. They say on average, 40 percent return after two years. They told me here at Pine Ridge we are at the average.[1]

There was lots of wrangling at the conference over legal jurisdiction in death for coroner cases and what the coroner can order a federal medical officer to do.

A mimeo slip passed out shows the Pine Ridge Agency had the greatest number of average daily census last fiscal year (1953), the largest total of hospital days, while the average length of stay of patients was average as compared to that of other reservation hospitals during the fiscal year.

Here on the Pine Ridge the Indians still make sweathouses out of willows, which are stuck into the ground, doubled over to make a small, igloo shaped hut. They cover that with blankets. They put hot rocks in a pit in the center of the hut. They pour water over the hot rock to produce steam. But they do not jump into the cold water anymore, as they used to. The huts average six feet in diameter at the ground.

November 8, 1953

Did I tell you a saying common among the Indians? The Black Hills are a sore point among the Indians. The fact that the white men have the area, that is. They are also sore at Chief Red Cloud who traded the Black Hills around 1877. In prolonged illness or for any illness that may bring them to the hospital and when referring to the immense cost to the government, they say, "Oh well, the Black Hills is paying for it."

When prisoners needing medical attention are brought to the hospital, they are not under guard during that time. But those we have had so far are all serving time for minor charges. One of the police said that if a murderer or some such criminal were brought to the hospital, they would keep a guard here for the prisoner.

I have $150,000 of a year's appropriation to spend, and I'm keeping pretty much to the budget that I have. Our spending is budgeted each three months, and while lots of hospitals in our Area are having trouble keeping within their budget, we are not. I went over my budget to see how I was doing, and I remember making a note here last week that I had around $150,000 to spend in a year's time. The figure is closer to $200,000, actually $193,000. That is a lot of money. Going by quarters, we are running even. Now if I can just keep the rest of the agency here from stealing our money.

This is deer season. I had some very delicious roasted deer meat the other night, last Wednesday. It was one shot by an Indian and given to the head of the Home Economics Department at OCHS. After dinner we went to the Legion Hall where the Indians were holding a powwow.

It is getting cool here as you may expect. The change of clothing is apparent. The men wear tight caps with bills. They have discarded the multicolored straw hats turned up sharply at the brims on the sides like cowpokes wear. But I did see some of these cowpoke hats, multicolored, and bright colors too, made of felt. Quite a number of men wear the fur lined caps, as do many of the children, with the ear flaps on theirs. Children coming into the clinic are now wearing underwear, which is often dirty and full of pin holes. Nonetheless they are warm. The ladies' underwear is no different, except they wear more underskirts. Of course, most all wear blankets or shawl robes.

I treated a patient this morning at 4:00 a.m. for lacerations of the left forearm going down to the bone and of the left arm through part of the biceps and of the right hand. She had been stabbed by her husband. We see few cuttings, but numerous cases in which women are beaten by their drunken husbands. But the women all go back when the husbands are sober. Sobriety frequently lasts only a couple days. One outpatient, the secretary of the tribal council, had an altercation with his in-laws. The in-laws got the best of it, hitting the secretary over the head with an iron pipe.

November 20, 1953

I had a meeting with Mr. Sande, Mr. LaCourse, and Miss Holden concerning the resignation of both our clerks. It seems now that Miss Kehna, who has resigned before, is again doing so to be closer to her home. So Emma Nelson, the hospital secretary, who is inclined to be antagonistic to many things, decided to resign at the same time, thus leaving the hospital in the lurch as far as clerks are concerned. Anyway, Miss Holden advised me that though Miss Nelson's resignation was voluntary, she would be sent out of the service with prejudice because she will go back into service again soon and others will have the same trouble with her insubordination, sarcasm, antagonism, and the like. Miss Nelson is smart and efficient, but she wants to exercise judgment and decision exceeding her authority. With Miss Holden's advice, I wrote my reasons for these opinions.

Superintendent Sande called us down to talk about them. Miss Holden said to hold my ground and not change my ideas. In the meeting Mr. Sande said Wednesday that we couldn't write anything of the sort without having first told Emma Nelson such in advance with letters addressed to her. He admitted his mistake for not writing one when an incident happened when she refused to admit a patient to the hospital on September 30. Mr. Sande said I should have written one to her. I did talk to her. So he said he would then get a new resignation sheet signed by her. I would leave off remarks, and then he'd write me a memo asking why Miss Nelson is resigning. I'd answer him giving all these reasons, since I had talked to Miss Nelson at the time of one offense and pointed out her mistakes. He said a copy would be sent to Area Office to be put into her files. Therefore I should send her a copy of my memo to him. Afterward Miss Holden said, "Maybe I advised you wrong." Perhaps she did since Miss Nelson did not receive notices of her conduct. But Miss Holden warned me that Mr. Sande was protecting the Indians again. Miss Nelson is Indian.

Today I had an entire afternoon in the offices of Albert Pyles, head of Education. Present also were Mrs. Elizabeth Forshey, representing Welfare and Health, and Mr. Alvin Zephier, head of Rehabilitation and Relocation. The Law and Order representative was absent. This is a meeting of Health, Education, Welfare, Law and Order, and Rehabilitation for adult education classes. We spent all afternoon planning a schedule for speaking over all the reservation. Each of us will carry the message about our programs and services to the outlying communities. I don't know how I can always participate, but guess I'm expected to do so. We decided on visiting eight communities: Red Shirt Table, Manderson, Porcupine, Kyle, Allen, Wanblee (which in Sioux means "eagle"), Oglala, and Pine Ridge.

Anyway, after lots of discussion, Mr. Sande was called in, and he told us we shouldn't start our meetings so early since it is near the primary elections for the Indians and we'd be charged as being partial and playing politics. I thought Mr. Sande was going to rearrange our schedule, but as he has not we will go on as planned.

Mr. Sande and I talked about apnea, since I had used the word in a letter to him. We talked about some medicine he wanted me to order for a white man being transferred to Porcupine to work. The man didn't want to go, and he used illness and lack of a certain medicine he needed in the winter for justification. Mr. Sande had called me and said Mr. McIntosh used hydrobeline and bilron and could I get it. I said I'd order it. When we said we would get it Mr. Sande told Mr. McIntosh, and his argument was lost. So the other day the medicine came, and I told Mr. Sande, who told me today the man doesn't really intend to get medicine after I've gone to the expense of getting it since he lost his argument and now has to move from Martin onto the reservation.

November 22, 1953

It was so crisp yesterday. Snow covered the ground with a very thin blanket. The wind had a biting tang. I previously went out to see Edgar Red Cloud, the great-grandson of the famous chief. Edgar took me across the hills over miles of "Red Cloud" land, as he called it. We went to the chief's home. It was a typical structure here, which reminds me of the slums of a big city. Anyway, I wanted to photograph the chief in his regalia. The chief said it was too cold and to come back tomorrow. So I did just that today. The chief got into his costume, and I got some very nice shots of him. It was warmer today, only about 40 degrees, but so windy that it gave the chief considerable trouble with his headdress. I nearly committed a federal offense. I asked Edgar if the chief liked candy or cigarettes. I thought I would offer a token for his trouble. Edgar said, no, but he liked beer and could I get him some? And as you know, it is not a federal offense to sell liquor to an Indian off the reservation, still you cannot even give it to them on the reservation.

Red Cloud is chief as in a line of accession in the family, but he has no power at all. He is recognized as the chief, and at all gatherings he gives speeches. After his death, Edgar will be chief. At the chief's home was a Yuwipi hut. There are two kinds of spirit religions here among the Indians besides the Christian religions. One is Yuwipi, and the other is the Native American Church, started about 1912, which is the peyote cult. The elder Red Cloud, the chief, is Yuwipi. In the yard were the sticks or willow poles made into the shape of a hut, or like an igloo, a half globe. These are covered with blankets or canvas. They are perhaps six feet across. In the center is a hole. The Indians get a special kind of rock. It is heated on a fire outside the hut. This rock, which is not supposed to chip when water is poured on after being heated red hot, is put in this hole and the water added. The steam has curative powers.

A medicine man must be present. All people get inside who are taking part. They are naked. They sing and chant a ritual.

The Indians who follow these Yuwipi practices are sincere believers. If one of the people there is sick, he is to be cured. If a child is ill, those present ask the spirit to heal it. Then it has other purposes. If you should lose something—for instance, a dog—you would have a Yuwipi ceremony and ask the spirit to tell you where the dog was. If someone had stolen it, the spirit would not tell the medicine man the actual name of the person who had it, but he would describe the place where the person lived or happened to be. The Great Spirit would tell the medicine man, for instance, that the dog was now at a house where there was a windmill. In other words, he would give a description of the location. Offerings are made to the Great Spirit. The offering is tobacco. A sack of Bull Durham was hanging on the willow hut frame, and around the bottom of the sack, going all the way around, was an item that looked similar to a rosary. On a string about every inch was a tiny piece of colored cloth wrapped around a pinch of tobacco. This small nobbing of tobacco was perhaps one-half centimeter across. Edgar says there are supposed to be five thousand nobbings of tobacco, but that can't be because there weren't that many there. Anyway, Edgar is going to get me one of the "rosaries." Edgar, incidentally, is a Catholic. He seems more of a Christian than most. Many Indians practice their own religions and go to the Christian churches as well because it affords a chance to meet, eat, and so on. Also the churches give them clothes and other assistance.

Edgar and his wife and family were taking beads off of a dress to sew onto buckskin. Edgar makes his buckskin by taking deer hide and soaking it in nothing but plain water for nine days, changing the water four times. After nine days the hair slips off easily. Then he rubs it with lime. He soaks it in oil for a day and a night. Following this he rubs it with white dirt, which the Indians find. This gives it the white color. Then the hide is rubbed and pounded with stones to make it soft.

One of the fellows down at the Armistice Day dance the other night was Charlie Yellow Boy. He is more or less the leader, or rather was the leader at that dance. He is a colorful old man. He was one of the original travelers with Buffalo Bill Cody. He has been in Europe and met royalty.

I was told by Mrs. Elizabeth Forshey about the Horse Dance. She was the only white person along with two of her friends who were allowed to witness one last summer up by Oglala. Whenever some maiden has a bad dream, which implies injury or hard luck, a Horse Dance is held. The Indians gather, and after they sing and chant to the Great Spirit, this girl gets on a horse and is hooded. The horse is then supposed to dance. Mrs. Forshey said that they had some real old nag, and it was all she could do to keep from laughing when the horse was supposed to be dancing.

I was invited to a peyote meeting tonight. Well, I just got back from the meeting. It was Yuwipi instead of a peyote ceremony. The meeting started at 6:30. I didn't start out until 9:00 p.m., so when I and an Indian got there the door was locked, and we couldn't get in. But the Indian fellow who went with me knew when we had found the right house before we heard the noise and confusion. All the furniture had been moved outside. The members sat inside around in a circle, and the medicine man, Plenty Wolf, led the meeting. He would talk and rattle a gourd filled with sand. Then he would beat a drum and lead the singing. Everyone seemed to know the songs, for they all sang together. There were other Indians outside who knew the Sioux language. I was the only white person there. They told me when the medicine man was smoking his peace pipe and saying a prayer, when he prayed, his speech was different. It sounded to me as if he were reciting a poem. I'm going out again some night when they hold another meeting and get there earlier and get in on the inside except it's so dark I'll never see anything and certainly not see what the Indians see, a light that will burn very dimly and increase in size and then get smaller.

November 23, 1953

The Indians are great readers. They are not illiterate people. Even the old-timers whom I presume had no schooling can read. They read newspapers, bulletins, anything they can. But the funny thing, and a thing that prevails among many people, is that as soon as they see something in black-and-white, then it is believed to be a fact, even if it's the biggest lie in creation.

The educated Indian who is ready to live with the outside world (off the reservation) does not like to be pointed out as an Indian. Alvin Zephier told me this. He is quite an educated person and like anyone else. I asked him why this was so. He told me that he considered himself as anyone else and didn't want to be pointed out as being something different.

Another member of the committee going out to give Adult Education lectures is Mrs. Elizabeth Forshey, head of Social Service. We discussed giving buffalo sandwiches or elk sandwiches to draw a crowd. So then Mrs. Forshey told us she was going to get thirty thousand pounds of beef to distribute to the needy this winter. Already she has gotten vast quantities of government cheese, butter, honey, and dried milk. Mrs. Forshey has decided this winter not to start doling out relief funds till January because people can still work, and it isn't too cold yet. A notice about this was published a month ago in the *Pine Ridge*, the agency news sheet. Not long afterward one big, strapping, healthy Indian gent came into Mrs. Forshey's office and said he had read the notice that relief wouldn't be started till January, and he wanted to apply now to get on the rolls for relief.

This is a note on the chief, Red Cloud. The present chief is Jim. He rides down to the agency or rather to town via a back road. He drives down in his wagon and with his team. He doesn't like to go around where there is too much automobile traffic so he takes the back way.

Beads were introduced to the Sioux back about 1890. Before that time their clothing looked just as decorated then as now with small intricate colored designs. Those designs were made with porcupine quills. The quills were first dyed various colors and then the quills were run between the teeth to flatten them. That gave them the right moisture. I asked Mrs. John Cornelius, who is an Indian crafts art teacher, why they couldn't be soaked and flattened in some way. She said then they would swell up like macaroni and break. No one practices the porcupine quill art anymore, and she would like to revive it. The original buckskin costume of the original chief Red Cloud is hanging in a museum here. The last time I went down to see it I took particular notice of it. The small intricate multicolored designs are done with porcupine quills. The present chief's is done in beads.

Other costume items were the large bibs and aprons of eagle leg bones traditionally worn by women. Now the Indians can't get eagle bones, so they make their aprons out of compressed rice flour. Those who can make especially intricate and delicate designs in their work carve designs so they look like bone. I don't know the exact name for that part of the costume worn.

I visited Andrew Standing Soldier in his home several times. He lives only a couple of blocks from the hospital. Here is a thirty-five-year-old Indian man who has been doing art since he was fourteen years old. He has a style of his own. He is good. Someday his art will be well known. He sells as far as Spokane in the Northwest. He is currently doing some stuff for a trucking company. He is truly terrific. But he is like so many of the Indians here. Though he is good, he doesn't stick to his work enough; drink interferes. Anyway, he did a large set of murals at the OCHS on the history of the Sioux Indian. This is fresco, he calls it. He has done some for a library at the Standing Rock Agency in North Dakota. He does Native Indian scenes and historical scenes. I asked him once to do a watercolor for me of the battle of Wounded Knee, and he is going to this winter. I'm anxious to own some of his things. Mrs. John Cornelius loaned us a picture by Andrew to hang in our house. It shows the Indian women loading little travois pulled by dogs, as the Indians used to do long ago. Not only do many of Andrew's pictures hang in the Agency Offices here, but I saw a couple hanging in the Bureau Office in Aberdeen. I also told Mr. Pyles that he should photograph the murals at the school and print a running commentary on the history of the Sioux.

I guess I'll go home and plant some grass seed and sprinkle some gravel in our driveway. We still have a pile of gravel in the driveway. I've shoveled out half of it or better. Got some grass seed and will plant it myself.

I was going to take some pictures Thanksgiving at the Legion Hall, but Indians didn't meet for a powwow. Instead they had modern dancing. We went to Dr. Joseph Walters's home for Thanksgiving and had a delicious turkey dinner.

November 25, 1953

Some notes on past tribal practices. Regarding childbirth: In the past when a young girl was ready to deliver a baby, it was routine that her mother-in-law delivered the baby. If the mother-in-law was not living or available, then the mother of the expectant mother delivered the baby. If the family was not satisfied with the qualifications of the grandmother, they called in a lady from the tribe who was supposed to be good at such matters. This specialist went through a ritual that included sticking her finger down the baby's throat, washing it thoroughly with water, and then covering the baby with the fat taken from large white owls, which have an abundance of fat. Then several marks with red or blue paint were made on the baby's face.

Regarding marriage: In earlier days when a young Indian male saw some maiden he thought he wanted to marry, he would first discuss the matter with his father. Next his father would discuss it with the parents of the girl. If the marriage was thought a good union, they would all agree. On the "wedding day" the young man and his family retired to the girl's family tepee. Now it was custom that the young man could not look his father-in-law or mother-in-law in the face at any time. So in talking to them he first talked to his wife who relayed the message; then they, having a message for him, would relay it through their daughter. There was no ceremony as such. All marriage consisted of was coming together, a feast, and an exchange of presents or gifts. The young man gave his in-laws a horse, and they might also give him one. The mothers exchanged gifts, and the fathers exchanged gifts, and the mother of the young man gave gifts to the bride's sisters, and the mother-in-law gave gifts to the young man's sisters. Gifts consisted of buckskin leggings, dresses, moccasins, jewelry, and so on. Usually the men exchanged peace pipes. Days later the father-in-law might give his daughter a bow and two arrows and say, "Tell your man to go out and kill a deer." Later, when the Indians had guns, the father would say, "Here is a rifle and one shell. Tell your man to go and kill a buffalo." The old man telling me this said, "They sure made it tough on a young guy," by giving him so little ammunition.

Regarding the practice of scalping: Long ago, during and after battle, warriors would gather scalps from the enemy they had killed. If you were a warrior and killed a man, you might not necessarily get the credit if you did not get the scalp. And the man who did the killing was not necessarily entitled to the scalp. It was the first man to get to the dead or dying body. Then when coming home the brave would carry his scalps tied to a long pole. He would be waving this as he pulled into camp.

At one time a woman might wear a corresponding number of horses' tails or other animal tails on her dress to signify the number of scalps her husband had gotten. Speaking of scalping, Mr. Joe Adams, an old man who is one of the maintenance men at the hospital, tells me his father had scalped thirty-two white men in battles in Utah and Wyoming.

When the Indians went to battle, they started off with meat only for food. The steaks of buffalo were dried and pounded until they were dry and soft. A piece of fat was taken, and the dried meat was wrapped around the fat so as to make a "meat ball." They might go off with thirty of these in a small bag. Some days of battle they would eat nothing and drink only water. And they might take along a young boy with them. The boy had to be fourteen years old before he went along to tend horses, keep camp, fetch water, and do chores in general. This is the way he learned to become a warrior, by starting from the bottom up.

The Indians used to paint streaks across the forehead and down the side of each cheek depending on the number of scalps they had gotten in a battle. The colors were usually blue and red. The wife, if she painted her face, painted it to correspond to that of her husband's painted face. The Indians made the colors red from a certain clay that they baked and mixed with a fat. Black was produced primarily from charcoal.

November 28, 1953

The present tribal council was originated in 1934 by the Wheeler-Howard Act in Congress. By this act the Indians govern themselves with an elected body and representatives. Before that time there was a council, but the leaders were chiefs and had influence. It was the chiefs who went to the Bureau officials with their complaints and recommendations. Now they have a president. The chiefs of the old councils were family descendants. Here on the Pine Ridge reservation only two chiefs' descendants are alive: Red Cloud, the most colorful, and Ben American Horse. Chiefs Little Wound and Bad Wound are dead, and none of their survivors are leaders. Primary elections will be held two weeks from Monday.

Yesterday we started the first leg of giving lectures on the reservation in eight different communities, scheduled to run over four weeks' time. The schedule as we drew it up was for the five groups, Health, Education, Welfare, Law and Order, and Rehabilitation, to meet at Red Shirt Table at 10:00 a.m. and Oglala at 2:00 p.m. Mr. Pyles sent out notices that said we'd be at Oglala at 10:00 a.m. and Red Shirt Table at 2:00 p.m. Arriving at Red Shirt Table at 10:00 a.m. didn't make our situation bad. It is a small community, and it took only a couple of men about ten minutes to assemble the seventeen people who live there. I gave my talk, and it was a good speech.

The meeting was worthwhile. I can see its purpose, which is to acquaint the people with the problems and program of the various departments. But when we got to Oglala at 2:00 p.m. we found there had been a large crowd there at 10:00 a.m., and it was impossible to bring these people together since they are too much scattered.

At Red Shirt Table the leader of the community seemed to be Stern Two Bulls. Red Shirt Table is full of Two Bulls. Anyway Stern, an old man, put forth several problems to the panel. Even before the meeting I learned that there had been a very large hail storm there in June that ruined all their crops. And apparently this community relies heavily on the vegetables in their cellars in the winter. Mr. Stern Two Bulls said, "We prayed for rain but someone else prayed for hail. It ruined all our crops." Mr. Sande, the superintendent, who spoke for Law and Order since that department chief wasn't there, asked, "Who prayed for hail? That's the ones you ought to get." Stern, who has a good sense of humor replied, "I guess it was those at Pine Ridge." His problem was directed to Welfare since he expected the community would rely heavily on that department this winter.

Red Shirt Table is a small community five miles from the power lines of the REA [Rural Electric Administration]. But REA wants a guarantee of $75 a month before they come in with electric lights.

We had a very nice lunch at the school. For the seventeen students, in all grades up through eight, there is one teacher, an Indian, Mr. Shaw. He lives with his wife and family in the top story of the school. Besides the day school with seventeen pupils where we met, there is a Catholic mission school with twelve students.

Our House: It is way too late to plant grass seed, I think. I should have done that a month and a half ago. But the agency said hospital funds would have to supply the grass seed, even though it seems to me Maintenance should do it. When I leave there is no promise another doctor will get this house. Well, a while ago I took some hospital grass seed and brought it over here. But no one ever got around to planting it. So I did it myself today. Then I took care of that last big pile of dirt, mostly, and a few rocks, and the lump sum called gravel. I got tired of driving around it so I just spread it around myself. So all in all I put in a big day of physical labor.

Five. December 1953

Mrs. Forshey has been giving help to a paralyzed man. She finally gave welfare to this guy's wife, thinking she'd stay home and care for him. The wife ran off to Nebraska with others. She is taking the welfare money, buying malt and cheap wine, and actually running a beer joint or tavern. The woman has people in her home each night, buying liquor. Now that Mrs. Forshey has found out about this, she is shutting off all relief to the family. These people are corkers. Give them money, and they spend it right away. Saving money or acquiring material objects doesn't appeal to them.

December 3, 1953

I went up to Wanblee, approximately a hundred miles from Pine Ridge, for a community services lecture. Mrs. Forshey, the social worker who gives the Welfare presentation, took me up. We stopped in Martin and picked up Mr. Lautzenheiser, the child welfare worker. Right now he has the assignment of establishing which children are enrolled in the Indian schools. Mr. Pyles, head of Education, is down on him because there apparently are kids in school who should not be there. They enroll anyone to keep up their census and get larger appropriations.[1] At Wanblee, there should have been a hundred people there. However, by the time we finished and the stragglers came in, we had eight people to talk to. Such a waste of time when I worked myself up sick trying to get my work done before I left. That included two major operations, which Dr. Walters did for me.

The heads of Health, Education, and Relocation talked. Mr. Sande usually talks for Law and Order because Mr. Swift Bird never attends these meetings. But Mr. Pyles, who heads all these meetings, was there but didn't give an Education talk. I don't know why. Mr. Sande didn't give his Law and Order talk today either.

The trouble with these meetings is that when questions are invited, they aren't of a general nature but become very personal. Someone wants to know why he hasn't gotten relief. One man who had been reviewed by medics and was refused by social welfare and state welfare, made the statement, "Well, I guess I'll have to take my family and go to Kadoka and go to work." Some fight like fury to get welfare. They are able-bodied men, but they'll do their best to get relief and not work.

Mrs. Forshey hates Mr. Sande. She says they have to work together. They apparently complement one another. Mrs. Forshey soft-peddles Communism and admitted that some of her best friends were Communists at one time. She comes from St. Louis. Naturally she hates McCarthy. But she doesn't speak well of Roosevelt. She speaks nastily of this administration. I can't figure out just what she might like. She seems like Gerald K. Smith.[2] She simply gives her disapproval of everything.

December 4, 1953

Mr. Allen J. Brands, chief pharmacy officer of the Public Health Service, allocated to the Department of the Interior, Indian Bureau, visited Pine Ridge today to take stock of our drug room. He says our drug room is about average with overstocked drugs and outdated drugs. It was interesting to learn from him that about four years ago the Indian Bureau had all civil service doctors, excepting 7 Public Health doctors, and now they have something like 126. Before that they had no health programs. Now they have definite programs.

What interested me even more is that the general rumor from Washington, where Mr. Brands has his office, is that the Indian Bureau hospitals will be taken over by the Public Health Service by July 1, 1954. He believes that the bill defeated last year will be voted on favorably by January 1954. The heads of Health, Education, and Welfare, Mrs. [Oveta Culp] Hobby,[3] and Interior, Mr. [James] Douglas McKay,[4] have gotten together on the costs of the transfer.

Since I never have received my travel pay to this station, Mr. Brands said he would do something about that because he knew about the problem in Washington. That surprised me because he is the chief pharmacist. Apparently they have to cut new orders on my orders, so I'll get my travel pay from Mabton and not from St. Louis. Mabton is farther, would net me more money, and especially since I am from there, I certainly want to be reimbursed.

Mr. Brands came over for dinner at the house. We got in a conference with Miss Holden and went way past 6:00. At the same time he asked me about irregularities at this reservation, in the hospital, and with the agency. So I made an appointment with him to go over some of the things tomorrow morning with my memos and notes on the various deals.

December 5, 1953

I couldn't for one moment forget to tell you about our buffalo meat that Edgar Red Cloud gave us. Without a doubt it is the best meat I have ever eaten. The flavor is like a really rich beef. Someone said, when I told them how we had enjoyed it, "Now can you understand why the Indians are so fierce that the white men came and slaughtered the buffalo for the hides, left the meat, and eventually killed off the animals?"

Friday morning, yesterday, we were to give our series of lectures for Community Services at Pine Ridge. This is the town on the reservation with the largest population. Not one single person showed up for the meeting. Not one. Mrs. Sande said if we had had it down in town at the Legion Hall where the Indians are used to meeting, that probably some would have come, and I presume she is right.

December 5, 1953

This has been a hectic weekend. I thought I'd perish from exhaustion on Thursday. I had two major operations scheduled. One had to be cancelled, and I had to do an emergency appendectomy. Then I had to go on to Wanblee and lecture so other fellows did the last operation scheduled. That made three operations that day, which is something for this place.

I hate to give lectures. I can't give lectures. Yet I must be doing all right for I've heard various compliments on my speech. Jeanne has carried home a few from people. And Superintendent Sande was so impressed with my speech that he sent a carbon of it to the Aberdeen Area Office.

December 10, 1953

There has been so much activity lately that I've not had time to make notes on our house. Since we have been here we've been told that the pipes for our water needed to be "winterized." But our water pipes got NOTHING. So they froze Tuesday night. Maintenance came, thawed them out, and left at noon. Jeanne came home and turned on the hot water. A pipe under the sink cabinet was loose, and water and steam flooded everything under there, including about $30 worth of fruit cake, powdered milk, starch, and so on. Such is life on the Sioux reservation.

Today we went to Manderson to present our talks in the Community Services program. Mrs. Forshey wouldn't ride in my car, said she was afraid it was going to stop any moment. So I drove her car up there. We had the largest turnout we've had so far. The meeting went over two hours. It was very stimulating for those people and for us. There were numerous inquiries about securing welfare and relief, even in those who had worked all summer.

They were disgusted during lectures about Law and Order that the bootleggers were getting many items often stolen from other tribal members to trade for liquor. One man was disgusted with Law and Order because his boy had ridden to one of the wild parties being held around Manderson on Thanksgiving night, and someone stole his saddle. He thought Law and Order ought to find the saddle. Mrs. Forshey and others in the Bureau have heard about it and believe the son, who is a good-for-nothing, traded it for liquor. This is a reaction typical of everywhere we've gone. Outsiders' preying on the Indians' taste for liquor has been an ongoing trend since the reservation was established.

Mrs. Forshey has been giving help to a paralyzed man. She finally gave welfare to this guy's wife, thinking she'd stay home and care for him. The woman ran off to Nebraska with others. She is taking the welfare money, buying malt and cheap wine, and actually running a beer joint or tavern. The woman has people in her home each night, buying liquor. Now that Mrs. Forshey has found out about this, she is shutting off all relief to the family. These people are corkers. Give them money, and they spend it right away. Saving money or acquiring material objects doesn't appeal to them.

We have our new eye doctor, Dr. Harley Quint, at the hospital now. I'm sure having my troubles at the hospital. Have a new secretary who isn't much of a secretary. I gave her some dictation that went, "The trouble with you guys is that you send us too many patients at one time." It came out, "The trouble with you guts . . ." And she transposes sentences and takes out of thin air stuff I don't even say. One sentence in a letter came out, "We don't operate on Health funds." How stupid. That is all we operate on.

Today I put an intramedullary nail in a man's broken leg. It is the first time any such operation was done here. This guy was injured in Rapid City a couple of days ago. There were pictures of him in the paper. So I asked Mr. Cocker, of Soil and Moisture Conservation, to come and take some pictures, and I'm going to prepare a demonstration of services rendered to people on the reservation and send it to Oveta Culp Hobby, the secretary of Health, Education, and Welfare, to show the work we are doing since there has been some question of abolishing the Commissioned Corps of the Public Health Service. The services would go on, but the doctors would be civil service.

December 11, 1953

Today I started out bright and early. I drove first to Porcupine or Pahin Santi (the Indian word for Porcupine Tale, the name of the town) and then went on to Kyle. Mrs. Forshey didn't go so I got one of my friends to go with me for company, Edgar Red Cloud. Ed also tells me what goes on in some of these meetings when some of these people talk only in Sioux. For one thing, a couple of months ago a woman was brought into the hospital. All I found out was that she had gotten drunk and gotten into a fight and came into the hospital with an injured eye. We sent her to an eye specialist in Chadron, Nebraska, Dr. Griot. She came back to the hospital and then signed out against medical advice. She may now be blind, but due to her refusal to stay and take the treatment. She is one of the cases here that is well known to the social worker because she is always drunk.

Let me give you an example of what a sense of humor Indian people have. Edgar the comic told me that he had an operation for his eyes at the hospital about eight months ago. One fellow told Ed he needed an operation on his eyes so he asked Ed what it was like. Ed told him, "Well, they took this eye out," pointing to his left eye, then extended his arm out, "they worked it over. I watched them with this eye," pointing to his right, "when they had it on the table." This was enough to scare this one person from the hospital. I thought Superintendent Sande would convulse with laughter at this.

And another thing I heard from Mr. Sande. It would help if one knew the local politics. Ethel Merrival is the local troublemaker. She does the Indians harm and tries especially to harm Mr. Sande. She was fired some time ago from a job she had with the Agency Office, and ever since then she has been fighting everything with tooth and nails. She criticizes everything. Nothing is constructive. She makes negative statements such as when Eugene Rowland returned from the Korean prisoner exchange, and she commented, "If he'd been treated as another boy and not an Indian, he'd have more clothing." Then she puts the meanest stuff in the newspapers all the time, reports she hopes and tries to make damaging, especially to Mr. Sande. Today there was an announcement over the radio that Indian politicians at Pine Ridge were handing out spoiled buffalo meat to the Indians.

It all started this way. Yellowstone Park personnel said since they were decreasing their buffalo herd that they would give Pine Ridge fifteen buffalo, each weighing about a thousand pounds. But the tribe had to send trucks and men. So the tribe donated $1,000 and sent two trucks and six men. They wired Mr. Sande last Saturday that they needed more money. He knew that these men must have had a party and probably were drinking liquor. He sent no money and told them to get home the best they could. What had happened was that they gutted the buffalo and threw them on a truck, whereas they should have then skinned them and hung them up to cool. Well, when the buffalo got here they were taken to a freezer and four quarters of them were deemed spoiled.

One of the men instrumental in getting the buffalo for the tribe was an Indian and also a friend of ours who comes to the house, Jake Herman. Ethel Merrival has been on the outs with him so she telegraphed Congressman E. Y. Berry that politicians were handing out spoiled buffalo meat.[5] So when the newspapers called Mr. Berry yesterday for news he told them this, and then the Rapid City radio put it over the air this morning. Mr. Pyles, head of Education, said that one-year schools were to get turkeys for school kids' meals. So when Thanksgiving came and the kids got none, a rumor was circulated that the school officials, the white people, were eating them. The truth was that the turkeys hadn't been distributed.

One thing that I learned from Edgar Red Cloud today was that many Indians believe in Yuwipi. They come to our hospital, but they practice Yuwipi before they come, or they leave the hospital to practice it. Medicine men, I have learned, are licensed by the tribe. This was a surprise. Guess I'll get a license. Except that I don't believe I could fit in. Ed once told a man relying on Yuwipi that he had better go back to the faith of his Christian church and get medical attention. The man died a few days later, not having gone to an MD. Edgar told me once he was ill in the hospital, and a group came to him from the other cult, the Native Church, and wanted to take him out and feed him peyote weed, but he wouldn't go. He told me several stories about people treated by medicine men. He told me about a man who had been to an MD but couldn't get well and who went to a medicine man who fed him sage, and then he got well.

The Indians have their troubles. The Health Department has theirs. These meetings are of benefit. The people do talk over their problems. We will at least have some understanding. And these people do have troubles. They have long distances to come. They have to wait in our clinics until late and then go back home, some of them a hundred miles. I feel sorry for some of them. At Porcupine I saw one of my patients who had been hit over the head recently by a pipe because he had been drunk and was mean to his wife. The FBI is on the case.

Oscar Bear Runner is a member of the tribal council. Today he was the first Indian I've seen who reminded me of a politician. He was as euphoric as the dickens. He came to give some of the departments hell, but he was considerate of Health and very pleasant to me. And after being in the hospital he understood some of our problems.

Today the question came up about some people paying their bills. Mr. Sande said most people would be billed, and if they couldn't pay it, they wouldn't have to. That sent a rumor through the room, all in Sioux. I learned about it later. Ed told me. They were alarmed. Mr. Sande shouldn't have said what he did. Only a few people are being billed from this hospital: those who have permanent jobs, and, of course, they should pay. Oscar Bear Runner was definitely the leader in this area. He interpreted for some of the people. But almost all Indians understand English. They don't need translators, but they do get them and rely on them. It is a characteristic they have.

I definitely feel Health is doing more to help their public relations. These entire meetings are beneficial for all departments in that the people get to meet the department heads. At Kyle we had a poor turnout, though we had the representative from the various districts around here. At Porcupine we had a fair turnout.

Before I forget it, let me tell you another story Ed told me. He said about two weeks ago a family got a letter informing them their son was coming home from Korea. So the family had a Yuwipi meeting for the soldier's good health and to wish him a safe journey home. The medicine man said the word he got from the Great Spirit that night was that the soldier was now at mid-sea and would be home in two weeks. So the family prepared a big feast that was to be tonight in the boy's honor. But yesterday they got a letter from him. He was still in Korea and was being delayed. So Ed says he has no faith in that stuff. It is "baloney." What right has a man to take a piece of bark from a tree, he asks, and give it to a sick man and think himself so mighty as to make the man well? Oh, Edgar is a funny person.

At Kyle, Welfare got the big kicks again. But, of course, there is money in that department to be given out. Thank heavens I have no money to dole out. Gosh, everybody wants some. If the allotment to Welfare for the year were handed out all at once, every person on the reservation would get about $11 and some cents. Commodities are given out, the honey, canned beef, cheese, powdered milk, and butter. One such commodity was sometimes used in unexpected ways. Because the agency received great quantities of powdered milk, it was used for lining out the baseball diamond instead of white chalk. The powdered milk was free, and chalk for the ball field would have had to be purchased.[6]

At Kyle the chairman, Mrs. Clifford, who said she was always chairman because she guesses she "gabbed so much," said that now that Kyle was given some commodities, they had difficulty getting someone to go after them, and why couldn't the Bureau haul them out? She took up a collection to pay for today's hauling. And the reason she came there was for that purpose. Mr. Sande and I put in a dollar. She surely must have gotten more than she needed. I didn't bring money and had to borrow from Mr. Sande.

At the school at Kyle where we met the people they were preparing for a school carnival. In all of these districts the school is the center of activity. The only phones for some communities are at the school. The school principal must solve problems and help the people with their difficulties. All community meetings are held in school buildings.

December 18, 1953

I have a real problem. Ethel Merrival, the problem child of Pine Ridge, has a niece she has planted in the front office as a secretary. She can't take dictation. She can't type. She can't spell. She can't do anything. She hasn't even the stimulus, the intellectual capacity, to look up a word in the dictionary that she can't spell. I found out Social Services was offered her services. They wouldn't take her. When we had one of our clerks quitting they pushed her off on us. I told Mr. Sande the other day I wouldn't sign her Form 52. I called Miss Wayne in Aberdeen, and she said she would send us a clerk. I told Mr. Sande when I wanted to send in the Form 52 for her, and he said, "Hold everything." So he came up to the hospital when I was operating and went into a huddle with Miss Holden, and Miss Mathews, the secretary, and it was painful for Miss Holden. Well, he gave her the Form 52 to give to me to sign, and I can't do otherwise since he is over me.

Yesterday we went out to Allen. I have such a rotten cold I can hardly speak, but I gave my talk. There were quite a number of Allen citizens there. We had a good meeting. At the last when things were breaking up and people were coming up to talk with different department heads, I was talking with two men who came to ask me some questions. Mr. William Fire Thunder, or Billy, as he is known, is the tribal secretary of the Oglala Sioux. Mr. Fire Thunder nearly got one of the nominations for president of the tribe, for the primary election to be held in two months. Allen happens to be his home, and he was there on vacation from the tribal office. So he attended the meeting. He was making some comments on a project of Rehabilitation involving coffins. So he was going on about coffins this and coffins that. All of a sudden there came a lull in my private conversations with the two men and I heard the word *coffin*, but I thought it was *coffee*. I immediately stood up and yelled, "Coffee?" He looked around and said "Coffins" casually. I thought Mr. Sande would bust laughing. We had been served coffee in one place and I thought someone had announced coffee and was going to serve us.

One woman's speech was the same as we heard in every community in which we visited. Her conclusions were the exact words we hear everyplace, only she said it with better emphasis. She complained about the lack of funds and said she can't go anywhere or can't get anything. She mentioned about the long lines, especially of Pine Ridge people so that, in her conclusion, "The Allen people, it seems like, just can't get anything. We can't get any help."

My cold is worse today. We went to Wounded Knee, and had twenty-five present for the community meeting. For the size of that small community that was a very good, almost a record, turnout. We were an hour late because Mr. Pyles and Mr. Sande wanted to go to a school program at the boarding school. I could scarcely speak, but my talk went over pretty well. I give the same speech every time. I feel like giving pieces of cotton to those members of this traveling troop for plugging their ears. They must be terrifically bored. But Mr. Pyles says he enjoys it more every time.

Today one of the court judges of the tribe, Mr. Moses Two Bulls, who is one of the nominees for president in the general election, was along. He presented the Law and Order story. Someone asked him to give his speech in Sioux, so he did, but he summed it up in English afterward.

Judge Moses Two Bulls said that by Indian standards practically everyone is related as an aunt, uncle, or in some way to one another so that they hinder justice by not telling on one another if one commits a crime. This is bad. Everyone is up in arms about the lack of Law and Order, they say. The Indian relationships are such that practically everyone is a relative so that when some of them do tell on another, they then go back to the court in a day and "take back" their complaint.

Six. January 1954

Circumstances for the Indians are becoming worse, you know. They are becoming more dependent all the time. Their morals degenerate with them. Some run Aid to Dependent Children into the ground. Unmarried women have children because it pays them. They get a check. Some people around here will undergo surgery only because they and their family can get checks during the time they are ill. Mind you, here are a group of seven thousand people. There is no work on the reservation, and with the present slump in employment on the outside they are desperate to get money. Then they do foolish things, like paying someone $25 to bring them all the way from Wamblee, a hundred miles away, to get a lease check that may amount to only $2.50. Actually this place is economically depressed right now. During the Depression they were well off. They worked at WPA and CCC projects, and Mr. Sande tells me they always had money to buy food and other necessities. This is the worst time now. If Mrs. Forshey handed out the money in her annual budget for Welfare to every Indian enrolled on this reservation in one day, they would all get only around $11.

January 6, 1954

Today Mrs. Forshey, the social worker, asked me if I'd heard when I was going to be fired. I didn't know what she was referring to. And she said, "Haven't you heard?"

"No," I replied.

"Well, then," she began, "Ethel Merrival is going to have you fired!"

"Why?"

"Because you're running the hospital to suit yourself and not the Indians."

I had wondered, after being here about three months, when I'd be next for Mrs. Merrival's attention. She has tried to fire Mrs. Forshey, Mr. Sande, and various others. But in addition to me she wants the firing of Miss Holden, the head nurse.

We were given a bum deal at the hospital when Darlene Mathews, the niece of Mrs. Merrival, applied for that civil service job last month. She was on temporarily at the agency. When one of our clerks quit work, they did a dirty deal placing Miss Mathews at the hospital. She was serving as a spy for Mrs. Merrival. But our books are open, and our record is clean. She can't get anything on us except that we are running the hospital to suit ourselves.

Well, the showdown came when Darlene could not even type or take dictation. I told Mr. Sande I wouldn't sign her temporary appointment for even one month. Finally he asked me to, and I had to. I wrote to the Aberdeen Office, without contacting him, to ask for another secretary. So we called the Aberdeen Office on one of those three-way phone arrangements. Aberdeen told us that we would have to relieve Miss Mathews since her temporary appointment was up. So after the conversation, Mr. Sande told me to tell her. I did. I asked her if she had passed her civil service examination. She said no, so I told her that was the reason she couldn't be given more than a temporary appointment and that she was relieved of her duties as of December 29. I think this started her war on us, especially after Miss Holden had to tell her off when Mr. Sande came up here once because I wasn't going to sign her Form 52. I was busy in surgery and couldn't talk to her.

The whole thing is that Mr. Sande and Mr. LaCourse did us a dirty trick placing her here when they knew she wasn't worth a damn. Now that she had to leave employment on order from Aberdeen, Mrs. Merrival has started to make war on us. She says we aren't working for the benefit of the Indians. The records show we are doing more surgery than has been done before, and we are hospitalizing more Indians.

January 8, 1954

I'm waiting to get letters from Congressman Berry. Mrs. Merrival will write him for sure. I am afraid to think what my reply will be. Thank heavens I don't have a political appointment.

Mr. Ryder, the boys' advisor at the Oglalla Community High School, asked me if I would play in the pep band between quarters and halves of the basketball game. I was a bit surprised he would ask me to play for the high school kids. Then he told me the band was made up of local talent recruited the way he was recruiting me.

I went down tonight. The band was composed of old men who worked for the agency. I was the youngest. The snare drummer was Cleveland Nelson, about my age. The rest of the men were in their fifties and sixties. There were only two other white men, Manning C. Ryder, the trumpeter, and Mr. Fairbairn, who teaches agriculture at the school. The bass horn was played by Waup LaDeaux. He is the municipal judge here in Pine Ridge. "Fish" Goings, the defense lawyer there, played alto with me. One of the trumpeters, a former circus musician, is frequently drunk. He didn't make it here tonight. Blue Horse was the other trumpeter. When I apologized for making so many sour notes, Mr. Rider said "Oh, Blue Horse is making them repeatedly." There was a drummer, bass drum, and a trombone. The trombonist sat next to me. He broke an ear stem on his glasses. So he perched them on his nose and every once in a while he would blow them off his face. We made noise though, and we had fun. ochs played Cheyenne and won.

Of course, I had already heard that Ethel Merrival was trying to have me fired. But Edgar Red Cloud, one of my friends who is at the Wakpamni District, came to me with the story. Edgar said she complained about me because I had cut visiting hours, and her complaint against Miss Holden was that the food at the hospital was no good. Then she tried to circulate a petition about the visiting hours. She was asking Edgar and several others where to send it. She ended up guessing she would send it to Congressman E. Y. Berry. Edgar told me he would keep me posted on proceedings against me by Ethel Merrival.

January 11, 1954

I was scarcely out of bed this morning before my phone rang at the house. It was my secretary telling me that Mr. O. Sande's secretary had called to say there would be a meeting of all department heads in Mr. Sande's office at 9:00 a.m. I just got there, ten minutes late. Mr. Sande announced that he was going to be fired. Or perhaps I should say transferred. He just got back this weekend from a four-day stay or visit in Washington DC. Mr. Sande laid the blame for his firing directly on Ethel Merrival. But in a huddle later with Elizabeth Forshey, she says it is not Ethel Merrival directly but rather his gross mishandling of so many situations here. Anyway, Mr. Sande blames it all on Ethel Merrival.

Jeanne and I paid a visit to the Sandes' home tonight. Mr. Sande is an interesting person. And we can commiserate now anyway since Ethel Merrival is after me and Miss Holden. Mr. Sande said there was only one person that could handle Ethel Merrival around here, but he is gone. That man was living with a woman who liked him and kept him. They had family galore. Then he took a fancy to a young eighteen-year-old high school student. This girl's mother beat up the man one night with a flashlight, but he came back and got the girl and eloped to Rapid City, got a car, and went down to Oklahoma. He didn't keep up payments on the car, so he was put in the penitentiary. "Too bad," says Mr. Sande. "We need him here to take care of Ethel."

Ethel Merrival has also been working on Joe Mast, head of Grazing and Forestation. The reason is because he has charge of the unit system. The land here will accommodate six cows per quarter section. That is all the feed there is for a year. So he takes several sections of land and calls it a unit. He rents it to someone on a sliding scale. At the present time it is $8.75 per section.

But Ethel Merrival is one of the few who runs cattle and has to rent land. She is screaming at him for the high prices of rent. She can't make a go of her cattle, and none of the Indians who run cattle can. The government started a program that gave the Indians money to buy cattle and start a business and to pay back that money in three years. The three years are coming due, and all these Indians are in debt. Mr. West, head of Extension and Loans, has been warned not to go and get the cattle to pay the debts since the cattle then would belong to the government and the Indians would shoot him. The man who would be sent out to get the cattle is Charlie Pike, an Indian in Extension.

Mr. Sande says today that Mr. Pike has a rare job if he goes out to get the cattle. He is the one that may lose his life. Oh, I tell you this is going to be a most interesting place around here. I'm anxious to see the developments under the new superintendent, who is to be Mr. Ben Reifel, a Sioux Indian enrolled on the Rosebud reservation.[1] He is a Harvard man, trained in sociology and anthropology, and he got a doctorate in administration only a year ago. Mrs. Forshey says Mr. Reifel believes the Indians should be made more independent and should try to get out and make something of themselves.

Circumstances for the Indians are becoming worse, you know. They are becoming more dependent all the time. Their morals degenerate with them. Some run Aid to Dependent Children into the ground. Unmarried women have children because it pays them. They get a check. Some people around here will undergo surgery only because they and their family can get checks during the time they are ill. Mind you, here are a group of seven thousand people. There is no work on the reservation, and with the present slump in employment on the outside they are desperate to get money. Then they do foolish things, like paying someone $25 to bring them all the way from Wamblee, a hundred miles away, to get a lease check that may amount to only $2.50. Actually this place is economically depressed right now. During the Depression they were well off. They worked at WPA and CCC projects, and Mr. Sande tells me they always had money to buy food and other necessities. This is the worst time now. If Mrs. Forshey handed out the money in her annual budget for Welfare to every Indian enrolled on this reservation in one day, they would all get only around $11.

Mr. West told me of another subsidy for the Indians. When they graduate from high school here, Indian students can go on to college and have their way paid for by the federal government. The students can pay this back with no time limit and at a very small rate of interest. But he tells me there are few who take advantage of it. He thinks the school system here is sadly lacking in some phases of its teaching. I have contended all along from my observations that the Education branch was working against WITHDRAWAL.

It is not *Withdrawal* anymore. Now it is called *Adjustment*. Mr. Sande says *Withdrawal* as such cannot come about simply because the Indian is too dependent. In some places the job and responsibility of the government, with conditions as they are, are snowballing and the problem of Indian dependency is becoming worse.

While I think of it, Mr. Sande said he could write very damaging letters about Ethel Merrival. For instance, he could question her behavior. In other words, he said he could fight this thing and write many things about her, but he'd have a fight and in his words, "I don't have the Air Force, Navy, or money to do it." Once Ethel Merrival resigned from the tribal council, Mr. Sande called the Executive Committee together and told them to accept the resignation. The next meeting, however, she was in her seat. When she went to get her travel money, Mr. Sande wouldn't let her get paid. The five members of the Executive Committee get $2,500 a year. The councilmen get $10 a day while the council is in session and 10¢ a mile for travel. They meet four times a year for three days at a time, but if they have extra money in the council's account they call meetings for no purpose other than to spend the excess of the council funds.

Well, Ethel Merrival then tried to get back on the council because there was some extra money. Mr. Sande told the Executive Committee they could rescind their acceptance of her resignation, which they finally did. Mr. Sande tells me that none of the Executive Committee likes her, but they are afraid of her.

Mr. Sande told me today Ethel Merrival applied for the vacancy at the hospital when her niece was ousted. Thank God for small favors; he told her I had made other commitments. The Area Office had this other girl ready to fill the position. I think that is why Ethyl Merrival is blasting the hospital now. Her whole effort now is spent trying to get a job. If Mr. Reifel doesn't give her one, she'll be fighting him. She wants to be on the inside to get ammunition to bolster her complaints.

January 12, 1954

Jake Herman, current fifth member of the tribal council, invited me to a powwow he and his wife are throwing. I learned that the council president and vice president are elected, and the president and tribal council then choose the secretary, treasurer, and fifth member. Since Jake is one of the two nominated for vice president of the new tribal council to start in February, I think it is part of a campaign stunt. There is usually a dance the first night the council meets, and today was the first day of the three-day quarterly council meeting. Anyway, Jake called me and told me to invite the doctors and to come down and take pictures. He said he told the Indians not to charge us. They do that sometimes, you know. Jake and his wife are serving them a meal at 11:00 tonight. People will come or go to anything if they are given something to eat.

In all the Indian dances around here I've attended I've never attended one before in which there were so many colorful costumes. At this dance they had Frank Fools Crow, Ben American Horse, Chief James Red Cloud, Afraid of Horses, and many of the notable people of this reservation. They even had a clown. Jake was in a circus at one time, and one of the fellows who went with him was Bear Shield from Manderson. Well, Bear Shield was there tonight as a clown, and what a clown he was. And what a fancy affair. Tonight they had two sets of musicians, singers and drum beaters. One pounded out a rhythm for a while and then rested while the other took over.

I had a call from Dr. Kurilecz at Rosebud, who let me in on some information. Miss Wayne and Mr. Kessis from the Aberdeen Office and Dr. Dean, surgical consultant and assistant hospital administrator from the Washington DC office, will be here this weekend. It was maybe ten minutes later when Mr. LaCourse from the Agency Office called to tell me Kessis had called him and gave him the dope.

Mr. and Mrs. Sande and the Walters were also at the powwow tonight. Jeanne and I took a walk around this lively berg after I had finished taking pictures at the powwow.

January 17, 1954

You can't beat these people. The other day I left the clinic early and came to the hospital section. A woman wanted to see me, so she followed me over. Miss Holden asked her what she wanted and why she wasn't over in the clinic. She told Miss Holden that I had told her that I wanted to see her in ten minutes in my office. I hadn't said anything of the kind. The patient didn't want to wait in the clinic just to get some insulin. She badgered Miss Holden, who told her to go to the clinic. Fifteen minutes later she was on the floor and asking her again. Miss Holden answered telling her to get out of there and into the clinic. The third time she wore Miss Holden out. You simply can't beat them. They'll wear you to a pulp. So the third time Miss Holden asked her where she came from. Chadron, Nebraska. How much did she pay to get over here? Ten dollars, she said. Well, didn't she know she could buy a bottle of insulin for $1.48? Yes, but this was government, and she was entitled to it.

We have a saboteur in the hospital: Margaret McGill, one of our nurses. She was the acting director until Miss Holden was sent here as director. So Miss McGill doesn't want to take a back seat. She can't organize or systematize her work. She runs her own program without helping us. She now is in cahoots with the only employee who is in league with Ethel Merrival, and I hope she stays that way. And we have a blue girl who is terrible. She makes comments like, "I'm not going to do that work and wear myself out."

Mr. Sande made a farewell address at a party given him by members of the tribe and agency offices. He said the complaint made against him in Washington by the main office was that he ruled with his heart and

not his head. Ethel Merrival encouraged employees, especially the Indian ones, not to attend the farewell party. But it was a huge success anyway. The Sandes got a check for $100 and numerous small gifts. Money
was taken up from employees. Jeanne and I went down. We lost some
silverware at the potluck supper. Jeanne took a plant. It was ten below
zero. The plant froze in the short time it was carried from the car to the
building. It has been very cold here, even too cold to snow.

Dr. Dean, the surgical consultant, Miss Resineck (phonetic spelling),
assistant hospital administrator from Washington, Miss Wayne, acting
area medical officer, and Mr. Kessis, the hospital administrator for the
Area Office, made a visit here, arriving last night. They will probably
leave tomorrow night for the Sioux Sanitarium. Dr. Dean asked me if
I knew of personality clashes at the sanitarium. I said no. I guess they
are having the same kind of problems as we are.

Well, we went through the Ethel Merrival deal. They told me to forget it. Miss Resineck said she had seen a bill for one reservation patient
to go through the offices of some congressman and the Bureau of the
Budget. Dr. Dean says the new commissioner of Indian affairs, Glenn
L. Emmons, is good, but his assistant, Lewis, from Idaho, is not so hot.
Emmons has been sold on the idea of autonomy for the medical service. Of a budget of $10 million for Health, nearly $2 million goes for
administrative purposes. Dr. Dean said estimates have been done to
show how Health could administer their own works with money left
over to hire more nurses and doctors where there are shortages. He's
not as confident as Brands was that Public Health will take over all together.

Then we got into the mess here at this agency and how other departments take our money and such. And he asked who besides me could
obligate money set aside for Health. I said, "You told me one, the politicians." But he meant on a local level. It should not be allowed, but
people in the agency use Health money terribly. He damns the authority and skullduggery of agency officials. He says they have too much

authority. The superintendent of the agency has more power than a mayor or governor with the Indians.

The main topic of interest to me was the business of eligibility for services. Who is eligible? He doesn't feel off-reservation residents are entitled to care. Indians who can should pay for medical service.

January 20, 1954

The gang from Washington and Aberdeen pulled out Monday noon. Miss Wayne asked me quite a bit about Miss McGill. She knew what sort of a character Miss McGill is. Miss Wayne has one place that needs a chief nurse but says they've had so much trouble there that she wouldn't dare transfer Miss McGill down there. Miss Wayne could send her to Cheyenne River Agency, but she hates to do that because Miss McGill is so bad she hates to send her anywhere. But I explained to Miss Wayne that wherever she sent her, there would simply be the problem of inefficiency and inadequacy, whereas we have that plus this resentment and sabotage because she resents Miss Holden over her. Miss Wayne is going to try to get rid of Miss McGill. Miss Holden feels she'd like to have Miss McGill's two hands and feet here. "I'd rather have her out because she creates too much unrest," she said. Miss Wayne told me Miss McGill was writing private letters to her asking for a transfer. Then not long ago Miss McGill said she didn't want to transfer. I think that Miss McGill thought Ethel Merrival could get rid of us and leave the place to herself. Miss Wayne told me that she had asked several nurses to come here and run this place. And that they refused to as long as McGill was here. One is the present chief nurse at Rosebud right now.

So Miss McGill is known generally for her terrible attitude. Miss Wayne said she was going to have a conference with Miss McGill Monday. Yesterday Miss McGill was off. Today she has been a perfect angel. I wonder how Miss Wayne handled her.

I was so ticked off yesterday. I had asked Lawrence Mickelson, principal at the school, if the home economist, Margaret Tallquet, could inspect our diets. Sunday he said Mamie Searles from the Aberdeen Office was here, and he'd ask her to come also. Then he came up here yesterday and said that since Miss Tallquet knew why I had asked for the inspection (because Ethel Merrival had raised a complaint about diets) that she didn't want to get mixed up in anything. I could have blown my top. Here is a woman, supposedly a professional in diets, who doesn't want to give an authoritative opinion on our diets. Yet I'm sure she calls on the doctors to give an authoritative opinion on medical things. So if she couldn't give an opinion on our diets, I think very poorly of her. I didn't ask for support. I didn't ask for a good report. I merely asked for an inspection and a report.

Miss Wanna arrived today from Sisseton to take the second clerk's position. Thank God Ethel Merrival didn't get the job.

January 22, 1954

I didn't get home for lunch today until 12:30. That is not so unusual. Going through town Edgar Red Cloud saw me, though I did not see him. I was home just long enough to sit down to the table when he knocked on our door before I'd taken one bite of food. Edgar told me he came over to see some pictures I'd asked him to view, some I'd taken of his father, the chief. But a little later he came out with something, and I knew then that was why he hurried over. Some women headed by Mrs. Joe Brewer, probably encouraged by Ethel Merrival, were visiting the council this morning with a petition to have visiting hours changed to every afternoon and every evening. Edgar told me that he signed the petition, but he said, "They told me they wouldn't vote for me for a councilman if I didn't sign their petition. So that is why I did. I wanted you to know that. Today is the last day's meeting, and it won't come before this council meeting. It won't come up until after election. Then I'll fight against it." But I know the Indians. Edgar being a friend has his loyalties divided. That is why he told me about it. But he did it because he is an Indian. I would have expected him to sign under the circumstances. Then when it comes up, if it does after elections next month, then I don't expect him to fight against it either.

The council is wrangling over the two nominees for president. Those two with the highest number of votes are Moses Two Bulls, quite a nice person, and Frank Wilson, who has caused difficulties to the tribe in the past, and who and was impeached and removed from the council several years ago, so they figured he was not a valid nominee. The third highest was Billy Fire Thunder, who is a very witty, clever person. Well, the two nominees are now Billy and Moses. Frank Wilson is suing over the election results. The charges and countercharges by Wilson's attorney and the council are that voting was done in back rooms. The main thing is that it was done after closing hours for the polls, that is, that voting went on after that time.

Apparently they were really after my friend Jake Herman. Edgar is sure sore at him. Edgar had four pieces of land in the gunnery range up north. Those Indians who had land there apparently got very little for it. But it was worth little to be sure. Anyway, Jake Herman and others borrowed one thousand dollars last year to go to Washington with the promise they would get more money for those people who had land in the area taken over by the government for the gunnery range. These individuals are getting letters now from congressmen that the proposal to increase the reimbursement for their land did not go through, so poor Jake is getting grief for the failed effort.

This is what makes my hair gray and gives me headaches. Eldon La-Course called about 2:30 p.m. to ask if we had a certain woman in the hospital. I checked, and the nurse said, "No." I told Eldon, and he asked me to check. I did. This time I learned we had a woman with the same surname. He said he'd call me back. Then Mr. Adams, the Agency lawyer, called me, but just after I'd gotten a call from Miss Wayne in Aberdeen. I couldn't hear her and said I'd call her back and try to get a better connection. Good thing too, because I wasn't up on what she wanted to talk to me about. Then Mr. Adams called and said this woman's husband had come in with some white man to check on a land sale of his. It didn't go through. He said he needed money for his wife. So, of course, he wasn't given any. What he had done was wire Congressman Berry in Washington DC and say that his wife was ill but couldn't be hospitalized here because there were no beds and that we said she needed medical care and that he needed money. But I didn't know much about this woman because she is Dr. Gasssman's patient. So I told Adams I'd check to be sure he hadn't recommended treatment elsewhere.

I learned that the tentative diagnosis was coronary occlusion on this woman. She came in yesterday. Then I knew she was the patient that Billy Fire Thunder and Jake Herman had rushed up to the hospital yesterday afternoon after she had an episode of chest pain during a pow-wow yesterday. This woman was examined by Dr. Gassman immediately. She was hospitalized immediately and has been in treatment. Nothing more could be done for her than the treatment she is getting.

But before I could call Adams back I called Miss Wayne. She said Mr. Cooper, the Area director, had had this inquiry from the congressman and wanted to know how to answer it. I told Miss Wayne we had a bed for the patient. The patient was getting all the care she needed and that nothing more could be done.

Then I called Mr. Adams and Mr. LaCourse to tell them. They had gotten to the bottom of the story by then. The husband had bought a car from this white man. He didn't have the money to pay for it, so he said he'd get some money, or rather thought he would, for medical reasons for his wife and finish paying for the car.

Look at the expense of telegrams and long-distance calls by the federal government. Consider the loss of numerous federal employees' time caused by such shenanigans. But this sort of thing happens all the time, everyday. The Indians are smart and cagy at figuring out how to obtain money.

It just happens that today we had two similar cases. One was a youngster who was discharged today. His mother wanted to take him home. Dr. Gassman said the boy would have to come back in two days to have a patch test done. His mother said she couldn't get here, and she would take him to a private physician. Then Dr. Gassman said if the patient had TB he would have to go to the sanitarium. The mother said she would take him to the sanitarium in Rapid City the day after tomorrow. Dr. Gassman said that was not necessary unless the baby had TB. So this afternoon, in comes the mother. She is separated or divorced, and some man came with her to talk for her. He said she wanted a letter to give to the chief at the Agency Office. He first said superintendent. We have no superintendent right now. Then he insisted it was the chief, by which I learned he meant the administrative officer, Mr. LaCourse. He wanted a note saying the kid had to go to the sanitarium and needed the money. I said if this kid goes to the sanitarium, he won't need any money since hospitalization is free there. In comes Dr. Bragg, to fill me in, since I hadn't known the kid. He told me all about it. In talking to Mr. LaCourse later, I asked if the family had been there. He said, "Yes." But he made nothing of it and knew better, so he hadn't called me. Very frustrating.

I'll never forget a veteran who had a well-healed burn scar on his chest. He told Social Services he had to go to a veteran's hospital in Hot Springs for an operation to remove the scar. They asked him to bring in his letter of appointment up there. He returned asking again for money for his family while he was hospitalized, but he didn't bring the letter, so they sent him up to me for an examination. He had some cicatrix over the anterior axillary fold, but no limitation of extension or other motions of the arm on the side affected by the scar. No doctor would have bothered with it now. So I called Mrs. Forshey to tell her. But the man went there again still without any letter for appointment with the Veterans Hospital and kept insisting he had to receive treatment. Of course, he could not have had such a letter. Some people do nothing but scheme to get money one way or another.

January 27, 1954

Last Saturday, on the twenty-third, someone shot my dog, Captain. He was in shock and lying on the back doorsteps of the hospital. I got him home and pumped him full of shots, gas gangrene, anti-tetanus, penicillin, streptomycin, atropine, and morphine. Then I gave him subcutaneous fluids and nothing else. He stood finally for a brief moment Saturday night. But he cried with pain. Sunday he walked some more. Monday we gave him milk to drink, and he wagged his tail and was alert to noises outside. Tuesday Captain went to town with Jeanne on a leash and enjoyed it. Today he was up to his old tricks and ran off again. Nonetheless I feel bad about it, and about any animal that is made to suffer. Guns on the reservation are plentiful and get into children's hands. One youngster shot into the air. The bullet went through a lady's shoulder. They knew who the kid was. It wasn't much later until he shot and killed his own sister. Nothing was done about it. The people seem unconcerned about such things on the reservation.

Ben Reifel, the new superintendent, is here. He came from Fort Berthold where he was superintendent. There he put out a daily news sheet. He put one out here yesterday. He announced the presidential candidacy of Frank Wilson and stated that Jake Herman told him that it was the first time in the history of this council that a white lawyer represented a person before a council trial, that some white lawyer from down near Mission was Frank Wilson's lawyer.

Ben Reifel came up and spent one and a half hours with me yesterday. Today everyone is remarking that they've only been able to see him and talk to him for minutes. I feel quite honored. He called to ask when he could come up to see me. That was considerate since I was very busy. I gave him facts and figures on the hospital and showed him around and introduced him to some of the personnel. I told him we had problems. I said there were certain matters of policy that I wanted to discuss with him, and that I wouldn't bring things up like that now but that I would like to have a fifteen-minute session with him weekly (as suggested by Miss Wayne). He thought this was fine if I had the time. He is a Rosebud Sioux Indian. A very straightforward chap. I feel sure the cooperation will be fine.

We went to Mr. Mast's home for dinner tonight. He is supposed to be under as much fire from Ethel Merrival as Mr. Sande was. Mr. Mast said once Ethel made a complaint that he had struck her. When he questioned her directly she said he looked as if he would. Mr. Sande asked for a written apology. She was frightened to death.

Mr. Mast said that today Ben Reifel addressed the council. He spoke to them in Sioux and translated in English that he expected to have to say no to them at times. He said he expected petitions would come for his removal. In spite of these expectations, he would labor away and always do what he thought was right.

Mr. Mickelson was at the dinner. He tells me that besides Mr. Mast, myself, and Miss Holden, now Mr. Adams and also Mr. Pyles are on the list for being fired. Mr. Pyles is a weak administrator. When Mr. Mickelson came, all the kids were getting into the movies and school games for free. Mr. Mickelson set it up so that the dormitory kids, or the more or less orphan ones, could get in for free, but kids who lived in town should pay. A damn good idea, I think. Somebody has to start somewhere to educate these people. Pyles told Mickelson, "No, don't do that. Don't antagonize them." Mickelson went ahead and carried out his plan anyway.

I learned something tonight. The Sioux often talk about white people in front of them in Sioux, but since there are some whites who understand Sioux they ALL use sign language. In school the kids do. And they say nasty things about the whites and even to one another. Instead of saying like a white person, "Ah, he said a nasty word about me," the student says, "He wiggled his finger at me." It is universal on the reservation, I guess.

Mrs. Mast says that Father Lawrence Edwards, who has been on the reservation for fifteen years at Holy Rosary Mission, is becoming more discouraged with the Indians. As Mr. Mickelson told us tonight, an Indian at Fort Yates said Indians are citizens plus. They have the rights of the whites plus so many other things. Mrs. Mickelson is teaching them in history class that history repeats itself and that all races and groups of people have all had things taken away from them.

January 28, 1954

I presume I've told you before that the full-blooded Indians have hatred for the children of mixed marriages as much as the Indians in general have hatred for the whites. At the school there was a very maladjusted Indian boy who figured out his difficulties quite well. He was half white. He said the white people didn't like him and neither did the Indians, so he was, of course, an in-between.

I see in Ben Reifel's newsletter of today that a nineteen-year-old woman died. She was admitted to our hospital a couple of weeks ago and was diagnosed as having meningitis. Her father signed her out against medical advice after she was here five days. I presume she got very ill, and her father took her to Our Lady of Lourdes where she died yesterday, I believe. What makes me so mad is when people go elsewhere like that, and they say we wouldn't hospitalize them here, and lie about the situation. And what some do is try to get hospitalization paid for with federal funds when they've gone elsewhere after refusing care here.

Emmaline Sauser, secretary for the superintendent, gave me a ream of printed matter. She said go over this in one hour's time, it was the only copy available, and be prepared to discuss it in the morning at a meeting with Superintendent Reifel at 8:00 in the morning.

This consisted of proposed changes by a committee designated by Commissioner of Indian Affairs Emmons some months ago. These citizens toured all reservations excepting the Alaska Indian Agencies and set forth recommendations. I notice that in their recommendations they suggest that Congress pass laws and legislate specifically "Who is an Indian." In other words, establish who is definitely eligible for services of the BIA. It would involve chiefly degree of blood and reservation and nonreservation residency and so forth. They recommend in their report that Health be transferred to the Department of Health, Education, and Welfare. Also, they recommend that plans be considered in the future for the transfer of Education and Welfare to that department also. Hurrah!!

Today Miss Holden told me many of the things that have been bothering her. She is forever after Miss McGill to get some work done and to quit evading and going around issues. She was sore at me for asking her to order instruments and supplies as their need comes up. She'd like to do it all at once. She is fuming at Mr. Bertsch of Maintenance because he won't connect a sink up for her without approval of the Maintenance Department in Aberdeen. She says Mr. Hunt, in that department in the Area Office, sits around, waiting for retirement in a year or so and won't go ahead with anything. He was down here a week and a half ago and looked over changes we'd recommended for knocking out a wall and doing so many nice things to improve this place. He bucked them all. And what's more, he fumed because we have a public address system in here since we have no individual phones. He hadn't known it was installed, and so he blew his top for not being told.

January 29, 1954

At the last tribal council meeting, held this month, Ethel Merrival presented a resolution that was passed by the tribal council to ask the BIA commissioner to pay, from our medical funds, the bill for a man who had surgery in Rapid City last August. Miss Resinick from the Washington office told me that the bill has been going through offices there. So Mrs. Merrival has already sent it in.

Mrs. Mathews called me yesterday afternoon to say she had a complete list of furniture the Carrs moved to their new house, the one Dr. Sheppard vacated. She had called me last week not knowing what pieces of furniture had been moved. I said I didn't remember now and asked for the survey list that is supposed to have been made last year when the order went into effect not to change furniture from homes. Since they didn't have one, they couldn't supply one. Well, Mrs. Mathews told me a few items that came out of there. Those she remembered because Mrs. Carr had sold them to her. I made a listing and took those few pieces back. It was an inadequate amount. The Carrs also took the refrigerator with them to the Sheppard house since the refrigerator there had been one from the Sheppard house originally since Dr. Sheppard brought his own when he came here. So Mr. Carr took that back to that house. A new family is supposed to move into the house this week.

It didn't occur to me to inquire as to how Mrs. Mathews may have gotten that list, but she told me. Mr. Walker, who is head of the Road Department, gave her the list. Later in the day I learned that the new employee coming is a road worker. Then I learned that the Carrs' former neighbors, or "residents" in that duplex, the Wilsons, who are also road employees, had sent Mrs. Wilson over to the Carrs on a "social visit." Mrs. Wilson wanted to see the whole house. She left soon and prepared the list and gave it to Walker.

I called Mr. Reifel last night. Mr. Carr told me he didn't think he'd stay here any longer. Told me even later he has written several places to inquire about job openings for X-ray technicians. I went over with Dr. Walters, and we told him some of the facts. Dr. Walters is without a refrigerator, and nothing, absolutely nothing, has been done by Maintenance except the usual thing, "Get Health to buy you a refrigerator." Yet damn it, when we furnish the houses with our funds we have no control of the furniture and cannot move it. It goes to someone else. Mr. Reifel didn't say much except to tell Lyman Carr we'd talk about it with Mr. LaCourse and Mrs. Mathews in the morning.

This morning we had a meeting at 8:00 with Mr. Reifel and all department heads. After I got back to the hospital I learned that Mrs. Mathews had called me even before 8:00 a.m.

At my private meeting afterward with Mr. Reifel, Mr. LaCourse, and Mrs. Mathews, Reifel started out, "Dr. Ruby told me he had a big problem. I thought perhaps it was until he told me. Then when I thought that after a person with his training and background has to be bothered with such trivial things it seems to me a waste of his time." Then he went into the problem during which Mr. LaCourse said all kinds of little lies and nasty things in a nice way. Finally, Mr. Reifel said, "If it comes to having a road man here or a technician we'll take the technician and forget the road man. We need medical personnel, and we are going to start treating our personnel with respect. Medical personnel are very hard to get." This man Reifel has real insight into the problem. I thought then if more people were like him there wouldn't be as much trouble getting medical personnel. He went on, "There are perhaps a dozen men that would come in and take my job. There are any number of people that would come in and take a road job. But there aren't any number who would come in and take the medical jobs. My own brother had a job with the BIA, and he gave it up. He thought to heck with all the nonsense he had to put up with. If we lost Dr. Ruby, we couldn't get another surgeon in here." Then he looked right at Mrs. Mathews. When I heard what followed I hoped he knew Mrs. Mathews was Ethel Merrival's sister. "And furthermore," he went on, "we aren't going to have a bunch of complaints and petitions out against our medical men, or we aren't going to have a Health program here if the people are going to start complaining."

What a man. What a giant of a fellow. What a person. Thank God for him. The meeting with department heads, which preceded this private conference, was for the purpose of discussing the Bimson Report or recommendations.[2] But most of Reifel's talk was about his idiosyncrasies, which he said he wanted to get across to people, because it might mean a promotion or the loss of a job.

He had four topics. He started out with these waiting for members of the council to be called. He says that in his staff meetings he wants members of the council present. But they didn't come in until the last ten minutes. Then all he said was that everybody was to take a look at the Bimson recommendations again, study them, and write an opinion of such on them.

The points he covered were these. One, he expected people to be at work at 8:00 a.m., work through till 5:00, five days a week, and stay later if there is work to be done. He does not like clock watchers. Of all the listings he gave I expect, and I expect others to follow, except I must talk to him and see if he is going to expect the doctors to do this. The doctors' average time for getting to work in the a.m. is closer to 9:00.

But the doctors work more than forty hours a week. They work nights. They commonly stay until 6:00 p.m. I usually take twenty minutes for lunch. Three take their hour. But anyway, the doctors, I feel, should be granted this privilege if he will allow it.

Point two was the care of government property. He expected all cars to be serviced and driven at the speed laws. Sixty-five miles per hour on blacktop during the day and fifty miles per hour at night, forty-five miles per hour on dirt roads. If he ever catches anybody exceeding the speed limit he will with no exception take the car away. Regardless of the job or work to be done, the patient, even if out on the reservation, will have to get a ride back into town the best way he can. I had heard about his particular idiosyncrasy before he presented it. Lights should be turned out when not in use. He brought up how surprising it was that at places where rents are being raised (as I've heard about and expect to occur here) and where people had to pay their utilities, how only one light would be burning when people had to pay the utility bill.

Point three was channel of commands. He expected no department head to go around him to the Aberdeen Area Office, and he expected no employee to go around department heads to him. If they did, he would keep the department head informed of the proceedings and refer this employee to the department head. When discussing point three, Mr. Reifel, a Sioux Indian himself, commented that we had to be examples to the Indians, whose philosophy was not one of saving.

Point four: liquor. He expected NO one to bring liquor on the reservation, and if anyone had liquor in the home or served it he would be arrested. He added, "But if you see me in Chadron, or any other place off the reservation where liquor is sold, don't ask me to have a bottle of beer because it will cost you the 25 cents for the beer."

Here is a man who, if he works as he talks and acts, and if he carries out what he says he will, will be a prince. He will be a service to the Indian people and a help to all department heads and employees in this agency.

Our house: Our furnace occasionally goes on the blink. Last Thursday evening it kept getting colder and colder until we were freezing when we realized the darn furnace wasn't working. So at 10:00 p.m. one of the maintenance men came over and fixed it. Water from condensation gets in the pipe, and water doesn't burn like oil so it discontinues burning.

January 31, 1954

Mr. Reifel told me that Indians buy peyote beans for $2.00 to $3.50 for a hundred beans. I had thought they cost more than that. He said that the man who ships them in here is being arrested and tried for income tax evasion. He apparently owes tax on $10,000. Since they can't for some reason get him for mailing them, which is illegal, they are going to get him that way. Now, says Mr. Reifel, those peyote cultists on the reservation who buy from the provider are trying to raise money for him to help him out in his trial.

Seven. February 1954

One of my patients who was in the hospital for a long time, now released, and who had both legs fractured when he was struck by a driver, told me the other day he was going to sue the fellow who had hit him. I said the government will put a lien against his bill for his hospitalization. He hit the ceiling. He had intended to buy a Cadillac. He couldn't understand why that would be done. I told him that people who could afford hospitalization now had to pay. He admitted a lot of Indians could pay for their bills. But he just couldn't understand why that would be done. I told him he was no different than anyone else. "Treaties. Treaties, Doc," he said.

February 3, 1954

There was a staff meeting of all department heads this morning on the Bimson Report. I had told Mr. Reifel I wanted to leave at 8:30 to do some surgery. So he excused me just before that time. I left the meeting and thought I'd better let him know what time I'd pick him up this evening. So I penned a message that I'd get him and Mrs. Reifel at 6:30 p.m. Tonight I picked him and Mrs. Reifel up at 6:20 p.m. after getting Jeanne and then Miss Holden and checking a possible surgical patient. Since I was ten minutes early, I talked with Mr. Holmes, the Area BIA attorney, who was visiting the Reifels.

We left the Agency and drove east on Highway 18, turned off for Wounded Knee, and then went on to Porcupine. All the way, I kept my speed at forty miles per hour on the good highway and then at thirty miles per hour on the dirt road. Mr. Reifel is death on speeding and poor driving. As a result, I've been driving very carefully lately. I tried to drive carefully tonight. But some chattering was going on. So once, when I turned my attention from the road, I hit a soft shoulder and pulled the car over. I don't remember ever having that much trouble before, but this time of all times I would have to have something happen to me. I was terribly embarrassed. Jeanne knew it and said, "Well, I believe you may have had a flat tire." I got out and checked. So did Mr. Reifel. Of course, there was none, and we knew it. But it broke the monotony of the embarrassment.

There were many people at the meeting. It is called an Education-Recreation meeting and takes the place of a PTA meeting. They meet in this district once a month and plan to have an Agency Department head come to each meeting.

The meeting began with the Pledge of Allegiance to the Flag. I can't remember how long it has been since I've done that. I realized it had nearly escaped my memory.

Then the Reverend Weston gave a reading by Robert Louis Stevenson apropos to doctors and nurses. Then he gave a prayer with blessings for medical personnel. Oscar Running Bear, who apparently runs things in Porcupine, started out on a big introduction of a great man being with us. A very wonderful person, and how fortunate the group was. I thought he meant Mr. Reifel, but then he said Dr. Ruby. So I got up and introduced myself and all those that were along. Dr. and Mrs. Walter were there, too. I gave my speech mainly on the topic of soap and water and its uses. I also spoke about diet, warmth, and cleanliness in general for both the prevention and the cure of certain diseases.

Then Dr. Walter got up and gave a plea for the mothers who are pregnant to come to the prenatal clinic. He cited the death of mothers last year at a hospital in Los Angeles where he worked. All the deaths were in mothers who had no prenatal care. Mrs. Holden got up and reiterated more or less what we had said and talked about bathing children. Then I got up with some finishing remarks. I then asked for questions. We had been invited by Mr. Schindlebower to talk on hygiene and sanitation. But none of the questions were on that subject. One was on visiting hours.

Then one fellow who turned out to be drunk, started the carping. He went on about a doctor in Kyle who quit because he didn't get enough money and he wanted to know why there was no clinic at that location. I attempted to explain that no nurses would go out there to live and that we did not have enough doctors at the hospital to send out. Every time we have to do an operation we tie up at least three doctors. The surgeon, the assistant, and the one who gives the anesthesia.

I explained the problems of limited availability of doctors. For instance the hospital was only supposed to do three operations a week, but this week we did three on Monday alone. We did one Tuesday. We did five today, and we're doing one tomorrow and possibly an emergency one tonight. I told him that doctors were not available. Then he went into how some doctors at the Veterans Administration had cut him out of a pension. That type of complaint we can't deal with. Miss Holden saved the day for me though. She got up and gave the best plea of the medical staff. Mrs. Holden afterward said to me, "That's what happens when you come to such meetings. These people crucify you."

Moses Schindlebower got up and said, "I'm the principal in this district. I've been here twenty years. This man doesn't even belong to our community. These people came out here tonight for a different purpose. If you don't confine your remarks to hygiene and sanitation, then there is the door." This guy got up soon after and left. The man who was working with Law and Order for the night followed him out.

Oscar Bear Runner thanked me and the hospital staff very profusely. Then he called on Mr. Reifel. Mr. Reifel spoke a few words in Sioux. He then translated it into English. He started out by saying in Sioux that we call doctors holy white men. "They are not holy," he said. "They are as you and I." "These people, where they come from, I don't know. But they have come here to work among our people, and they have come all the way out here tonight to talk to you and tell you a few things. They have asked you to use soap and water, eat proper diets, and provide warmth for your children. Yet they take children into the hospital, feed them, get them built up, and send them home and they come back in the same condition not much later. The Sioux race is going to die off if you, the people, don't do something about it. Use that soap and water, which is so easy to get. My mother was a poor woman. But she had soap and water, and she raised five boys. You can do it. But if you don't, there is no one that can raise your children for you." He said why don't you people send your kids to school, make sacrifices, and keep your kids in school and make doctors and nurses out of them? They would come back and work with their own people. He cited Indian nurse aids at the hospital and pointed out they were as good as any.

There was a moment when he talked about the great service we had done for these people tonight that I felt very humble for a minute. Then I felt I'd done a very poor job of trying to get something across. Ben Reifel, of course, is very educated. He believes in education. He recognizes that the Indian is going to have to pull himself up by his own bootstraps. The Indians should be thankful that there is someone who would take the time from such a busy workload and come and talk to them. But still, if they don't take the advice, they aren't going to be successful because there is no one who can do for them what they must do for themselves.

It was one of the most wonderful speeches I've heard given. Of course, he is Sioux and can perhaps reach them better and also tell them things that whites couldn't. It is what they need. A report in the *Omaha Herald* said that Mr. Reifel was the first Sioux Indian agent here and that perhaps it might help matters since no other superintendent has been successful here. I think the man is wonderful, his approach is good, and his ideas are important, vital, and great. I don't know if he will succeed here—time will tell. These people are stubborn. They are bent on doing as little as possible. But if he can get his thinking across to them, it will be for their benefit.

Oscar was profuse once again in his thanks as soon as Mr. Reifel got through. He then asked for a standing vote of appreciation. Everyone stood.

After the meeting there were several questions by those who crowded around. They are stirred by the idea of paying for health care, a little germ of an idea that Mr. Sande helped to spread. Mr. White Bull from Porcupine told me Joe One Feather had said he paid for his hospital bill on one of his family members. I told him that was not true, because federal employees are billed. Then he told me that in Wakpamni District a petition was circulated to have clinic more often. I told him I didn't know about that one. But it was more constructive than the one asking for more visiting hours. We had a lunch. Minced ham sandwiches and coffee. Good coffee. After which we journeyed back to Pine Ridge.

On the way back, I was tense to keep the car on the road. Mr. Reifel wanted to know if there was some way to get the germ theory across to the people. They drop a baby's bottle in the dirt but put it back in the kid's mouth. Germs and filth mean nothing to them. Since there are germs on the skin at all times but it is nothing they can see, they do not take stock in it. I told him I thought one way would be to take Petri dishes of agar out and have someone put their dirty hands on the agar. Then have the person wash well with soap and water and then touch a different agar plate. In a few days, they could see the difference in growth on the agar plates. He liked the idea. I believe it might help them to know about germ theory. He said they carry their ignorance over into peyote, where they think peyote cures all.

Mr. Reifel told me one man's explanation of how he cured himself of tuberculosis with peyote. Tuberculosis isn't caused by germs, the man told him, but by a bad condition in the blood that backs up in the blood. The blood backs up in the lungs, comes up into the throat, and suffocates a person. But by taking peyote, it purifies the blood. There are two cults of peyote, the Half Moon and the Cross Fire. One uses the Bible; the other does not. The two factions are competitors.

February 4, 1954

I remember that last night, after Mr. Reifel's speech, that I was sitting next to Mrs. Reifel during refreshments. I told her that hearing her husband talk about the doctors and nurses and what they were doing and the great service we had done last night at the Porcupine meeting that I really felt ineffective, and that I'd done little for the people. She said, "Oh, he likes to blow his top every once in awhile."

I was told a funny story the other day. There are quite a number of the Indians who go into the Black Hills each summer during the tourist season and make more money than they do in their usual jobs for the same length of time. One of these is Charlie Randall. He is the assistant dairyman at the school. His wife cans food in the fall. They have a nice clean neat house. They come to the square dances. They live and work as anyone else around here. But Charlie has archetypical Indian facial features. He dresses in a war bonnet and such, and he pitches a tent at Keystone along the Black Hills highway. He lives in the tent with his wife (who detests living that way) during his vacation time in the summer. There he poses for tourists who tip him for letting them take his picture. He makes good money.

One day a lady pulled her car to a halt breathlessly when she saw this Charlie there all decked out in feathers. She rushed up to him and started a conversation. She started out, "Me from Pennsylvania," and so on and so on. After telling all about herself as though she were talking to a most uncivilized person, she started in on him. "Where you live?" Then Charlie explained in large words and good sentences, that he lived on the reservation. And he was familiar with her part of Pennsylvania, because he used to drive a truck there. The lady didn't say another word. She sneaked off to her car. Charlie laughs and laughs when he talks about it.

I have a patient in the hospital now, a Catholic, who lives at Manderson. He got sick five or six days ago. Finally he went to Wounded Knee where his mother lived. He left his wife in Manderson. There his mother called in a "Witch Doctor," or Indian healer, who gave him peyote. When he came to the hospital, he was comatose. But he soon snapped out of it. He does have some underlying organic troubles, which apparently accounted for him going to the peyote doctor, or his mother saw to it he got to a peyote doctor.

Then we had a woman in the hospital who was a terminal cancer case. She was nearly dead when her folks took her from the hospital to get her home so that they could give her some peyote. She actually listed her religion as "Native American Church" upon entering the hospital.[1]

A group of hospital people interested in Indian folklore and in tribal government met tonight at the hospital for our first meeting. The meetings are not official by any stretch of the imagination. We served refreshments afterward and had cookies and coffee brought from the homes. Tonight Mr. William Fire Thunder, who is the present secretary of the tribal council, spoke to us. He and his wife drove in from Allen this afternoon. In two weeks Jake Herman is going to talk about sign language. Mr. Fire Thunder told us about tribal government. He started way back and told us about everything including the Wheeler-Howard Act of 1934, which allowed the tribe to elect their own officers every two years. Deep down the Indians have the same motives and drive as any people. But on the surface, they are completely different.

The tribal elections were held today. The unofficial returns show Moses Two Bulls is ahead of Frank Wilson for president. That is excellent. They show that my friend, Jake Herman, is trailing his opponent. The four councilmen ahead are Moot Nelson, Ethel Merrival, Bud Mills, and Jim Wilson. Jim Wilson continually opposes Ethel Merrival.

February 6, 1954

On February 2, Miss McGill handed Miss Holden a letter of request for transfer, and Miss Holden handed it on to me. I approved and signed it and passed it on to the higher ups for action. I guess Miss McGill figured she'd never be able to get a hold of this fortress, so she decided to transfer and asked for Alaska.

With this operation tonight, we did eleven, I repeat, eleven, operations this week. Three of the operations were strictly emergencies. Two were ruptured appendixes, and one was a gangrenous bowel case where we resected fourteen inches of gangrenous bowel in a patient.

I see in the last issue of the *Pine Ridge* that Cordelia Red Owl, a senior at ochs, has been invited to ride in the court of Miss Indian America this coming August. Cordelia was a princess in the homecoming celebration at ochs last fall.

I took a refrigerator from the hospital and gave it to Dr. Walter because his went on the blink. Then it also went on the blink. So I have to give him another from the hospital until Mr. Reifel gets another for him. But in order to give him one from the hospital, it means a great deal of doubling up on refrigerated things at the hospital. Poor Miss Holden started to bawl when I asked her for one. She just has too many little problems. And, of course, Mr. LaCourse wouldn't help her one bit by getting us one.

One of the nurses is giving Miss Holden fits by not showing up for work. So Miss Holden drafted quite a letter to send to her, stating that her performance is rotten and that she will get a very poor efficiency rating unless she snaps out of her bad habits of not showing up for work.

February 7, 1954

I saw Douglas Horse today and asked him if sometime he'd take me to a peyote meeting. He said yes, if I'd eat peyote. I told him I didn't want to do that. Then he told me how upset he'd been to have the doctors say that his father had been poisoned by peyote. So I called him to my office and told Douglas that there was something wrong with his father. He was ill. He had things wrong other than too much peyote. Then I told Douglas that we give hospitalized people different medicines that, if we gave too much, would poison them. He insisted his father wasn't poisoned by peyote. He said he'd been rejected by the army because of tuberculosis, and he took peyote and was cured so that he didn't have to go to the sanatorium. I then asked Douglas who had cured him, God or the peyote? Well, he guessed God, but the peyote was the sacrament.

Douglas told me he is Cross Fire. They use the Bible. Half Moon uses the peace pipe. In the Cross Fire they have high priests and ordained ministers, Douglas told me. They pray to God for strength and for help. Douglas told me he used to be a real tough guy. He drank heavily. He used to steal. And he was always fighting. Since becoming a member of the Cross Fire, he doesn't do these things. He prays to God for his guidance and help. He says God helps him.

I've never before established such rapport with an Indian as I did with this fellow. He does have a real faith. In fact, I wonder how this problem should be attacked without uprooting such faith these people have in peyote, a drug, if they can eliminate it.

They have four songs that they sing over and over. They pray. Their meetings last all night. They believe in the God of the Bible and Christ. Douglas doesn't condemn other religions. They have peyote meetings on the birthdays of children to thank God for keeping them going that far in life. They have peyote meetings for any occasion to thank God through prayer.

I heard that the drum of the peyote cults is different or has a different sound than the usual tom-tom. So I asked Douglas about the drum. The minister doesn't beat the drum. A special person does the drum. Is the drum like those they play at these dances? I asked. "Oh, no," he wanted me to know. "It is nothing like the one used for that foolishness."[2]

Douglas said that if his father gets well, he is going to have a big meeting of thanks and prayer and a big feast, and he would invite me. I had wondered if he was giving his father peyote while he was in the hospital. He told me that he was not.

One of my patients who was in the hospital for a long time, now released, and who had both legs fractured when he was struck by a driver, told me the other day he was going to sue the fellow who had hit him. I said the government will put a lien against his bill for his hospitalization. He hit the ceiling. He had intended to buy a Cadillac. He couldn't understand why that would be done. I told him that people who could afford hospitalization now had to pay. He admitted a lot of Indians could pay for their bills. But he just couldn't understand why that would be done. I told him he was no different than anyone else. "Treaties. Treaties, Doc," he said.

Miss Holden looks pretty worn out. She works long hours. Says she can't stand it much longer. She doesn't know of another place where there is more work to do. Her hip bothers her. She asked me if I would get her a medical discharge. I am sure she is entitled to one on the basis of the trouble she has. She will go to her private doctor first. That will be Dr. Crum. And then on the basis of his findings, the discharge can be initiated here. I told her though, that I want her to stay here until I leave this service, which will be early this next winter.

February 9, 1954

We certainly got a swell plug from Mr. Reifel in his daily newssheet dated February 8. He cited that we'd had 2,288 admissions since July 1. I can't believe it myself. Anyway, he cited the tremendous amount of work being done by the hospital and that he requested people to please adhere to the visiting hours. The cooperation that we are getting from him is marvelous. Edgar Red Cloud dropped over to the house at noon. He comes over frequently. He made a remark when I asked him about Mr. Reifel. He said, "We can't pull anything over on him because he knows us."

One of the patients at the hospital has been Henry Black Elk. He is newly elected as a councilman from the Wakpamni District, this district. I think he got some idea of the work that is done up here and he probably will help us in meetings.

There was a note sent to Mr. Ben Reifel on an episode about two weeks ago. The letter was from the Area director and stated that the constituent's call to the congressman was motivated by outside pressure from a white man and that his wife was being cared for here at the hospital.

All of the various sensations and beliefs told to me by Indians who have attended Yuwipi meetings follow. A Yuwipi meeting is conducted in this manner. Those partaking sit around on the floor. The lights are on. Two men tie the medicine man up with sinew. His hands are placed back to back behind him. The two helpers tie his hands by weaving the sinew around the fingers. Then they hood him with a blanket or animal skin and with a rope tie him at intervals down his body. The medicine man is laid down on the floor, face down. The lights are turned out. In what seems like two minutes, the lights are turned on, and the medicine man is sitting up on the floor as anyone else with the sinew and rope rolled in a nice ball. Before any of this begins, any pictures or statues of a religious nature, and any jewelry or silverware in the room or anything else made by white men are taken from the room excepting pictures, which are turned around with the face side to the wall. They just do not have any white-man-made stuff in the room.

After the opening ceremony, in which the medicine man gets himself out of the ropes and sinew, the ceremony begins. The man to be "healed" is placed in the center of the room. The lights are turned off. The others are sitting on the floor. There is a noise I'd describe as a drum spinning around the room as it beats. Then there is a general noise and confusion for a period of time. Doors sound as if they opened and shut yet don't move. The Indians see flashes of light through the room near the ceiling. They believe it is spirits flying around the room.[3] The medicine man goes rapidly about the room and taps people on the shoulders and head. Yet you do not hear him as he moves about. Gourds are rattled at various points faster than a person could run around the room to give the effect that the gourd is flying through the air. No person is heard running about the room as the effects appear. Drafts of air swish through the room. I wonder, did they use a pot of hot rocks, and pour water over them to make steam, probably somewhat as in the sweat bath. Yet that seems impossible because the rooms I was in were very small.

Before the lights are turned off the second time a particular sage-weed is put in the hair. This prevents evil spirits from invading the body. This same sage-weed is ground to a powder, with each person taking a small bit of it in his hands. He spits on it and rubs it on his face and hands. It is rubbed on the hands so that anything good coming his way can be grasped.

After the lights come on, singing and prayers begin. The peace pipe is passed around. Each person receiving it says "How" as he gets the pipe, puffs on it, and passes it on. Water and a dipper were passed as well. I did not put the pipe to my lips, but made the motions as if I did. And I did not drink from the dipper, but made the gesture as if I drank from it. After the ceremony, dog meat is served. I did not eat it.

February 10, 1954

Today at a staff meeting at the hospital Mr. Reifel came up for our meeting. So instead of discussing a portion of the manual I had each one introduce himself to Mr. Reifel and mention or discuss his duties. It was very successful. As I had wondered, some might be reticent to talk, but he questioned them, making it very informal and putting people at ease. Then he discussed, at my request, his idiosyncrasies as he calls them: liquor, speed, working hours, and so on. Then he was interested in Mrs. Olinger's introduction of herself, which focused on the role of the Public Health Service in the field. She told him she didn't think the people were ready for such service. That surprised him. But she added the people were not prepared for it. They didn't understand what a Public Health Service nurse does. People there in Kyle expected her to be a doctor and push pills, to be a flunky and haul them and their things around, and to be an ambulance driver and get them into a hospital. Her program is preventive medicine, what to do to prevent many problems before they occur.

Then Mr. Reifel told about a meeting he'd attended in Oglala yesterday. He discussed peyote. He said he was Episcopalian and believed in wine as a sacrament. But if his brother got ill, he didn't go buy a gallon of wine and force it down him. By the same token this is America, and the people are free to worship as they please and to worship whomever they please. Perhaps if peyote was a sacrament, it was okay to take a piece but not a great quantity of the beans. He told about one meeting where a hundred people were assembled, and due to a shortage of beans there were only five hundred beans, which went like "hotcakes." Mr. Reifel used humor all along.

Then Mr. Reifel discussed discrimination. He mentioned various meetings he attended in Nebraska and stated he didn't think there was a discrimination problem over there. He mentioned the importance of cleanliness for Indian children because there was apparent discrimination against dirty, ill-fed, and ill-clothed little kids in schools. He directed comments to Indian employees in the hospital, telling them their job was a big one. They were the ones to get to the Indian people on this reservation. They must spread the word about the germ concept of disease. And he said Indians are as responsible for discrimination as the non-Indian folk. It is a two-way street. They are always yelling "white man" and "half-breed." He said these in the Sioux language. Also, Mr. Reifel made it clear he is sick and tired of people yelling about treaties, and how they aren't being kept. The Sioux people have had a lot given to them, and it could be made into a lot more, but they haven't utilized it.

My impression is that here is a man who is not only going to sit in this office as superintendent and administer the laws; he is also going to do something for his people. He has progressive ideas and is going to press them. He has scheduled many meetings over the reservation next week and asked me to attend as many as I could and talk to the

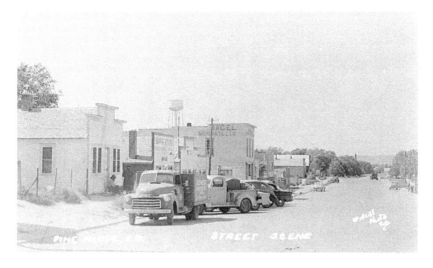

Street scene, Pine Ridge, South Dakota, ca. 1940s. Svara Store and Hagel Mercantile Company are visible left foreground. Electric power lines can be seen on the right. There are no sidewalks or street lights. The appearance of the town is similar to what Dr. Robert H. Ruby experienced in the middle 1950s. Courtesy Cheryl Hemingway, personal collection.

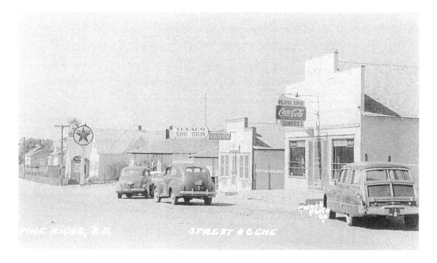

Street scene, Pine Ridge, South Dakota, ca. 1940s. Pejuta Teepee, a small diner, and Hemingway Texaco are visible in the right foreground. The street is unpaved, and wooden walks front some structures. Courtesy Cheryl Hemingway, personal collection.

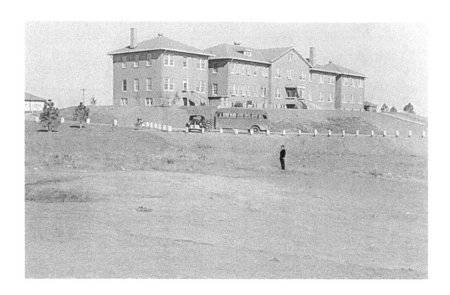

Early southwestern view of Pine Ridge Hospital. The center portion of the building housed the main hospital. The left wing functioned as a day clinic. Today the structure still stands but is no longer used for medical purposes. Courtesy Cheryl Hemingway, personal collection.

(*Opposite top*) Dr. Ruby titled this shot simply "Our House," taken in September 1953 shortly after the Rubys arrived in Pine Ridge, South Dakota. Jeanne Ruby is posed in front. Like many BIA employees, the Rubys lived on the west side of Pine Ridge down the hill from the hospital and near the agency headquarters. Courtesy Robert H. Ruby, personal collection.

(*Opposite bottom*) Dr. Robert H. Ruby in his navy uniform, with Captain. Photo taken outside the house in which the Rubys lived at Pine Ridge, South Dakota, in 1954. Robert H. Ruby, personal collection.

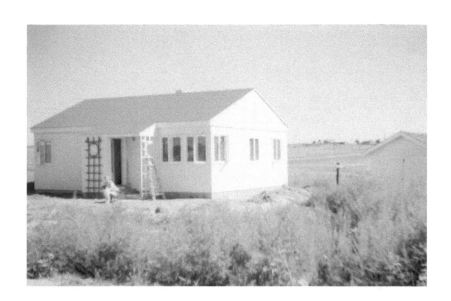

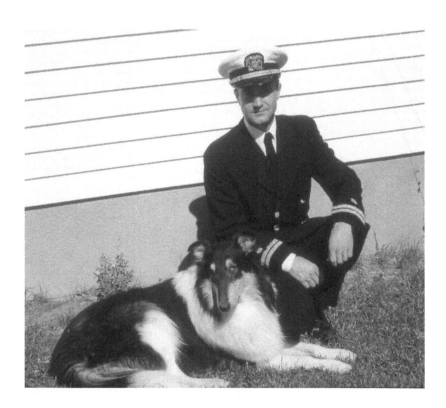

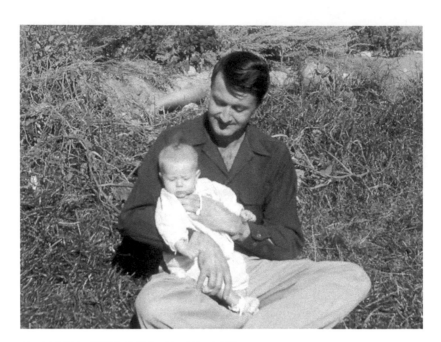

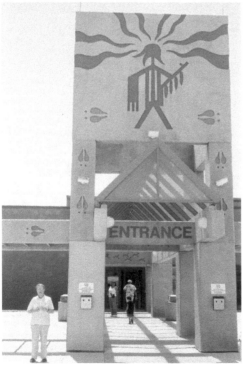

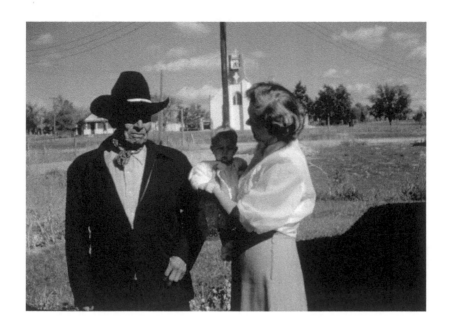

(*Opposite top*) Robert H. Ruby and daughter, Edna, 1954. Dr. Ruby believes that Edna was the first white child to be born in the Pine Ridge Indian Hospital. Robert H. Ruby, personal collection.

(*Opposite bottom*) Dr. Ruby in front of the new Pine Ridge Hospital, Pine Ridge, South Dakota, June 23, 2006. Charles V. Mutschler, personal collection.

(*Above*) Charlie Yellow Boy and Edna and Jeanne (holding Edna) Ruby. Pine Ridge, South Dakota, 1954. Looking east from the Rubys' house toward downtown Pine Ridge. Robert H. Ruby, personal collection.

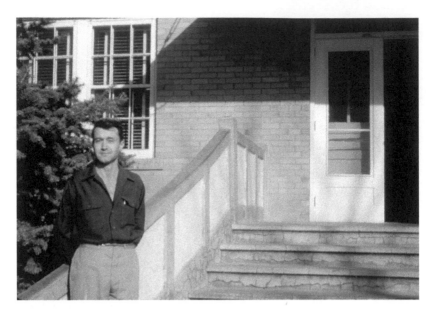

Dr. Robert H. Ruby on the front steps, Pine Ridge Indian Hospital. Taken in 1954, when Dr. Ruby was the chief medical officer in charge of the hospital. Robert H. Ruby, personal collection.

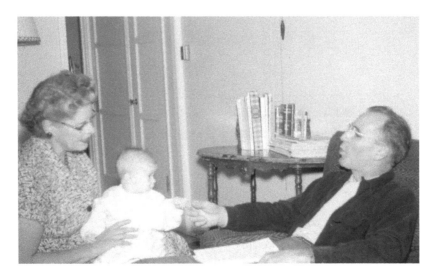

Lillian and Lawrence Mickelson with Edna Ruby, Pine Ridge, South Dakota, 1954. Lawrence Mickelson was one of the teachers on the reservation. The Mickelsons were Edna's godparents. Robert H. Ruby, personal collection.

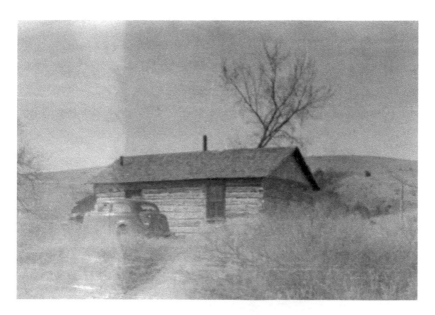

Typical reservation housing at the time Dr. Ruby was at Pine Ridge. Taken near Manderson, South Dakota, 1954. Robert H. Ruby, personal collection.

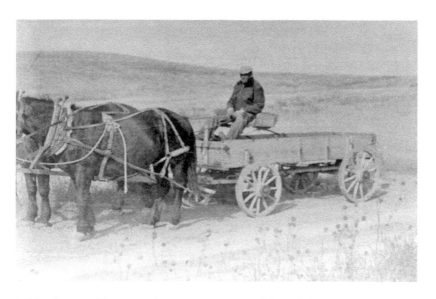

White Coyote with team and wagon, 1953. Many of the Oglala Sioux still utilized horses for transportation in 1953. Dr. Ruby remarked on this early on during his tenure on the reservation. Robert H. Ruby, personal collection.

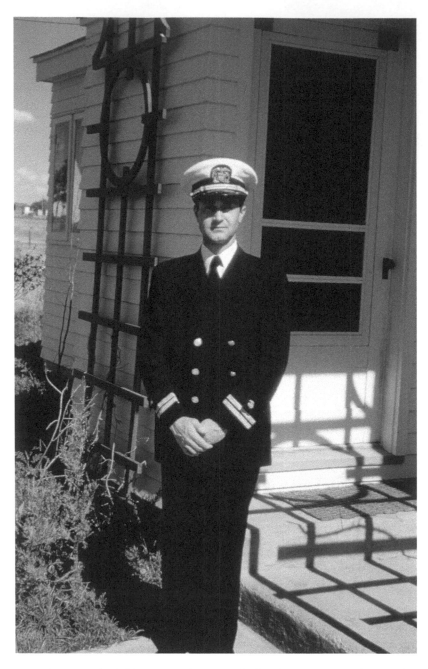

Dr. Robert H. Ruby in his navy uniform outside their home in Pine Ridge, South Dakota, July 1954. Robert H. Ruby, personal collection.

people. I want to do this. He came up to my office afterward, and we talked about off-reservation medical care and those eligible here.

February 14, 1954

Edgar brought us a Yuwipi "rosary" the other day, with the tiny bits of tobacco, the size of a pea, wrapped in pieces of cloth. They are used in the Yuwipi religion. These little pouches of tobacco are tied onto a string less than an inch apart. At the end is a buckskin pouch of the medicine man's medicines. This one that Edgar had made for us has headache medicine tied in a piece of buckskin, which is soft and white. When the medicine man visits a sick person to heal him, that person has to make the rosary. When the medicine man hands him the medicine to heal him, the sick man ties this in the buckskin and ties it to the rosary. When he leaves, the medicine man takes the rosary to a sacred high hill and asks the Great Spirit to heal the sick man. The rosary is an offering to the Great Spirit.

Edgar told me that the head medicine man here is from Rosebud. He called a meeting the other night to bring in all medicine men. He said he was going to take their authority and power away from them. He wanted them to stop for awhile. He predicted great storms this spring, about the time the grass gets green. The significance of this I don't understand yet.

Tonight Edgar took me to the sweat house ritual of a Yuwipi meeting at Chief Red Cloud's home. Indians sweat before going to healing services. Plenty Wolf, the medicine man, didn't exactly like me being there. Because Edgar is Catholic, Plenty Wolf isn't sure of him. When we got there, White Whirlwind, who stayed outside and did the scout work, told Plenty Wolf on the inside "Two white men are here."[4] Then he told who we were. Chief Red Cloud didn't mind our being there. He invited me back after the service. I'll tell you about the ceremony that followed the sweat.

It was about an hour before sunset. There had been a strong wind all day, but now it was quieting down. Red Cloud came to the sweat house with Plenty Wolf. They carried big bundles of tarp, old quilted blankets, and even a piece of old carpet.[5] Elk Boy tended the fire. He cut some pieces of wood from a tree trunk and threw them on the fire. White Whirlwind sat on a piece of wood. Red Cloud started throwing the pieces of tarp, blankets, and carpet over the sweat house. Elk Boy stirred the rocks over the fire. They were becoming hot. White Whirlwind got up, said a few words, and went toward a hose that was nearly a hundred feet to the west. Presently he came back with a pail of water. Plenty Wolf had a peace pipe and a tobacco bag. It belonged to Red Cloud. By now Red Cloud and Plenty Wolf had the sweat house covered except for one small section to the east where the fire burned brightly. The medicine man, Plenty Wolf, laid out four old tomato tin cans full of dirt near a small pile of rocks that were not being heated. On the top of two of them were some sage leaves. Red Cloud and Elk Boy sat down on the south side of the sweat house and took off their clothes. Plenty Wolf took off his and laid them on the north side. Meanwhile White Whirlwind carried the hot rocks by means of sticks to a hole in the center of the sweat house. The naked men crawled through an opening into the sweat house and sat down on the ground around the heated rocks. White Whirlwind then took the pail of water and threw it on the rocks. The tarps and blankets were held down by rope around the sweat house and by several planks leaning against it, except for a flap above the entrance that White Whirlwind now pulled down over the opening. The clouds of steam that rose from the hot rocks were now trapped in the small sweat house. He then laid the tobacco bag and long peace pipe down on the rocks.

White Whirlwind was the helper. He sat outside and tended the fire. The medicine man prayed. He shook the gourd rattle. Then he started to sing. Elk Boy and Red Cloud sang with him. The spirit of the Great Spirit descended and made noises similar to that which an owl makes. I heard them. The medicine man prayed as the Great Spirit descended on these groups of people, to bless them and care for them, to keep them from sickness. The peace pipe was left outside for the Great Spirit to smoke. The cans of earth are the invitation for it to come down to earth.

Presently it got a little hot in the sweat bath. The medicine man stopped the worship service. The audible tones of conversation were heard. White Whirlwind opened the flap of the sweat house. A blast of cool air cooled down the inside. The wet naked bodies shone from the moisture on them.

The sun had set, but it was still quite light. It was going to be a nice night. The moon was high in the sky. White Whirlwind put the flap down. The singing started. The medicine man rattled the gourds. The second verse. The third. I heard the sound of the Great Spirit. It sounded like an owl. The fourth verse. Then the medicine man prayed. Another song.

The ceremony was about over. The medicine man called to White Whirlwind to light the peace pipe. White Whirlwind took a pinch of tobacco from the long leather sack. He untied the leather binder at the top. The fringe of leather at the bottom moved with the breeze. After he put a pinch of tobacco in the pipe bowl he took a burning stick and puffed on the long stem until it burned. Then he passed it to Plenty Wolf. White Whirlwind pulled down the flap. Once more Plenty Wolf prayed. He puffed on the pipe and passed it to Elk Boy. "How," said Elk Boy as he took it. After puffing, he passed it to Red Cloud. "How," said Red Cloud and puffed. In his prayers Plenty Wolf told the Great Spirit that now they were offering up tobacco to him.

The ceremony was over. Plenty Wolf came out. The chief came out. Elk Boy came out. They dried with towels and dressed. Mrs. Elk Boy came from the house with a small black and white dog that had been bought in Nebraska. She painted a red stripe across the nose. Then she painted a red stripe from the nose to the end of the tail before the dog was choked to death. Since all animals have spirits, it is necessary that they go to the happy hunting ground. And if the painting, a "baptism," had not been done, after the dog's spirit had reached the Milky Way the old lady who guards the two forks would have pointed in the direction of the short fork. The dog starting out would have been on the fork that goes to "hell," or earth again. As he got to the end of the fork there is no turning back. The old lady would have pushed him over. But with the "baptism" having been performed, when his spirit got to the Milky Way, the old lady who guards the two forks would point to the longer fork, which would take the dog's spirit to the Happy Hunting Ground, or "heaven."

As soon as the dog was choked to death, Mrs. Elk Boy threw it on the fire that White Whirlwind had built up. The dog's hair singed. She scraped it off with a stick. She turned the dog over on the fire to burn the hair all around. She scraped off the singed hair with the stick. This she repeated until the heat drew up the legs, the hide cracked over the joints of the legs, and the belly started to bloat from the heat. Next Mrs. Elk Boy took the dog and dragged it through the grass to scrape off the remaining hair. The chief, Red Cloud, had brought a pail of water to the sweat bath after taking the tarps, blankets, and carpet from the structure and rolling them up. He threw the water on the fire to put it out. Everyone repaired to the house. Mrs. Elk Boy gutted the animal, leaving the tail, head, legs, and hide on. She threw it in a kettle of boiling water after washing it in water. As soon as the food was ready, the worshippers ate it. Plenty Wolf ate the head. The dog had been cooked with nothing added, no vegetables or such.

The party repaired to the house about one hundred yards north. Here Grace Shield had taken all her earthly belongings from her house so the worship service could begin after the feast.

February 16, 1954

About ten days ago Eugene Rowland, the recently returned Korean War veteran, was married to a Black Feather girl. The general announcement and wedding dance was held last Friday night. Rowland, his wife, and Bob Poor Bear and his wife overturned their car. We kept Rowland's wife in the hospital until Sunday and wanted to keep Poor Bear as well, but he wouldn't stay.

Today I finally decided to leave for the Kyle meeting in honor of Mr. Ben Reifel. Yesterday he was honored at Wanblee and will be honored at various places all this week. I probably won't get away anymore. I took Edgar Red Cloud with me. Edgar asked me if I would take Charlie Yellow Boy, so we stopped to pick him up. Mr. Reifel passed me this morning going to the meeting. Thank heavens I was only going thirty miles per hour. He is so against speeding. Edgar told me that yesterday Julie White picked a fight with Mrs. Black Feather. Over what? I wondered. Eugene Rowland. Edgar said that Rowland was to marry Julie's girl but then married the Black Feather girl. He said the fight happened right there in town yesterday. I didn't think anything about it until it dawned on me that I had tended to a woman with a split head yesterday. Mrs. White, I believe she was, and she told me she had been fighting over a man. Edgar said before it was as though "twenty women were fighting." He said when they fight they pull off clothes, bloomers, and then grab each other's hair and hang on for dear life so that no one can hit the other or get away.

The meeting at Kyle was very fine. There were three hundred people there. Mr. Reifel called on all branch heads to speak. I took the opportunity to tell the people they were luckier than other communities. They had a Public Health nurse, and other communities did not but wanted one. Then in line with Mr. Reifel's thinking, I asked them not to abuse the privilege, but said that the nurse was there for preventive medicine. That meant keeping people well and not being a doctor and treating people without orders from a doctor.

The branch chiefs explained their programs, except Ed Coker, head of Soil and Moisture Conservation. He said he noticed the pride of the people, that one of their own had returned to govern them. Then he implored them to do as Mr. Reifel directed. Mr. Coker said Mr. Reifel couldn't raise everyone up by their bootstraps, but he would tell them how. Then, as everyone on the program before had been preaching, Mr. Coker asked them to hang on to their lands. He cited the great Sioux Uprising before 1876 when the Sioux fought the white man to keep their lands. Now they were giving it away for a few pieces of silver. What a strange turn of events. First the white man took the soil, and now they were asking him to keep it.

What I learned was that an average of one-half section of land was sold to whites every day. That would mean that in five years there would be no more Indian land. It wasn't pointed out to them, but the Indian pays no tax on trust land. So when they do give up their lands, they then will have nothing concrete to put their hands on.

Mr. Reifel was his usual self. I too have noticed the pride of the people, in him, as their leader. I ate with the Reifels and with Ben American Horse, a colorful senior chief, Andrew Fools Crow, from whom I've ordered some moccasins, Ed Coker, and Mr. Mast. Mrs. Reifel told me she didn't wish to come today, but she had gone yesterday, and Ben thought she should come today so the community wouldn't feel slighted. She told me about an experience they had when they visited here fifteen years ago. They encountered people whose car got stuck, and Mr. Reifel took their eighteen-year-old girl ten miles on to Kyle to visit friends. When they got there it turned out the friends had a kid with Scarlet Fever. Fortunately none of them came down with it.

Charlie Yellow Boy traveled with Buffalo Bill's Circus and Wild West Show. Once he broke his left leg on a bronco in Chicago, and he later broke the right one and had to stay in the Pine Ridge hospital for that. Charlie had a medicine man and a Yuwipi meeting at his home last night and said he was having another to treat his wife and other people tonight. Edgar asked him if I could go, and he said yes. So tonight I picked up Edgar and Mrs. Forshey, and we went off to Charlie's home. We were there perhaps an hour before they started. Sitting around, Edgar was talking to Silas Yellow Boy, one of the medicine man's helpers. Edgar told me later that Silas said, "Looks like we are mixing more and more with white people." Edgar told him his wife was half-Indian and pretty much white, and so she had no more business being there than we did. Edgar said when he arrived, Chief Red Cloud gave him the dickens for bringing us out there. Edgar told him Charlie invited us. The medicine man came up and said he was glad to welcome us and asked Edgar to take him to us. Edgar had told him we brought some cigarettes and money for him. He talked to us with Edgar as interpreter. He told us he was glad for us to come. He said he had treated many white people in North Dakota, South Dakota, and Nebraska. He said one father came looking for him all over the reservation to treat his boy who was paralyzed, and that he was able to cure the boy. Tonight three women and two men were being treated. Mrs. Charlie Yellow Boy was being treated for cramps in her feet and legs. Hazel Shields was being treated for headache. There were more people in this little log cabin than came to many of the community service meetings at which I spoke in various places on the reservation.

The building was perhaps thirty by ten feet. There must have been thirty people there, all Yuwipi believers except Mrs. Forshey and myself. The medicine man was George Poor Thunder from Allen. After he welcomed us, the chief told him that he had been only kidding, that it was all right for us to come. But Edgar said the chief really was upset with him at first for bringing us. Before the service, the medicine man told us his power comes from the thunder and lightning, power given him by the Great Spirit.

Blankets had been put up over each window and the door. All the furniture had been moved out. Around the edges of the room there were mattresses and blankets for squatting on. Those to be treated, the visitors, and those who followed the Yuwipi religion assembled and sat around the room. The medicine man, George Poor Thunder, came in. He was about six feet tall. Thin. His face was lined deeply. His braids fell down low on each side. Wisps of hair fell over his forehead and face. His lower lip came up over his upper lip. It gave him a mean appearance, but he was a gentle old soul, about sixty-five, I presume. His helpers were Silas Yellow Boy and Flesh, both medicine men.

Charlie Yellow Boy, at whose home the meeting was held, carried in a pail of hot rocks that had been heated on a fire outside. From a pail of water Silas poured some water over the rocks, producing steam. He brought "flags" and placed them above the pail of steaming rocks so the steam would reach them. There were four large flags and four small ones. The larger ones were on sticks about two and one-half feet high. On one there was a yellow cloth, representing the sun and the moon. On another there was a red cloth, representing the red man. And there were two white cloths, representing purity. The four smaller flags were the same colors. The sticks were eight inches high, and the pieces of cloth smaller. The sacred alter was made at the south end of the room. It consisted of two small cans of earth, one on each side of a large can of earth. At the north end of the room were two more cans of earth. Silas put the two white flags at the back, one in each can of earth, and on the alter he put the yellow flag in the can of earth to the east and the red flag in the small can to the west. He stuck the four small flags in the large can at the center. And in this he put a large stick perhaps three and one-half feet in length. Then he carried in a large bundle of sage and laid it down before the altar. This was rolled in a tarp. Silas Yellow Boy handed a branch of sage to each person in the room. Then he took a large branch of sage and lit it. The fragrance permeated the room. He laid it on the floor and stepped over the burning branches.

The medicine man went out and brought in his doctor's bag. He opened it, took out the peace pipe, and laid it on the altar. He laid out a small piece of paper, a foot across. He took four feathers and smoothed the dirt he took from a small mound to make a nice pancake of it on the piece of paper. Then he took feathers and tied them to each large stick put in the center can. Meanwhile, Silas had carried the bucket of water and put it on the altar. A package of Bull Durham and an unopened package of Lucky Strike cigarettes were laid on the altar. In Yuwipi, an offering of tobacco is always made to the Great Spirit. Then Silas took a long "rosary" and tied it to the stick in the white can in the back on the east. He continued stringing it along the room to the stick with the yellow flag, across the altar to the stick with the red flag, back to the white flag on the west at the back of the room, and then to the one on the east, making a perfect rectangle. The medicine man handed small "rosaries" perhaps a foot long to those being cured, three women and two men.

Silas took branches of sage and gave one to each participant. These they put in their hair. Then the medicine man took a quilted blanket from his suitcase and handed it to Silas, who hung it at the back of the room. Next he took a particular kind of weed, and while it burned or smoked he let the smoke go through the blanket by waving it around. Then he took this sprig and went around the room, making an arch over each person there. Behind the altar was Richard Elk Boy, the drummer and main singer. There was only one coal oil lamp burning. This was moved from its perch to the altar. The medicine man closed his suitcase after taking out some rope, perhaps the size of clothesline rope or a window sash.

The ceremony was ready to start. The drummer started his drumming and sang. All joined in. A large woman came forward and tied the medicine man's fingers together with his hands behind his back. He had first taken off his shoes and sweater. She got the quilted blanket and threw it over him. Next she took the long piece of rope, tied a hitch around his neck, then around his chest, and around his waist, thighs, and below the knees. Then the medicine man began singing. His voice sounded muffled as he sang to Wanka Tanka.

The coal oil lamp was still burning. The woman took sprigs of sage and tucked them in each loop of the rope behind the medicine man. Silas Yellow Boy and Flesh were at the back of the room, poised. The medicine man turned after singing. The men rushed up and laid him face down. They sang a song before the lights were put out. I presume the ceremony with the lights out lasted approximately one hour or better, probably one and one-half hours. All during this time the medicine man talked with a muffled voice as though through the blanket. Various songs were sung. There was conversation between songs. The gourd flew about the room. It makes a noise of loose shot inside a dry gourd. It traveled around the room very rapidly. Visible sparks would flash starting at one end of the room and going all the way around.[6] These were the good spirits. Toward the end of the ceremony there were really loud noises and many flashes of spirits. These were the evil spirits leaving the room. After this a very tender song was sung. Before this the singing had gotten louder and louder. But as the bad spirits left, or after they left, a very comforting song in comparison was sung.

Between songs, some of the conversation with the person being treated was carried on by the medicine man in his muffled voice. Then during the next singing the gourd would be heard mostly over in the direction of that patient, who told all about his symptoms. Then there were flashes of the spirits. Next was a song when spirits would disrobe the medicine man. After this the lamps were lit, and he was sitting up. The medicine man got his peace pipe and handed it to a lady, who lit it and puffed and said "Taakuessen." "How," responded everyone. Then she passed it on. The next person puffed and said "Taakuessen." Everyone responded with "How," and so on, all around the room. Finally Silas got the pail of water and handed everyone a dipper of water. After each person drank, he or she also said "Taakuessen" again, and everyone responded with "How." "Taakuessen" means we are all one, or we are all related. Then everyone got up and stretched, for a break, and then assembled to eat dog. After the lights came on, the "rosary," which had been strung all around the room, was gone. On the flat pancake surface of dirt were marks left by THE GREAT SPIRIT. They were a message to the medicine man.

I can't figure out how the medicine man or the helpers performed the service. The medicine man was tied in a blanket all during the treatments. He had a muffled voice. But it seems to me that at times he sounded not quite so muffled. The room was so small for that many people sitting around with their feet stuck out that I do not see how a helper could travel around that wooden floor with so little space, so rapidly, and not trip over anyone or get across the stage at the end without it creaking. Before the ceremony, if anyone walked on the stage, it creaked. Then when the spirits were seen in the dark above the people, I think something was hit on the floor to produce that sound. But I don't see how all this was done without brushing against someone.

Before we began the service, the medicine man told Mrs. Forshey and me that this was not like a motion picture. This was serious. Treatments would be given. Then he asked Silas to make comments to us, during the ceremony. When Silas did, he sounded as if he were sitting at the place he was before the lights went out. So if he helped, and actually I could hear the medicine man's voice, muffled, at one end of the room with the gourd noise at the opposite, then I don't see how Silas got back there so quickly. And the other helper, Flesh, couldn't have done all that in the dark without knocking over something at the altar. Then he asked Silas to ask me if I knew the treatments were being made. I said, "Yes, I saw the spirits around the room." I heard some muffled talk, but Edgar said that was the right thing to say. When the ceremony was done, the medicine man was untied, and the lamps were lit. The "rosary" that had been strung all around the room was then gone. I can't figure it out. We didn't smoke the pipe. The medicine man said, "Touch the pipe. All my friends do." We were handed water, and I just pretended to drink. At one point the medicine man interrupted his service. He told Silas to tell the Waswicu that the spirits told him they were glad we (two white people) had come to the service.

February 17, 1954

I took Edgar home late last night after the Yuwipi meeting, and his wife was not feeling well and wished to be in the hospital where she could rest. She had five teeth pulled a couple days ago and was feeling miserable. So I ran her up to the hospital and admitted her. She complained of numbness on the left side of her body, though there was no indication of any cerebral vascular accident. She was upset from having her teeth pulled.

Andrew Standing Soldier, who has promised to make me a watercolor of the battle of Wounded Knee for over three or four months now, hasn't done a thing. His excuse kept being that he couldn't get to Rapid City to get any paper. So when I was up there recently I got some. So I guess I'll go over Saturday and see what he has done.

At the meeting in Kyle, Mr. Reifel kept making remarks about Red Cloud's people. Edgar, who was at the meeting, told me that a lot of people didn't like that since they wanted recognition of other chiefs and subchiefs in the Red Cloud band.

Mr. Reifel called a meeting of department heads tonight. He read his final recommendations made for the Bimson Report. That man is the smartest and most clever person in an intelligent way. His recommendations for transferring Health to the Department of Health, Education, and Welfare were super. He said an established organization such as the Public Health Service had better facilities and recruitment of personnel, and that recommendations they would make for reservation care would be those made for other people, and this should be of benefit to the Indian people. I had made recommendation for this, but not in the nice way he put it. He did a very wonderful piece of work on his report. Then he invited everyone over to his home to participate in eating all the welcome cakes he and his wife had gotten out on the reservation.

I went to the hospital to do some paper work on some cases. I was stuffed, having just eaten dinner at the Carrs' home. But one of Dr. Walters's cases, a pregnancy, was bleeding, and he was afraid he would have to perform a Caesarean. The woman finally delivered spontaneously; Dr. Walters had to come over to the hospital. He is ill, and he screamed horribly at Miss Holden. She came downstairs to me practically in tears. I calmed her down. And then very nicely, Dr. Walters came down on his own and apologized to her so she felt so much better, which made the evening perfect. PERHAPS. The woman delivered but is still bleeding. He treated her for that. I hope we will not have to do any hysterectomies tonight.

Those in the peyote religion here in South Dakota have a charter from the state to practice their religion. But there is nothing in this charter for the Native American Church that allows or condones the use of the peyote bean. The church is not recognized as legal in the probate court for the Bureau of Indian Affairs. For that reason, there is a backlog of troubled estates when someone has died who was a member of the Native American Church and was married in that church. As such, probate does not recognize a surviving woman as married to the deceased. Billy Fire Thunder is the lawyer for the Native American Church.

February 18, 1954

Ben Black Elk talked to a group of interested people tonight at the hospital. He is the son of the famous Black Elk who has written three books on Indian religion and customs. Ben spends all summer at Mount Rushmore coining money from the tourists, has appeared on television and spoken on radio, and has met President Eisenhower.

The phrases or words in quotes are my own spelling of what Mr. Black Elk told me tonight. In speaking, the Teton Sioux use "La," as in Lakota. The Yankton use the "Da," as in Dakota. The Santee use "Ne," as in Nekota.

Both Jake and Ben had given a lecture at school earlier in the evening to teach Indian lore to kids so they can tell others and will know it.

February 20, 1954

The Week in Review:

Sunday eve. I went to a sweat bath Yuwipi service. I didn't go into the sweat bath though.

Monday. Doctors had a conference in evening.

Tuesday. I went to Kyle, spent all day there, talked a couple minutes during the ceremonies for Mr. Reifel. About three hundred people there. At night I went to a regular Yuwipi meeting where they doctored patients. You'll get the particulars in my next letter. Not this time.

Wednesday. Jeanne and I went to dinner at the Carrs' home. Dr. and

Mr. Quint also invited. I left early and went to a staff meeting that Mr. Reifel called.

Thursday. Jeanne and I went to a meeting that one nurse and I started where we get Indians to come and talk to hospital personnel who are interested.

Friday. Jeanne gave a tea for Mrs. Reifel, complete with silver service. I surprised Jeanne and sent to Chadron Floral for flowers. They sent a dozen big yellow daffodils. Gosh, they were pretty. Then that night they gave a dance for Mr. Reifel here in town. We went over and took pictures as usual.

Today. I've given you a rundown above. Nothing but work, work.

February 23, 1954

Douglas Horse, a member of Cross Fire Peyote, said first in response to my question of how many "beans" would he eat in a night, "As many as I can get." Then, when I pinpointed him he said, "perhaps sixty." He does not crave the drug when not able to go to a meeting. This is in keeping with articles I've read on peyote. It is not habit forming. So it is not a narcotic. The more "beans" eaten, the greater the mental response.

Ben Black Elk tells me that Yuwipi and worship of the Great Spirit used to be practiced in broad daylight many, many years ago. He doesn't think much of the present form, thinks it's a perversion of the old, and indicated he had grave doubts that it was real, meaning that the spirits were what make the flashes of light, and so on.

The funniest thing ever, I think, was Friday night. Jeanne and I and three other doctors went to the dance at the Legion Hall given for Mr. Reifel. Edgar Red Cloud came up to me and said, "Do you know that George Poor Thunder, the medicine man from Kyle, is one of the dancers?" I told him that I hadn't recognized Poor Thunder as one of the feather-bedecked men out there dancing. I asked Edgar to tell him to come over and that I wanted to photograph him. Edgar went over and talked to Poor Thunder for the longest time. Then he came back and said Mr. Poor Thunder didn't want to be photographed, that he was a medicine man and not a dancer. I know that he must have been horribly embarrassed, because he maintained such a professional air at his home.

Last Wednesday or Thursday, there was a message on my desk to call Joe Swift Bird, the chief of police. I did later, but he was gone, so I never did call back and figured it wasn't important since he didn't call me back. Well, today at the Agency Office I met him, and he said, "Say, last Tuesday I heard there was going to be a meeting out east of town so I went out there during the night. I saw your car there so I turned around and left. The windows were all boarded up and it was dark. I couldn't get in." I said, "Joe, I've turned Yuwipi, and Mrs. Forshey was out with me." I sure had to laugh.

But another thing about the dance for Mr. Reifel at Legion Hall last Friday night, two boys were creating a disturbance. They wouldn't get off the floor when asked. So Mr. Reifel took one of them by the knap of the neck and booted them out of the building. Being Indian, he can do it and get away with it. Mr. Sande or anyone else should have been able to do that, but being a white person they can't get away with it.

Saturday afternoon Mr. and Mrs. Reifel visited the hospital. It was 4:10, and Mr. Reifel made the remark it was after visiting hours. So he guessed he'd better go. Before that I told him about our money plight. I haven't been worried because I know we have to have food and drugs, and the federal government will just have to dig it up. Mrs. Reifel told me she enjoyed the reception held in our home for her the day before. She said when she entered she thought she was back in civilization again and not out in the sticks.

Saturday evening I went over to see Andrew Standing Soldier. He has started my painting of the battle of Wounded Knee. He said he'd worked on some other painting, but mine is going slowly and that he wants to get it done nicely. I notice he has painted three Hotchkiss guns on the hill that shot down on the people. The history I've read so far states there were four. But he said he'd been talking to his grandfather, who was there, and that most of the Indians wore white tops over their clothes as part of the Messiah craze and they had a red streak across each shoulder and down the front. He even told me he'd made a trip to Wounded Knee to see the lay of the land. But I think he was blowing smoke.

On Friday, Mr. LaCourse called to say we had received a telegram from the Finance Department in the Area Office saying not to spend another cent of money. We have no money left for the rest of this quarter, which runs to the end of March. Mr. LaCourse called Aberdeen today. Mr. Kessis hadn't even known we'd been sent a telegram stating that we had no finances left this quarter. He didn't know we'd spent our allotted money. Mr. Kessis said Dr. Robert Bragg's brother was interested in coming here as a dentist. He wanted to know if we'd take him. I said yes. I told Bob a couple of weeks ago to have his brother tell Washington he wanted to come here. He has a wife and no children so they have a duplex reserved for him.

A copy of a letter sent to Mr. Brust in the Area Office from an Eva Nichols concerning Victoria Ashley upset me at first. I thought the social worker in Omaha had let us down. But the letter said this woman was walking the streets, and that the social worker at the Salvation Army had no time for Indians and so on and so on. Then when I took it to Mrs. Forshey, she said, sounds as if the complaining woman has a chip on her shoulder. But she didn't know her personally. I did some more sleuthing. I learned from Emma Nelson that the complainer is "another Ethel Merrival." So my suspicions were wrong, and Mrs. Forshey was right. We had provided authorization for medical care, a trip to Omaha, and payment for board and room. Are we supposed to breathe for them also? Two more cases today, wanting something, saying the hospital here had no room. So much bunk.

February 25, 1954

Today I got up early and went out to Slim Buttes to attend the meeting called for by Mr. Reifel. Stanley Walker and I arrived first. Then Mr. Brown Eyes, in charge of the community, started his meeting late and apologized at length. Moses Two Bulls, the new president-elect, talked. He asked for cooperation of the group of the council, not to come and buck legislation, not to make it political, but to make the council what it is supposed to be, an economic organization to work together for the good of the people.

There was a recess before dinner. Mr. Reifel called a cabinet meeting since all department heads excepting Welfare were there. He said we would "throw some things around" until it was time to eat. Mr. Reifel said working together was fine, but it had to start with individuals working. He had seen a poster in the school of European-American culture of people who had worked, worked to get where they are. He said the Indian people wouldn't necessarily have to go through a period of serfdom, that could be disposed of quickly. But he said they would have to work. Some of his ideas were to make a map of the reservation and plot each family, and then to see what families were willing to farm or raise chickens. Other families should be encouraged to move from the reservation. He had no ideas yet what to do with the majority of people who live a welfare existence from hand to mouth. He thought families who could be self-sustaining should do so.

Mr. Reifel is interested in finding out the percentage of women to men on the reservation. There are apparently more women than men, and this is a bad situation. He says the women can demand what they wish whereas if it were the other way the men could demand what they wish and therefore demand greater morals in women. He pointed out that the death rate has been lowered drastically. He cited recent troubles—such as one man living with a woman, not married, and having four children. Then when he was being forced to marry, he ran off and married another woman. And now he has five children with her, and in the meantime he has been back with the other woman also and has four more children with her. This one woman with eight children is getting Aid to Families with Dependent Children. Mr. Reifel feels some plan should be worked out to get more women than men off the reservation through the relocation program. He pointed out that some women are bearing all the children that they can. There is one woman in the hospital now who just had her sixth set of twins, and she has had two single births also. She is only thirty years of age. Her most recent delivery made news.

Mr. Reifel has many far-reaching plans for changing the social order and economic order to make these people self-sustaining. I wish I could work with him more. And I was terribly upset when I had to leave then and come home because I was nauseated. Gastroenteritis again. And I was supposed to have talked this afternoon. I wanted to tell these people something about the germ theory of disease. I see Mr. Reifel made reference to it in his news sheet of today. But I just couldn't stay. There were council members there. I wanted to tell them about hospital visiting hours.

Tonight I was invited to a dinner of council members. On my way home I found Vincent Red Cloud with car trouble and gave him a push.

February 28, 1954

I found out the name of the grass used in the Yuwipi meeting for burning and "purifying" the room. It is called sweet grass. The flattened blades are braided.

There is no word for time in the Indian language. Consequently they have no conception of time. The word *time* now in the Indian language is "the little hand on the face of the clock." They have a word for minutes, which is "by the big hand of the clock." Everyone has heard the expression "by Indian time," meaning the characteristic way in which the Indian keeps appointments and accomplishes tasks, walking in just whenever he gets there. There is no hurry, no fuss, to start on time. So meetings start late and run late. A single task to be done is not looked at in its entirety to see when it might be completed. The Indian enjoys the moment in which he lives. He doesn't have in the back of his mind tomorrow, where will I be tomorrow, and what will I be doing.

Nebraska borders the reservation at the South Dakota–Nebraska borderline, so this provides easy opportunity for Nebraska to recruit for harvesting the farmers' crops. Those farmers even built a separate "shantytown" for Indians in one small town to house the laborers. These families gradually began to stay and live in Nebraska towns more and more. Those who are residents and those who stay only a few months out of the year spend practically all of their money in Nebraska, paying state and local taxes. BUT the minute one gets ill, Nebraska wants to shove them back to the reservation hospital. This is discrimination. These people who have established residency there should be entitled to the community services of the place in which they reside. We have had more and more of this problem. In one case lately a young Indian lady who became ill is in the hospital in Nebraska. The social worker told our social worker quite frankly they wanted to get rid of her when our social worker mentioned some way in which one of her family also residing in Nebraska could probably pay for her bill.

Nebraska wants to send two kids with tuberculosis here for their hospitalization and work-up. They have lived in Nebraska for seven years. Now, in Gordon, where the shantytown was built, the town is thinking of uprooting that. That would send all these people back to the reservation. They would have nowhere else to go. Labor will be hard to get now with so much unemployment. So they plan to get rid of those who they needed at one time.

The house. It has snowed and "blowed." When it snows it keeps a continual puddle of mud and sand in the house. When it blows our dirt turf keeps a continual stream of sand and silt filtering throughout the house. But I do believe I'm going to get a fence built around this place. Maintenance superintendent Otto G. Bertsch was over to see about making next year's budget for Maintenance. I told him I wanted a fence now, and he has some wire Health paid for that is left from another home. He wanted to put funds into his budget to fix nurses' houses out in the field. I told him nix. We wouldn't have nurses to put out there. I suggested he move some of those houses in here to be used by doctors.

Eight. March 1954

Father Buechel likes the Indians. They are his friends. He has every bit of patience with them. He's been with them a long time. I wonder if others could spend as much time here as he has and have the same feelings. Most people working with Indians are government people and spend only a few years with the Indians. The average government employee has little patience with the Indians for being so resistant to change. Father Buechel says the Indians have progressed greatly in the past fifty years. He believes the white men do not have enough sympathy for them. He says he has seen Indians die from the adoption and use of the white man's ways.

March 3, 1954

Jeanne and I were just like the Indians last night in that we had to go see the movie *The Great Sioux Uprising* at the OCHS auditorium. The film was about Red Cloud and his band, the Oglala Sioux. The movie had more to do with horse thieving than the Sioux. One night a week, usually Wednesday, is movie night. This time, they showed the film both Tuesday and Wednesday nights. Guess they had a full house again tonight. It was interesting to see how the Indians would react. Each time Red Cloud uttered some Sioux words, they would laugh uproariously at the attempted use of the Sioux language. Once, when Red Cloud said "The Oglala votes for peace," there was a big clapping of hands. But when horse thieves stole their horses after this, and they were pursued by the Sioux warriors, and as a Wasicu [white person] was killed, they clapped. People here are very fond of movies in general, and they especially like movies on Indians.

Before going to the film last evening I had an appointment with Mr. Reifel. I had read in the news sheet that he would be in Rapid City on Friday to talk with officials there about Indians in Rapid City. So I called for a conference. I wanted to tell him about all the people that were coming down here for treatment who were Rapid City residents. I showed him some of my files on those people. He is going to visit the sanatorium also. So I showed him five recent AMA [against medical advice] tubercular patients' summaries from the sanatorium. Things are so much lighter at the hospital this week. Less work and less rush and straining of nerves. I am home earlier in the evening.

Ben Black Elk, son of the famous Indian philosopher and historian and himself a showman, came in to the hospital today. He caught his finger in a fan belt this morning at Manderson when he volunteered to go and get a casket for Sara Looks Twice's family. He fractured a bone and pulled off a tendon. I sutured it back and put on a cast with the distal phalanx of the middle right finger extended. He sure won't be dancing and talking now. He has two upcoming speaking and dancing engagements. Says he'll just do the talking. I've seen him at many dances around here.

March 6, 1954

Charlie Yellow Boy, the man who invited me to his place to see a Yuwipi meeting, is in the hospital. He came in a couple of days ago with symptoms of cardiac failure. I asked, "Charlie, didn't that medicine man help you?" Charlie responded, "Oh, he helped me a little but not enough." In spite of this, people continue to have their faith in their medicine and their religion. The fact that the medicine man didn't cure Charlie's heart trouble doesn't make him lose his faith. This morning I asked Charlie how he was feeling. He said he was very much better.

March 7, 1954

Joe Swift Bird, the chief of police here, called me a couple of hours ago. He said someone came up to tell him late this afternoon a child was sick. Joe went over to the place about 6:00 p.m., and the little girl was dead. He called me about 7:30 or shortly after and wondered if I'd go see the child. He said to meet him at the police station. But I wasn't dressed and I hadn't eaten so it was fifteen minutes before I got there. So a young man named Romero told me Joe had gone over, and he would show me the place.

When I got to the one-story shack on the south side of town, I walked right on in. I saw Joe, who said, "Come in here." At first I only saw a woman I've seen in clinic and about six kids there. Then I saw on the table a half dozen pint bottles, liquor bottles, empty, and two beer bottles, empty. I went on into the next room. There was an oil stove that had the room heated nicely and two beds. There was another room extending from this, but I didn't go in there. The beds were covered with dirty, ragged, torn patchwork quilts. Joe pulled a portion of blanket down, and there was a two-year-old girl, dead.

I looked over her body. She had bruises and abrasions over all her body. On her left arm were teeth marks. When I turned her over there were dried bread crumbs in the bed. There was a table or a bureau of some sort. I couldn't tell. It was covered with heaps of dirty ragged clothes. The wallpaper was torn. There were calendars and pictures cut from magazines on the wall. A portion of the plasterboard between the next room was broken through. I looked up to someone standing behind me. It was Mr. Reifel. I hadn't seen him in the kitchen when I walked in. I was embarrassed that I hadn't seen him. I told Joe I would take the body to the hospital. We wrapped it in a piece of blanket, and I carried it through the kitchen. I saw a table covered with more piles of gray dirty clothing, a table on which sat the bottles and dirty dishes. There was a low cook stove and some cupboards. There was no covering on the floors. The woman sitting there and the children started to cry as I carried the wrapped body through the room.

Joe told me that the mother has two children, both illegitimate. The dead girl was the youngest. The woman's brother came over this morning, and his wife was with him. They were drunk and started fighting.

The bereaved mother jumped in, and I guess it was a free for all for awhile. Joe told me he has heard that from time to time the woman gives her children liquor to shut them up when they will not sleep. He wanted me to see if there was any liquor in this kid.

He called the FBI. George O'Clock said he'd come down from Rapid City in the morning. He told us to call the coroner in Hot Springs. Joe Swift Bird called him. I hope that gets me out from doing an autopsy. And I'm sure it will. Such a hovel. Such filth. How can children be reared under such conditions? How much better if they had gotten clothes or food with that money.

At noon yesterday Sarah Holden called to say Louie Rosseau was there. He is a hospital employee, who has been out three months sick. She had really laid down the law to him. He finally said, "Well, guess I'll go talk to Mr. Reifel Monday and see about getting transferred somewhere else at the agency." We hope that he will do that.

Rosebud sent us six patients Friday plus one they dumped on us. They carted him over here just to get rid of him. He is an old man enrolled here, but he had been staying over there.

I just finished reading *McGillycuddy—Agent*. This is a book about Dr. Valentine McGillycuddy, the first agent at Pine Ridge, written by his second wife. It is a book that one year ago would not have been interesting to me, but today I was absorbed in it. I read it Friday, and Saturday I completed it. It is all about people I know. I was intrigued. And I reveled in McGillycuddy's circumstances because I find myself in them.

That impressed me more than anything else. I don't think these people have changed one bit. McGillycuddy remarks in chapter 1 that the troublemakers were always making complaints to congressmen and higher ups in the BIA, just as they do now. Numerous investigators were sent out from time to time. This is all so true, even today. These people haven't changed one bit. On page 103, he quotes Red Cloud as saying, "Father, the Great Spirit did not make us to work." Later on he says, "The white man can work if he wants to, but the Great Spirit did not make us to work."

March 9, 1954

Mr. Reifel put in his news sheet for today all about the death of the little girl two days ago. Since then several people have asked me about it because they saw I was called in by the police. The FBI men investigating it, George O'Clock and Lynn Smith, down from Rapid City, came to the house here last night to get my write-up for them. They told me then I'd be called, probably in June, to testify about it if they could get it through the Grand Jury in the next couple of weeks.

The Mickelsons were here to visit us tonight. They told us all about the murders at Fort Yates where they were employed before coming to Pine Ridge, and said that there were many at Rosebud. In fact, they told me Mr. Reifel's mother was said to have been murdered at Rosebud. Anyway, they say there is much violence. And there is, even here on this reservation. But there is too much of that stuff going on, and no one brought to justice. The FBI men told me that last night, and they said they were for sure going to bring this one to trial. It might serve as an example to a few.

The FBI men told me last night when they were here at the house that the coroner, a layman in Hot Springs, got a doctor at the Veterans Administration Hospital in Hot Springs to perform the postmortem examination on the little girl and that they had already had a call and the girl had a "split liver." I told those FBI men when they were at my office earlier in the afternoon at the hospital that I'd be willing to bet that the girl died from a ruptured viscous. She had so many bruises on her abdominal wall. This fits in with the history they got. Someone who went to the girl's home to care for the children said the girl complained of pain in her abdomen. She collapsed when they set her up to the table. Later she revived slightly after they laid her down. They fed her and she vomited. So she was beaten earlier when the drunken brawl was going on.

March 10, 1954

Seven months ago, just shortly after arriving in Pine Ridge, I heard about Father Eugene Buechel, a Jesuit priest now at St. Francis Mission on the Rosebud reservation. I've heard that Father Buechel is an interesting person. He compiled a book of the Lakota language. I wanted to meet and talk to him, and today I had my chance. I visited with him this afternoon and went through his museum.

Father Buechel is a friendly person. He looks his eighty years, but he has much more energy and enthusiasm than a man of eighty and is perturbed that many of his churches have been taken from him. He now has two churches on the reservation that he visits. Father Buechel first came to the reservation in 1902. He left to study for the priesthood and returned to take charge of the Holy Rosary Mission in 1907. He stayed there for twelve years. Then he was sent to the St. Francis Mission, where he was in charge for years.

Father Buechel took us to a separate building, which was built for his collection. A New York appraiser once appraised his collection of Indian artifacts at $16,000, he said. He says he is so glad that he collected many of the things that are no longer seen, certainly no longer used, and perhaps some items that have not gotten into other collections and are no longer in existence. I thought this would be a rapid trip through the small building. I soon learned that if I had let this man talk without pulling him along myself, we'd probably have been there yet.

Father Buechel likes the Indians. They are his friends. He has every bit of patience with them. He's been with them a long time. I wonder if others could spend as much time here as he has and have the same feelings. Most people working with Indians are government people and spend only a few years with the Indians. The average government employee has little patience with the Indians for being so resistant to change. Father Buechel says the Indians have progressed greatly in the past fifty years. He believes the white men do not have enough sympathy for them. He says he has seen Indians die from the adoption and use of the white man's ways.

Father Buechel started his collection from the Indians years ago. He bought the items from them. He says they charged him prices they would charge one another. He was proud that no one has ever charged him, to the best of his knowledge, what they would charge other white men or tourists, which would be a higher price than for things bought and sold to one another.

In the museum was paraphernalia used in dances. There were buffalo heads with the long train of eagle feathers and staffs with eagle feathers all down the side. There were tomahawks. I saw some Ghost Dance shirts. This intrigued me. I had heard from Andrew Standing Soldier that his grandfather said the Indians wore the Ghost Dance shirts and in his picture he painted for me they looked like cloth but for some reason I thought they had been leather. They were not. They were of calico and flour sacks, decorated with red dye as Andrew had related. Father Buechel had several of these.

He asked me if I'd noticed how Indians do not like to leave their children at the hospital. He said it even used to be worse. They want their children with them when they are ill.

This was a most interesting afternoon. I'd have been there yet if I hadn't stopped Father Buechel from talking. Dr. R. L. DeBenedetto, a medical officer from Rosebud, accompanied me. We had cookies, ice cream, and coffee before leaving the mission.

March 11, 1954

One of the frequent patients about the hospital is a woman with three children. The youngest is two months old, wrapped in dirty clothing. She has constipation, but her mother uses very basic language in explaining about bowel movements. The woman was married in 1948 to a wounded war veteran. In 1949 she developed epilepsy. In 1950 she fell on a stove and burned her face during a spell. She told her troubles to me. Her husband gets $30 a month, gives her $15 to use for food and clothing. He takes $15 for himself and buys liquor. She says he is drunk all the time, and she doesn't have much work. She lives with her mother-in-law and her grandmother-in-law. "Who does the cooking and washing?" I asked. She said that she did. "You don't know much about Indian ways," she told me. That much is expected of her since she and her family are living with their in-laws.

March 12, 1954

We jumped out of bed this morning expecting it to be as any other day. I could hear the wind howling around the house. When we opened the shades I could scarcely see more than fifty yards. Everything was white. We ate. I went out to drive to the hospital. Both our cars were covered with snow. It had drifted in over the yard so that next to the house there was no snow and out five feet there was two feet of snow. I could scarcely budge my car. The nurse called and said she'd send a car. Guess she figured I'd start out about that time. But all morning there was no car. It was nearly one o'clock when Dr. Quint came to get me in the jeep, which is the dental car. We put it in compound low and plowed our way to the hospital. There were two cars stranded along the roadside in that short distance. Dr. Quint had traveled to the hospital on his skis.

I had many calls to make this morning. So I got most of that work done from home. Part of that was finishing up work I spent two hours on yesterday trying to determine a person's eligibility for health care here. This included investigating through social service, Mr. Reifel's calls to communities on the reservation, and investigating done by personnel in the front office. I called a Dr. John J. Feehan in Rapid City and told him that after exhaustive research, we would assume the responsibility for the care of a patient who is being cared for in Rapid City now. Then yesterday a man, working as a committee with the mayor in Rapid City, called me to take two patients. Neither was eligible. One family has lived off the reservation for years. He kept arguing. So I luckily had gotten the call in Mr. Reifel's office, so he took the phone and set the Rapid City man straight. He told me later the guy is a local man's brother.

Then Mr. Shaw, the principal at Red Shirt Table, was shoveling coal this morning, got a quick sharp pain in his back, and fell to the floor. He had to be helped to the basement. So a great effort was made to get out to him. Not one doctor wanted to go. It was a mess. Dr. Walters called Mr. Reifel, who politely told him he wanted someone to go. We drew straws. Dr. Gassman got it. Dr. Walters decided to go with him. They started out with a Road Department snowplow leading the way by clearing the snow. They got only a few miles beyond Oglala, they told me tonight, and turned around and came back. Dr. Walters said the wind was shifting the snow about so furiously that they couldn't see more than a few feet in front of the car, so they couldn't tell if they were on the road or not. The wind blew the snow in so hard under the hood that the engine kept quitting on them.

This was a clinic day. But as might be expected, no one came to clinic. We had only one patient all afternoon. A boy fell from the porch at Holy Rosary, and Father Lawrence Edwards brought him in. He was all right.

Mrs. Mickelson just called. Mr. Mickelson is caught up at Rapid City, stranded by the blizzard. Predictions are for worse weather coming this way from off the Black Hills. The wind is noisy. The sting of the falling crystals is like a million little spears striking your face. Visibility at times is nearly zero. A shroud of white envelopes everything. As fast as the walks are swept, the wind whips snow to cover them.

March 12, 1954

Mrs. Forshey acquainted me with the agency vault. In the locked vault in the agency is a complete record of all people enrolled on this reservation. Copies of all letters concerning them go into this. This came up during investigations yesterday on the Rapid City patients, whom doctors and various others want to send here.

Mrs. Forshey told me about the fabulous file on one man. It is about two feet thick. These files are fabulous as social histories on these people. For instance, this gent's first wife was Delia. So after she died there were many letters signed Delia. He had his second wife's name changed to Delia so she could sign for land and allotment checks for the former Delia. She says there are records to show he cheated his brothers and children, even, out of land. Mrs. Forshey says he is a very smart old fellow.

Another person I've heard much about here is Henry Standing Bear. He was a prominent person making speeches for Withdrawal. I see in a book, *The Wounded Knee Massacre* by James MacGregor, that Henry acted as interpreter along with Bill Bergen for the survivors of the battle of Wounded Knee when in the 1930s they each told their stories of that battle. What a horrible book. It is the most non-objective book I have read. It is all pure sentimentalism.

Some people you see frequently at the hospital, such as a man from Allen who was in the hospital the day before yesterday with several splits in his face and scalp. This guy is in for one reason or another frequently as a result of drunken brawls. He's a friendly, likable chap when he's not drunk. But I've seen him so many times I couldn't count them. Mr. Reifel is publishing daily the list of those people jailed. About eight out of nine are for drunkenness. He asked me the other day about publishing the names of those people who sign out of the Sioux Sanitarium AMA with tuberculosis. I said that I know I'd appreciate it because I'd steer clear of such folks. He didn't think it would have the same effects on these people as that. But it would eventually make the public conscious of the disease, conditions, and the harm likely to come from such individuals. He said he wasn't sure if he could shame the individuals. He added he has been told by lawyers he can print anything in his sheet that is true. He has good progressive ideas.

Andrew Standing Soldier finally brought me the watercolor he did of the battle of Wounded Knee. It is superb. I wouldn't take $500 for it. It is correct in detail, excepting he has three Hotchkiss guns trained on the Indians. History says there were four. One thing bothered me at first. There was no snow on the ground in his picture. One of the accounts I had read said there was snow, but it is a book full of misinformation. The research I've done since indicates there was no snow on the ground at the time of the battle. It snowed there the next morning. The Indians are in Ghost Dance shirts, as they really did wear then. He has painted lots of smoke in the air from those first shots. It is a wonderful picture.

March 14, 1954

It was a fierce night Friday. We got a call again that this time Mr. Shaw, the teacher up on Red Shirt Table, had broken his back. Two doctors and the road crews started up to the table to get him. A road plow kept ahead of them, but as fast as the roads were opened the snow drifted in over the road in piles.

Once again the party turned around just after they had gotten up on the other side of Oglala. The wind drove the snow through the hood coverings of the cars and filled up the inside. The next morning (yesterday) we had three feet of snow and more where it had drifted. There was no wind. It was not too cold but snow, snow, was everywhere.

So this morning the snowplow started out with a car containing the road crew and the hospital ambulance with Dr. Walters and me following. The roads were blocked with snow. Cars sat where they had been abandoned the night before. They were so deeply covered in snow that they were barely visible. The road crew stayed on the road pretty much, but there were no marks or guide posts to tell them when they were on the road. When we got up on the table there was less snow. There the high winds had swept the snow over against the hills and into the lowlands. There were even bare areas against the northeast sides of hills and on flats. When we got to the school, Mr. Shaw was in good shape. He had a ruptured disc. No broken back. But he had to be moved with caution for the least little jar would give him excruciating pain.

We had not been back to the hospital long, perhaps three hours, when a man called from up near Porcupine and said his wife was in labor and that the roads were not open. What could he do? Dr. Walters, our obstetrician, gave him instructions. About 6:30, the father called me again to say that the head had come but the baby would come no farther. He had walked two or three miles through heavy snow to get to a phone. We told him to get the roads opened. We'd come up with the station wagon. He got Mr. Pourier, a road man in that area, to plow the road from Porcupine up to his house.

Dr. Walters and I started out. One chain on our car kept breaking. We wired it first and this worked awhile but after that this one wire kept breaking. We made it up. The swath made by the snowplow was not wide. The banks of snow many times were higher than the car. We had to be careful not to plow into these and get trapped.

When we got to the small road leading to the man's home he was out shoveling more snow away. When we went into the home, it was dingy, lighted by a kerosene lamp. We found his wife. Only a hand had come, and a piece of the umbilical cord, which was now clamped off so that it was inevitable that the baby was dead. The head was way up and stuck.

We loaded the woman in an ambulance, on the stretcher of the station wagon, and were off. Our chain on the right side kept breaking at the wired area so much that we took it off. The roads were passable enough, thanks to the road plows. We hurried on out to Highway 18 and on into Pine Ridge, then on up to the hospital on the hill.

The woman was in fair shape. Dr. Walters took her to the delivery room and tried to help the dead baby to come. The head was stuck. He'd have to do a cesarean. While the operating room was being prepared, the patient suddenly developed pain in her abdomen. Her pulse shot up to 140. Her blood pressure started down. Her respirations came in grunting strides. She looked pale and shocky. We suspected that she had suffered a ruptured uterus. We hurried her to the operating room.

Quickly Dr. Walter and I started to operate. Sure enough, when we got inside, her uterus had ruptured. There was lots of blood in the abdominal cavity. Before this we had some blood typed and cross matched. She was an "A" type. We had none on hand. One of the maintenance men donated his blood while the jail brought up prisoners who were type "A" to also donate blood. We started blood. Our patient was ghostly in appearance. She barely responded. We clamped the big vessels to the uterus after having taken the baby from the uterus and abdominal cavity. Quickly we separated the tissues from the uterus and the rest of the pelvis. We closed the defect. After she was in bed she began to respond. She gradually got better. It was 4:00 a.m. when I went home to bed.

This morning at 10:00 I came to the hospital. It wasn't long until a transfer came from the Rosebud reservation. They hadn't called us. It was a five-and-one-half-month-old child. A pretty baby. It was distended like a drum. Its abdomen was as hard as a drum. Fecal material and vomitus was rolling out of its mouth. The child was pale as the snow. It barely breathed. Its eyes rolled back in its head. I started to work not knowing when its last breath would come. I put down an oxygen tube, put a tube in its stomach, and started to draw off some of the bowel contents and gas. I took a long transparent polyethylene tube and put it in a vein in its arm. The vein was the size of two strands of thread. It was difficult to get my tiny tube in it. I succeeded. I started some blood. In two hours the baby looked like it would live. The problem was to get the child in shape first so that we could operate.

About 6:00 the child's color was better. It was breathing better. It could focus its eyes. We used local Novocain. Quickly we opened the peritoneal [abdominal] cavity. The ileum [part of the small intestine] was sucked up into the cecum [pouch at the beginning of the large intestine], it was an intussusception [intestinal obstruction]. I reduced this. The bowel wall was good color except for only a rounded area. I sutured the ileum up along the side of the ascending colon, hoping to prevent any recurrence. I put a colostomy tube into the large bowel and out a stab wound in the flank. Then I opened the ileum and ran it over the suction tubing to decompress the small bowel. I closed that. I put streptomycin in the abdominal cavity and closed the wound.

The baby is back on the floor. He looks fine now compared to three hours ago.

[At this point Dr. Ruby's letters were not actual letters mailed to his sister. Marion Johnson and her two sons came from McCall, Idaho, to visit Robert and Jeanne Ruby. The entries for March 22 to April 8, 1954, are more accurately described as journal or diary entries, rather than correspondence—Eds.]

March 22, 1954

All last week it was dark and dismal. My sister informed me that she would arrive in Cheyenne Friday night from McCall. We expected to have a nice trip down Friday since the train arrived at 6:40 p.m.[1] But by Thursday afternoon it was windy, and snow was flying. After the experience from the weekend previously, we knew it was possible that by Friday morning there would be so much snow that we'd never get through.

We started out Thursday, getting to Rushville, Nebraska, about twenty miles south of Pine Ridge. Then we remembered that a burner was on the electric range with a pan of water for moisture. We called back to the agency to shut this off. After leaving Rushville, we had no visibility at all. Then we got hung up on a drift outside of Bridgeport, Nebraska. The truck behind us couldn't get enough traction to pull us out. A car came and was going to push us out, but he got stuck. We shoveled until we got out. I went equipped with chain, shovel, and extra clothing and blankets. Mr. Reifel had suggested to all at the agency that whenever traveling, take these extra things, and boy did they come in handy.

The snow was cold and particles pounded into my forehead, but we were freed. The roads were covered with sheets of ice like glass. Finally we got into Bridgeport and stayed there for the night. We got into Cheyenne the next morning. We spent the afternoon getting the car serviced. Picked up Marion and her two kids, Craig and Brent, and got home Saturday at one a.m. The roads back were mostly dry and clear.

Saturday I drove Marion, Craig, and Brent out to Wounded Knee to see the monument and mass grave. We went to OCHS and got stuck. Charlie Randyall went to get a tractor to pull us out, but it wouldn't start, so he took a pickup and pulled us out backward. Mud thrown from his car covered our car with mud so you wouldn't even know it was a car.

The next day, Sunday, we went out to Slim Buttes to visit with Mr. Jamruzka, who is a teacher out there. He showed us pictures he'd taken of the Sun Dance last year. Going out we got on a wrong road, got into the "axle grease," and went flying down a hill whipping from right to left.[2] The farther we went, the faster we went. Jeanne hollered, "Take your foot off the gas." I told her it wasn't on the gas. So Marion hollered. "Take your foot off the brake." I told her my foot wasn't on the brake either. Finally we whipped completely around.

At Slim Buttes, Mr. Jamruska told me about a boy who is so eager to go to school that he studies during noon hours. He rides a horse from the state line, miles away. He has never been late or missed a day at school. In this last blizzard, the one we got caught in going down to Cheyenne, his horse got loose and got into a drift and smothered. I felt sorry after hearing this story. First thing I did this morning was to call Mr. Reifel and ask him what could be done to get the boy another horse since the family is poor and do not have more horses. I told him that my wife and I would like to help in getting another horse for him.

When the Indians have it nice they gripe and are more reactionary. Mr. Sande "ruled with his heart instead of his head." As such, he extended leases on Indian property the past five years. This took the lands out of competitive bidding. However, it was what the Indians wanted, so Mr. Sande would grant it. Now with Mr. Reifel here, this is no longer allowed. Though it is really better for the Indians, they don't think so because they want the extra money. Anyway, I'm sure many are now sorry they gave Mr. Sande such a hard time because he was attentive and considerate to *their* wishes. Mr. Reifel is more concerned with adherence to the written laws and regulations. He doesn't permit attacks on department heads. Whereas Mr. Sande would listen to the tales of woe and call department heads on the carpet, Mr. Reifel will listen and then send the complainers to the department heads saying the department head's decision is final.

March 24, 1954

The Public Health nurse at Kyle had an altercation with the Boss Farmer, a full-blood Indian, the other day. He had thought Mrs. Olinger had reported him for drunkenness and cohabitation. So, in a drunken stupor, he went over and quarreled with her. She filed a complaint, and so this is being investigated. But the Boss Farmer has a circle of friends that are now circulating vicious gossip about Mrs. Olinger. She is upset, and so she came in to see me again the other day, one of the numerous visits about this affair. I went down to see Mr. Reifel. I asked if we might send Mrs. Olinger to Wanblee, though I knew she wouldn't want to go to this one isolated place on the reservation. Mr. Reifel said to tell her to forget all about the vicious gossip. He said the only time for her to do something is if someone files a complaint against her, then investigate it.

Mr. Reifel said there are already petitions out to get rid of him. He hasn't even been here three months. This type of activity is a typical pastime here, however. Since Mr. Reifel came I haven't heard a thing about the petition to get rid of me or to increase visiting hours.

I never did get any copies of the *Pine Ridge* bulletin last month, even after I contributed $100 for paper on which to print it. So I went and begged a copy. Mr. Reifel put in the paper that Jeanne and I had gone to Cheyenne to pick up Marion and her sons. Numerous people have read it and asked or inquired concerning Marion. Mr. Reifel's daily news sheet is a fine sort of publication for circulation of news. He is not only publishing those arrested but those with tuberculosis out on AMA.

Mr. Reifel told me we were to get a new Public Health nurse. She is reportedly an African American. So now maybe we'll have someone to station up in Wanblee. They expect the nurse up there to be a doctor and expect her to treat and diagnose disease, thus saving them long trips to the hospital. We have to go to Wanblee and explain to the people the purpose of a Public Health nurse. If they will accept her under the conditions, one will be sent there.

Going out to Wanblee there was lots of snow on the road. Coming back it had melted and rained. We started up one hill. The car came to a halt and slid all the way back down. I tried it again. And this time the car slid in the greasy gumbo sideways as well as back down, getting stuck. Mr. Olinger came by on his way to town. He hooked on a tow chain, and he had sawdust tires so pulled me out. He pulled me up the hill, down another, and up another. So then on to the highway, Mr. Olinger led, and a pickup followed. It was a ten-mile-an-hour trek for about fifteen miles over greasy gumbo.

When I got back, I went to the Holy Rosary Mission to see Felix Walking. He got his artificial leg prosthesis. It is a trifle long. But he was up walking on it. Felix has been carving out long pipe stems for peace pipes. He is going to carve one for me.

Dr. Paulson from Rapid City called and wanted me to take a woman from there as a patient. Rapid City pulled that on us once with that same patient, a resident there for seven years. I said absolutely not.

March 26, 1954

I have spent all day in conferences or dictating letters except about fifteen minutes that were spent seeing patients. First of all, a bulletin from Mr. Reifel's office did not reach my desk in time, so I didn't make it to a staff conference in his office on Community Services at 8:15. He called me and found me at home, and I went over. This morning we discussed the problems caused by families leaving the reservation for seasonal work. The result is difficulty keeping their children in school and determining what benefits they can expect such as medical expenses. No definite conclusions were reached before we broke up at 11:00 a.m. Many ideas were tossed around, and so Mr. Reifel says he and I will get together now to write up something definite that the person or family head can take with him when he goes out to work.

About a hundred families will leave in April, another hundred in May, and two hundred in June.

Mr. Reifel says this morning it may prove useless to call on Health, Education, and Welfare and on Law and Order to help correct so many existing discrepancies in conduct around the reservation, if his theory about the cause is correct. He feels that there are many more women on the reservation than men, leading to increased immorality. If this is true, no amount of help will correct existing immoral and bad conditions until there are more men than women.

He cited pioneering days, for instance. When a few women, not the hussies, he stated, went into a community, their conduct commanded respect and chivalry on the part of the men. But when there are more women than men, morals break down. When women are fewer, their morals are better. That must be so to obtain a man, and this requires better morals in men. He uses the term "scarcity value," commenting that it is a poor term when speaking of human values, but nevertheless it applies. He was told that on the Rosebud reservation there are two females for every man.

He is now doing statistics on this reservation to ascertain the percentages of the sexes. More men leaving the reservation makes the situation worse, such as men going into the service or more being sent out on relocation.

Mr. Reifel says that he is going to do more to help women leave the reservation. Circumstances being equal, he'll offer aid and help to girls over boys. Help girls through school, and help them leave the reservation.

I had other conversations with Mr. Reifel. He told me about a family which gets $1,000 lease money a year and other income. They blow it all in a matter of weeks. The house they live in is in shambles. They come back for relief. He says that he got a member of the family to file a complaint to the tribal court. It is the only court in the United States that can judge a man incompetent to handle his affairs, and his money then can be budgeted by the superintendent.

I had a talk with Mr. Mickelson. Apparently Mr. Reifel broke down the teachers' morale at school last Tuesday or Wednesday. He went over and found fault with many things, especially dirt. It happened to be a muddy day. Mr. Mickelson reported to the teachers in conference later. They took it personally, and now they are all hopping mad. Mick (Mickelson) thinks poorly of Mr. Reifel. He feels Reifel came over with a chip on his shoulder that morning and immediately put himself on the defensive.

March 28, 1954

Yesterday morning when we all got up at 6:30 it was sunny. There was barely any snow on the ground. Then, before we could get ready to leave for Mount Rushmore, it was cloudy. But we left home about 7:00 a.m. After we left Oglala, there were skiffs of snow. Before we pulled into Hot Springs, the snow was almost blinding. There was perhaps three inches on the ground there. Having Marion's two little boys in the car, we decided to take no chances. But on inquiring about conditions in the Black Hills, we were told there was to be no wind (blizzard), only light snowfalls. So we decided to go on up to Custer and find our Uncle Orrin.[3] Going up through the game reserve past Wind Cave, we looked for buffalo for Craig and Brent to see but found none. We saw some antelope. In Custer there was some snow. We got coffee, shopped, and asked where Orrin Holmes lived. The post office told us to take Route 85A up; it went right by his home. He lives across the road from the Horsethief Inn, not far from Hill City.

We found Uncle Orrin. He lives comfortably in a large house with an inviting rock fireplace. He had made a blueberry pie. We shared our lunch of fried chicken, and he furnished other things. After lunch Uncle Orrin said he would drive us up to Mount Rushmore. By the way the crow flies it was only four or five miles to Mount Rushmore.

Uncle Orrin drove us through the old mining town of Keystone and then to Hill City. Then we drove out on Highway 16 to where they are working on the monument of Crazy Horse.

Uncle Orrin said that he knew Henry Standing Bear. He is the one who promoted sculpturing the monument to Crazy Horse. Standing Bear died in the hospital here about five months ago. Uncle Orrin owns several hundred acres of land around there, and he said Korczak Ziolkowski wanted to use a large granite mountain on his place to carve the monument, but Uncle Orrin didn't want to sell the land. So Henry Standing Bear suggested another granite mountain.[4] Ziolkowski actually outlined the figure at that place, but then he chose another mountain, where the sculpture is today. The rock is less satisfactory for working, Uncle Orrin says. After six years of blasting and working, they do not yet have a surface on which to outline the figure.

Back at Uncle Orrin's place we got warmed up and had blueberry pie and coffee again before we started on our way home. The sun then came out gloriously, and we had dry roads all the way home. The boys' mission when driving through the Black Hills was accomplished after all. We saw some caged buffalo.

March 29, 1954

I stopped to see Mrs. Forshey at her home yesterday regarding a patient hospitalized at Our Lady of Lourdes in Hot Springs. The female patient's name didn't sound familiar to Mrs. Forshey. She had come in as an emergency case and delivered her baby. Now the hospital wants authorization. I checked this morning with the agency, but there was no account of her there.

I learn more bad things about Mr. Pyles all the time. Now he is peddling nonsense to Mr. Reifel that he has no say-so at the boarding school, that Mr. Mickelson does, and as a result Mr. Reifel is blaming Mr. Mickelson for lots of things. Mr. Pyles is responsible because he is over Mickelson and his outfit. I know for a fact that Mick doesn't do things without Pyles's approval. And I know that one drunken employee gives them lots of trouble and should have been fired. Mick set up things to have him dismissed, but it didn't happen. This is only one of many examples. Pyles softens things so as not to create any animosity with the people of the reservation who will always be here. What he does is make things bad for Mick. Pyles is so afraid of his job that he is the biggest willy-nilly I've ever known. He is dumb in some ways but smart in other ways, such as spending other peoples' money. Mr. Pyles, for one thing, told Mr. Reifel that it was always his understanding that he has had no say-so or that he had no authority at OCHS. What could be farther from the truth?

In a conference this morning Mr. Reifel talked about special adjacency. The Extension Program here is thrown at the people. They are brought together with no relationship between them but just as a group of objects carried by the wind to an area. As a result, cloth has been handed to the people, and they were asked to make a dress for themselves and maybe a dress for a school kid. That is forcing labor. You could go out on the street and tell a man, "Here is a sack of potatoes; go plant them and give me half of what you raise." That is not the philosophy we need. What should be done is not induce people to do things by giving them something, but go into well-established groups such as the women's groups, and there are many of them. They are well-organized descendants of war heroes and warriors.

Today we are a government of pressure groups. The Indian commissioner has made definite stands on state support of Indians. But what happens? A rich state like Minnesota, with no reservations, does not want to support orphaned Indians. So pressure groups get Congress to pay them for that care. He asks then, with a poor state like South Dakota, is not Minnesota better able pay for that sort of thing?

March 31, 1954

First sunny day we've had in nearly three weeks, with sun all day long. It is certainly welcome. Made for a nice trip today to the Rosebud reservation. I went over to check some patients at the Rosebud Hospital that were surgery patients of mine here. I took Jeanne, Marion, Craig, and Brent. Afterward we drove over to St. Francis, to the mission, to see Father Buechel and his museum. They enjoyed it, but the museum building is not heated, and so it was cold in there.

Jeanne gave a dinner last night for Marion. We invited the Mickelsons, the Masts, and Margaret Talcott.

Nine. April 1954

Monday morning we went to the inaugural program for the new tribal council at the OCHS auditorium. Moses Two Bulls was installed as president. I saw Ethel Merrival there. She was dressed in buckskin and sang the Indian Love Call. Jokingly I told folks afterward that she was singing that for me. Mr. Reifel gave some remarks. He pleaded with the new council to look! look! look! into the innocent faces of the young high school students there from Holy Rosary and OCHS. There lay "the hope of the Oglala Sioux people," he said. Then he asked, "Were we going to allow liquor on the reservation to degrade our people?" Then with a "look!" he yelled, "Did you look?" to one of the members of the new council who had a tie vote, so he was sitting on stage. The man he called out to is the biggest bootlegger on the reservation. With such public shaming that guy is liable to shoot Mr. Reifel. There was ghastly silence. Mr. Mickelson, seated in the balcony with us, peered around to me over his glasses with a smile on his face.

April 2, 1954

Harley Quint said that people all over have been asking him about Mr. Reifel. He had just returned from two days at Mission on the Rosebud reservation. He was refracting eyes over there. People asked him if it was true that some had gotten petitions out against Mr. Reifel. Eddie Coker, who was there also, said Mr. Reifel had gotten threatening letters all right. And, of course, Mr. Reifel told me there were petitions out against him. All his reforms to help the Indians to help themselves are unpopular. I wonder how long he will last.

It is warm and sunny today, the third day of sun now after all the weeks of blizzards and snow. Butch Stoldt, my neighbor, was over and wanted me to admit a pregnant woman to the hospital. I told him just to take her up. He said her people were out fishing. On the way up to the hospital I saw many kids out playing with no coats. Craig and Brent have been playing out all day in the burned-out house next to us that is being repaired. They had been over to the neighbors, the Stoldts, with all those kids yesterday.

Yesterday at noon Dr. Walter went with me, and we talked before the Extension Group at the home of Mr. and Mrs. Harris at Denby. The group was made up entirely of white people. We talked about cancer since this is cancer month.

Miss Holden has all her letters and data to try for a retirement for her back ailment now. She is working hot and heavy on that now.

April 3, 1954

Last night I had asked some people to the house for a little get together for Marion. The Quints, the Walters, and the Cokers came and helped by bringing food. Then there were Edgar, Reno, and Mary Ann Red Cloud; the old chief, James Red Cloud; Blue Horse and a woman who I believe was a Blue Horse; Charlie Yellow Boy, and Brady Richard, a Cheyenne Indian from Lame Deer, Montana, who is visiting the Red Clouds. Elk Boy brought the old chief down and wondered if I would take him home and, of course, I did afterward.

All of the Indians brought their bright costumes. They went in the bedroom to change into them. Then we had a regular powwow. Edgar and Blue Horse played the drum and sang. There were several dances, one honoring the returned prisoner of war, Eugene Rowland. They did the Rabbit Dance. In this dance, both male and female dance together, a forward and backward sort of step. I danced with the women. Others danced with the ladies. Then they did the two-step and mixed. There were two solos. Reno Red Cloud, who performs the Hoop Dance all over the country, danced for us, first with one hoop, then with two, then three, and then four. It was very good. Then the Cheyenne Indian,

Brady Richard, did a solo. Elk Boy sang a solo, a love song. Blue Horse sang a song from Yuwipi. And the old chief sang a song to his grandfather, the original Chief Red Cloud, and he used the gourd.

Edgar told a story for the chief. Once there was a chief who thought it was time his young son picked out a wife. He knew of a pretty young girl in a tent nearby. So he started going over regularly to talk with the girl and with her folks to prepare them and the girl for his son. As was custom long ago, when a boy went to court a girl, he took a blanket and threw it around himself and girl as they talked. Lots of times there would be a line of boys waiting to throw their blanket over a girl. Eventually this chief began preparing his own boy for "catching the girl." But soon the old chief got interested in the girl himself. One day he noticed another fellow in a blanket with the girl as he waited for his turn to wrap her in his blanket. He wandered off a ways, and when the young man came out he noticed it was his son. The old man was now jealous. Then he went to his son and told him that he'd found out through their relationship that the girl was his sister, and so he'd better leave her alone. The boy lay on his bed for several days not talking. Finally the boy's mother got him to tell her what was troubling him. "I can't understand, mother. You are my mother, aren't you?" She said she was. Then the boy said, "Well, father told me that the girl over there was my sister. So the girl's mother must also be his wife, or the chief's brother's wife." Just then the chief was coming up to the tent and heard his wife tell the boy, "Son, I'll tell you something. The chief isn't your father." When the chief heard this he stopped and listened. "Someday I'll show you who your father is. I'll go like this," said his mother. She made a gesture with her hands. The old chief saw it. He spent the rest of his life watching for his wife to make the gesture so he could see who the father of "his" son was.

The evening was wonderful. Marion enjoyed it immensely. We all had lots to eat: Spanish rice, beans, cheese, macaroni, bread, coffee, cake, carrot sticks, and celery. Everybody there took gobs of pictures. I made three trips to the garbage with worn-out flash bulbs. We ran out, and Dr. Quint tried taking pictures with no bulbs, but they will be no good.

Little Craig and Brent were so impressed by all the feathers and the dancing. I took them and danced with them once. The Indians wore some of their best costumes. I thought they wore more beaded stuff than they usually wear.

Red Cloud told us he had been photographed with every president from McKinley on up to the present time and even with Eisenhower. The old chief always gives a speech. Last night he brought out the point that the red man was in this country long before the whites. Never before had any white people in Pine Ridge invited a group of Indians into their home for food and recreation. The doctor had pity or felt sorry for the Indians. The doctor would like to be an Indian. The agency keeps the Indians poor. But people like the doctor want to help. And the doctor's wife. Soon there was going to be the inauguration of the new president, on Monday, April 5. He was going to tell the Indians about their friend and the other people here at the house. He was going to call them all brothers and sisters. The doctor was going to wear an Indian suit. What that remark meant, I don't know.

The best of the evening was when Chief Red Cloud and Charlie Yellow Boy gave Marion an Indian name. It was "Graceful Woman." The chief wrote the words for her in Indian. It is Wau-si-la-win. When they do that they honor a person. I thought that was nice.

April 7, 1954

I had a big day planned for last Saturday, April 3, which included a trip to the Badlands from Red Shirt Table. But it seems a virus made its rounds. Marion stayed in bed and rested, felt better that evening, and she and Jeanne went to the movie at Holy Rosary Mission. So Sunday we crowded in a little of everything. We took a picnic lunch to Red Shirt Table. It was a nice day. Took pictures. In the late afternoon Marion and I went riding on OCHS horses. Got back and went to the Mickelsons for dinner. We then brought the kids home and put them to bed, and the Mickelsons came to our house and we played cards.

Monday morning we went to the inaugural program for the new tribal council at the OCHS auditorium. Moses Two Bulls was installed as president. I saw Ethel Merrival there. She was dressed in buckskin and sang the Indian Love Call. Jokingly I told folks afterward that she was singing that for me. Mr. Reifel gave some remarks. He pleaded with the new council to look! look! look! into the innocent faces of the young high school students there from Holy Rosary and OCHS. There lay "the hope of the Oglala Sioux people," he said. Then he asked, "Were we going to allow liquor on the reservation to degrade our people?" Then with a "look!" he yelled, "Did you look?" to one of the members of the new council who had a tie vote, so he was sitting on stage. The man he called out to is the biggest bootlegger on the reservation. With such public shaming that guy is liable to shoot Mr. Reifel. There was ghastly silence. Mr. Mickelson, seated in the balcony with us, peered around to me over his glasses with a smile on his face.

Mr. Reifel has been carrying on a vigorous program to rid the reservation of liquor. He told us at the inauguration that Sunday morning he had found whiskey bottles lined on his yard fence posts. He said he was going to leave them there until someone took them away, until some Indian removed them. He said that when people visited him he would tell them that some Oglala Sioux put them there. It would be a symbol of the degradation. He really gave it to them.

We went down to the Legion Hall for the inaugural dance at night. It was packed with people. I took some pictures. The kids were spellbound. Ben Black Elk made recordings of the music and singing. Then he called various people at times such as Moses Two Bulls and Superintendent Reifel to say a few remarks on his tape recording. I was nearby so he called me over, introduced me, and asked me to say a few words. Mr. Black Elk told me that these recordings are going to be spliced into a program to be broadcast on the radio.

My friend Chief James Red Cloud asked me to take him home. I told him I would, but it would have to be soon because I was about ready to leave. But it was only ten p.m., so he didn't want to go home so soon. He said his daughter-in-law would take him.

We rose with the birds Tuesday, yesterday, and got the party off for Cheyenne. Jeanne and I had planned to stay overnight in Cheyenne since Marion's train did not leave Cheyenne until this morning. But then we got her situated in the Down Town Motel, only two blocks from the station. So Jeanne and I decided to return last night. We made the trip back in five hours. We fairly flew, going eighty miles per hour for awhile. The wind came up, and it was very dusty. I'm glad we came back last night. I got a sack of flour for old James Red Cloud. Took it out to Edgar's home this morning and told him to take some out of the sack and give the rest to the chief for me. This was a mistake. I should have given Edgar some and then taken the rest to the chief.

April 8, 1954

Felix Walking came over to visit with me tonight. He wants me to go to a peyote meeting with him. He explained the differences to me between the Cross Fire and Half Moon branches of the religion. His sympathies are certainly with the Half Moon. There they have a chief who conducts the meeting. They do not have the four designated chiefs as they do in the Cross Fire (Cedar, Road, and so on). They burn a fire of cedar. The cedar he compares to the incense used in Christian religion. And as in the Christian religion, the dove denotes the Holy Spirit. In the Half Moon, the water bird is the corresponding symbol.

Felix is carving me a peace pipe. I knew that he was carving on it but I didn't know until tonight that what he is carving is the symbol of the Half Moon peyote cult: the tent, which incorporates the water bird, the eagle, and the turtle.

In this religion the water bird's tail is represented by the four poles in the carving. The flaps at the top are the wings. The opening down the front to the entrance flap makes the neck and head. On the entrance flap is painted a turtle reaching up to the head of the water bird. At the level of the water bird's neck are three strips colored yellow, red, and blue. These represent a rainbow. Above is blue with spots or a storm. With the rainbow the storm stops. So below the rainbow there is not a storm. But below the rainbow on one side is the eagle (thunderbird) with lightning stripes above. The eagle is all powerful. It can create or destroy. On the other side is the shield that the eagle uses to protect itself.

The story is that the eagle wanted to create a human being. But it couldn't get down in the water to get mud with which to create man. And the water bird, which can live in and on water, could not get to the bottom to get mud. So the turtle went down and brought up mud. The turtle gave it to the water bird who gave it to the eagle.

The meetings in Half Moon are much the same as in Cross Fire except that the Bible is not used. Each member participates by singing four songs. Felix has attended peyote meetings in Texas, Oklahoma, and Nebraska. He says that the Half Moon and Cross Fire feud. He says people practicing peyote rituals are upset their marriages are not recognized in the tribal court.

Felix says Mr. Reifel is sure tough. He said the Sioux people are really tough, aren't they? I told him that they were, but that they had one of their own leading them and could fight like they can.

Felix's entire purpose for his visit, of course, was to borrow some money in advance on the pipe. I knew he wanted to buy liquor so I let him have only a couple of dollars, but no more. That is a typical characteristic around here. No more money till I get delivery on the pipe.

Felix said in the Half Moon sect they sign to Christ and pray to Christ. They call Christ "Peyjuta," which translates to "medicine." He says we know that when we get sick Christ will pick us up, raise us up, and cure us. So they use the word for Christ as medicine.

I asked Felix if he thought peyote would have cured his leg when he got run over. He said, "You guys didn't know it, but I had four peyotes after that happened." I have my faith. I asked him such a leading question and with such doubt in my mind that he would commit himself, but I could see he thought that peyote would have done the job.

[At this point Dr. Ruby's sister, Marion Johnson, and her two sons returned to their home in McCall, Idaho. The entries dated from April 10 through December 1954 are copies of the letters Robert Ruby wrote to Marion—Eds.

April 10, 1954

About one week ago a man was hit in the head with an ax wielded by his common-law wife. He was hospitalized in Rapid City but was transferred here Tuesday. He had a fractured skull. Tonight, out near Oglala, the Half Moons are holding a peyote meeting for him. I was going to discharge him today but then decided I'd better wait until after the peyote meeting.

Medicine men on the reservation are Mrs. Dan Young Bull Bear, who goes by the name Mrs. D. Y. Bull Bear, Jess Steed, and Andrew Fools Crow (who no longer practices, so I was told), all out near Kyle. From Allen is Poor Thunder. Near Pine Ridge are Willie Wounded and Plenty Wounds.

Wednesday evening (April 7) I could see from the south a huge cloud of dust covering the horizon. I finished my work at the hospital and was ready to start home just as the cloud reached Pine Ridge. It enveloped us and stayed practically all night. The visibility was practically nil. The fine dust sifted through the house. It has been windy many of the days. The head medicine man predicted storms this spring, but I guess that was a safe bet since I understand the springs here are rather stormy.

Mrs. Forshey is on the rampage. Her investigations show that the Education Branch here gets $729 for each child enrolled in the school. That is why the children's social workers refuse to take Indian children at this school who live off the reservation. The school takes them anyway, and the $729 is to board the youngster for a year. It is free of operating expenses or teachers' salaries.

April 13, Saturday night, I was at the Mickelsons and heard about all the rumpus when a young man, home from the Marines, tried to break into the girls' dormitory at the school with three other men. They were arrested and were in the jug. One of them slugged a policeman. Mr. Reifel tells me today that he can't do a thing about it. The FBI says there is not enough evidence.

Mr. Reifel asked me last night if Mrs. Reifel could ride to Pierre with me tomorrow when I go to Aberdeen. But he told me this morning she won't be going since he will take annual leave and drive her up there himself on Thursday.

I asked Mr. Reifel to put a piece in the news sheet about school kids, who, it has been determined by Welfare, can buy their own glasses. So far quite a few students and families have been given the prescriptions, but so far none have gotten glasses. I called all superintendents yesterday to check and see. Not one student who has been given a prescription has gotten glasses.

I talked to the local American Legion club last night on the subject of cancer. It was held at the Boy Scouts club building, a log cabin on school grounds.

April 13, 1954

I attended a staff meeting this morning with all department heads. Mr. Reifel has asked the members of the tribal council to join in these staff meetings so that they can see what goes on and carry the messages and ideas back to the people. Only a few showed up, and they were an hour late. Mr. Reifel had a real plan. He stated that what usually happens is that the tribe passes resolutions, which are then printed up, and it is two months before they reach the superintendent's office for action. A council meeting of three days has just been completed. Mr. Reifel asked the council to come today with the resolutions so that as they applied to the various departments they could be acted upon.

He called on Jake Herman. Jake said the tribe was wondering how it is that patients from way up in North Dakota and various other places can come down here and be hospitalized. Were funds transferred from the other agencies to this agency when they come here for care? Then he started on a real tirade about how the tribe wanted more money for something. Elizabeth Forshey took her pen and wrote the word MONEY three times. She passed it over to me. I made three exclamation marks after "money." That is all these people want, more money.

Mr. Reifel immediately cut that off, agreeing with Mrs. Forshey that what the tribe needed was not more money. I interrupted him and said to Mr. Herman that no other agency in this area has the hospital and the doctors we have here. I told him that doctors were going to be harder to get. This hospital was set up to take referrals of patients from other reservations. I told him that if it were not here, it would be elsewhere. Which would mean that the facilities and the complete staff that are available to these people here, and readily accessible and so near them, would be located elsewhere.

Then Mr. Reifel added that much money has been appropriated by Congress for this area, but not just for our hospital. He explained that the Area Office budgeted the money, and when making the budget for Pine Ridge additional money was appropriated and that needed to be taken into account.

After a recess, Mr. Reifel did most of the talking. The main topic could be headed Law and Order. What these people need, as Mr. Reifel says, is not more money but in my words: "A CHANGE IN ATTITUDE." Mr. Reifel cited that Fort Berthold Indians six months ago received $4,800,000, nearly five million dollars, for oil. And so what? Not one single Indian is better off. They are not dressed better. They do not eat better. Because the money goes for old cars and liquor.

The Indians, it seems to me, are demoralized. At one time in their history they had a strict set of morals that were admirable though not applicable to today. Virginity was respected, and a woman who went behind the tepees was ostracized. Stealing within one's own tribe was not done, though stealing from other tribes was honorable. I told this to Mr. Reifel. He believes that social patterns have carried through but are not applied to the individual and not to the tribe or to families alone. In earlier times, when a family had some food, anyone was welcome to come and share. As a result, today if one family gets welfare, another family believes it also is entitled to welfare funds. And even if all welfare funds were distributed, each person would get only a few dollars. But actually that would make the people happy.

These people have to develop new concepts. They are confused and are in a changing set of social values. They are reticent to accept the modern practices being forced on them. There is vandalism. There is crime. A man from Kyle had his house broken into last night. He was kicked by the drunks doing so. His head was split open. His children were in the home. He filed a complaint. What happens so much is that people are afraid to file a complaint. Or after they do, they withdraw it on the promise of receiving something from the offender. Their relationship patterns cause them not to file complaints. There is another trouble as pointed out today. The judge here is a local man who is reticent to fine or sentence people who violate the law. A good idea would be to have a judge who is not native to the area.

April 17, 1954

I started out before 6:00 a.m. on Wednesday (April 14) for Aberdeen. I started early so as to get all per diem for the day. Eldon LaCourse, our administrative officer, and Dr. Gassman, each took turns driving. Mr. LaCourse is a Umatilla Indian from near our home.[1]

We had a nice meeting the following day, then conferences yesterday. Many bits of suggestion and information were tossed about. But it all seems rather needless since in this service nothing happens for "generations," it seems, when change or clarification on matters is needed.

I had a conference Friday with Mr. G. H. Hunt, the head of Maintenance. He agrees with all my suggestions for improvements to the hospital and said he would prepare them and send them to Washington. Even though that could seem encouraging, it could mean nothing. But he did say he would try to get some of our tribal council to put pressure on congressmen for changes as soon as Washington prepares the cost of such remodeling. Eldon LaCourse and I talked this over, and he thought Moot Nelson, a tribal member, would be a good one to write Washington on our behalf.

Eldon told me on the way home that soon after Mr. Reifel came here he had a conference with Ethel Merrival in which he laid down the law to her. At the time she had a petition to increase visiting hours. I had felt since she hadn't been attacking us at the hospital and others that he had put the kibosh on her. Eldon said he told her the hospital was not for socializing and that the visiting hours would stand as they are. That was the end of it, apparently.

At the meeting on Thursday Mr. W. O. Roberts, the new director of the Area Office who replaced Mr. J. M. Cooper a few weeks ago, addressed us. I was interested in his remarks since he talked about the present trend in the BIA. The current term is not *Withdrawal* but *Rehabilitation*. I was glad to hear him say the BIA was flexible. Not all services to all Indians are the same. Where some are able to take care of their needs, others are not, and in those cases where they are not, the government has a moral obligation to continue offering needed services. Some senators were for abolishing the BIA altogether. But he felt there was a need for certain services in certain places. The trend is, where it is possible, to turn over to state and local services those federal services that have been carried on for years by the BIA.[2]

He said in 1921 that Indians had to be forced to visit doctors. At that time there were more medicine men practicing for Indians than white physicians. The big trouble is the state social services do not want to accept Indians in many instances. In North Dakota the welfare services for Indians are horrible. Families renting and owning homes around Devils Lake are not accepted by the county for aid for medical expenses even though they have lived in the community for four to ten years and some have paid taxes.

Mr. Roberts said that where state and local services are available, such as schools, the federal government does not owe the Indians school-ing. Since 1924 Indians have become citizens of the United States, and the Constitution does not allow special privileges or discrimination. They are individuals with the same rights now as others, and thus for progress the Indian families must be treated as others. There is oppor-tunity for all, and a firm-minded view must be developed with objec-tives for all people alike. There is a need for public assistance in the United States, but not for a race of people. It should be for unfortu-nate individuals only.

April 18, 1954

Easter Sunday. I took communion in church this morning. The Mick-elsons came over, and we had a huge turkey dinner that Jeanne fixed. While the women were putting dinner on the table, Mick drove me over to the barns, and there we got a huge sack of wheat grass seed. Since the grass seed I planted last fall isn't going to come up and since I won't get more seed like that, I decided we'd plant this wheat grass seed. We certainly need something to keep down the dirt and the mud around the house.

After the rain started to loosen the brick hard soil, I planted the seed after seven p.m. tonight and then raked it all after dark. It will have to be sprinkled daily to keep moist and soft enough to grow.

When in Aberdeen, Dr. W. R. Carey from Fort Yates, who is a friend of the Mickelsons, got word that his brother in Wyoming had died. The only other doctor at the meeting, Dr. William K. Carlile from Standing Rock, had to go to Denver for a physical. So I called Dr. Bragg, and he said he would go over to Fort Yates for a week. When I called, he said that Mrs. Fools Crow finally came in to the hospital for treatment of a long-standing problem. Mrs. Olinger had called me about her be-fore I left for Aberdeen. She wouldn't come into the hospital. I pre-sume, since Andrew Fools Crow is a medicine man, that he has been working over her. Even on Mrs. Olinger's recommendation to come to the hospital, she wouldn't. She must have gotten so bad that they did bring her in when I was gone. Today she isn't doing so badly, but she sure isn't good.

One of the things we talked about so much in Aberdeen was transportation. Dr. Carlile said that people who called for an ambulance are wrong in eight out of ten cases. What he meant was in eight out of ten cases ambulance service wasn't necessary. At some other places they said the ambulance calls were wrong in 50 percent of the cases. I wanted to say the doctors were fishing around for a directive from Aberdeen on transportation. But it was my opinion we didn't need that for Pine Ridge because we have Mr. Reifel, who backs us up on all we do.

That reminds me so much of last Monday when the boss farmer, Mr. Allen from Oglala, called for an ambulance for a woman who had fallen the day before and said she had a broken leg. I refused. With that the woman appeared at the hospital before she could have, had I dispatched an ambulance to transport her. X-rays revealed she had no fracture. She was in the hospital as an eye patient of Dr. Quint not long ago. She saved her wieners and bread in her drawer after a meal. Said she was saving them for her husband because she just knew he wasn't eating while she was gone. The nurses had to watch her like a hawk.

Dr. Walters told me Friday that while I was in Aberdeen someone came for an ambulance. He refused. They went to Mr. Coker, who was acting superintendent. Coker called Walters. He refused again. Walters said about ten minutes later, someone called to say the patient was dead. Our answer to this is that the ambulance would not have gotten her here soon enough. Also, more likely the person was dead, and the family wanted the body removed. If it is an accident case these people can always get a car and get in here in a shorter time than the time it takes us to drive out to get them and bring them in.

April 22, 1954

I spent an hour listening to Charlie Yellow Boy talking tonight about the past. Charlie is in his seventies. He was in Pine Ridge during the early days and remembers Agent McGillycuddy.[3]

This is interesting. I think. Mr. Reifel is really hitting on the alcoholism here. "Old Peg Leg" Red Cloud wrote to President Eisenhower about it. The president told him he had signed a bill permitting the Indians to buy and drink at the discretion of the local area.

These Indians liked their old method of obtaining liquor. They bought it from the bootleggers on the reservation. They paid twice as much. Nevertheless they liked that. But Mr. Reifel is making it tough even for bootleggers. They are leaving the reservation. And he is right because the reservation people voted not to allow liquor on the reservation.

Jim Red Cloud used to like Mr. Reifel but seems irritated by him now. Whereas Mr. Sande had him sitting in his lap, Mr. Reifel just looks past him as if he is one of the Indians when he is in the outer office on days with no scheduled office hours.[4]

Well, what happened today is that Mr. Red Cloud made a speech to a crowd that gathered on the street. They are writing to the Canadian government to ask if they can all move up to Canada. There is a group of Sioux up there.

This reminds me. Yesterday I was preparing a patient for surgery. The orderly, Louis Mosseau, said to the patient, Philip Iron Cloud, "You don't have much hair." I added, "That is a characteristic of full-bloods. You must be a full-blood, Philip." "Yes Sir!" he replied with vigor, showing how proud he was of that fact.

Mrs. Forshey is upset about all the work she is given to do, reviewing names of people who were examined for eye glasses to determine their eligibility as to whether or not the individual buys them or Health or Welfare does. She says we need a medical social worker. Amen! That is certainly true. For instance, people being billed for hospital care should be those employed by the federal government or tribal employees.

Mrs. Forshey wants teachers to supply information on families. She wants to circulate a form on people to Bank, and Extension, as Rehabilitation has done asking for family resources when a family needs a casket. If funds are to be available or the person has money in an account, the casket will be paid for out of that. Anyway, it is something we have to work on this summer.

Twice now Red Cloud has cornered me at the Agency Office, saying he has a deal and will be over here to the house in the evening, but he has never come. Instead he sent his daughter, Mrs. Elk Boy. She came with a pipe to sell. I told her I would loan her ten dollars and keep the pipe as pawn.[5]

Yesterday an extremely intoxicated man came to the hospital wanting to take me to a peyote meeting tonight. I took him back to the Holy Rosary Mission where he stays. Not three hours later, when I got home for supper, he was at my door again wanting a donation. For gas, he said. It was probably for beer.

Mrs. Olinger called me from Kyle last night. She said two kids were brought in there. Each had lacerations on their foreheads. They said they bumped into each other. She thought it was fishy, so she sent them on to us. They didn't get in before midnight. I called Joe Swift Bird. Richards and Martin came over, too. I guess the kids could have gotten their injuries by bumping into each other, but it is unusual. Both had two centimeter lacerations from the forehead down to the bottom of the skull.

April 25, 1954

Felix Walking was going to take me to a peyote meeting at the home of Joe Running Hawk, but he got stuck in Alliance and got home to Pine Ridge too late. About 10:00 p.m. he wanted me to join him, but it was too late. However, I drove him out to Stiff Tails, where they were holding a Half Moon meeting. I left Felix and listened to the beat of the drum and the praying for a short while from my car; then I came home.

It was wonderful out today. I got some more hose and a sprinkler from the hospital and soaked all the dirt around the house. Jeanne and I dug up some iris and some smelly leaf plant from the yard of the burned-out house next door that is now being repaired. We planted the plants around the house and around an area that is going to be an outdoor fireplace. We are going to line it with brick torn from the chimney next door. We raked up a bunch of weeds and old grass that contained bones and burned those.

We were going to do some more yard work tonight, but I had to run over to the hospital to tend to a girl from Porcupine who had been beaten. I ended up getting sidetracked. I went to the Walters' for coffee after that. Then I went home and played some two-handed bridge with Jeanne.

April 26, 1954

Our lawn: I planted grass seed last fall but too late. This spring the earth was tan with the wheat grass seed on it that Mr. Mickelson had given me. Then half blew off. Next we had a torrent of rain and lightning that flooded the place last Sunday night. The rest of the seed washed off and lies in big puddles off the terraced area. The huge deep ditch in front of our house is filled with water yet. It rained so hard it washed off the top hard crust of soil into the roadway. So again I got more grass seed and strewed that around. Damn wind blew that off. It is impossible to rake the stuff into the hard ground. We thought that by running water continuously from the faucet and sprinkler we could keep the earth soft enough for the stuff to start to grow. There are two water systems in town. One is fit for drinking in homes. But due to shortage there is another pipe system for outside home use. Since they didn't give us outside water, we got a hundred feet of hose and hooked it to the house faucet to use outside.

April 27, 1954

Mrs. Blue Bird, who was at our house the night of the dancing, is the mother of a son who is in the army. He sends home a $25 bond once a month to his wife, Julia Blue Bird. She gets the bond at one post office window, takes it to the next window, cashes it, and gets her $18.50. She can't understand why she doesn't get the $25. She thinks somebody is gypping her of the rest. She doesn't know what saving and interest are or what the benefits are of saving the bond for ten years. She has never heard of such a thing.

Wilson Brady, who has visited at the house, is a member of Cross Fire. There is a case in the court that was to be tried today but wasn't. Brady is supposed to have given Mrs. Afraid of Bear of Slim Buttes some peyote for an illness. The family now claims she is off her rocker and has been queer ever since she got the peyote to eat. Vincent Red Cloud posted bond for Brady. Edgar was going to the court case. He got Vincent over there so he wouldn't have to be jailed.

Edgar has posted bail for someone before, and on three occasions the person who was bonded did not show up. So Edgar spent time in the jug each time. That is the way they work their bonds. Since no one has the ready cash, a person posts their bond, and if the accused does not show, then the person who posted the bond serves the jail sentence.

One family has been living in Chadron, Nebraska, for quite some time, long enough to be considered residents. They were kicked out of Chadron and went to Slim Butte. And now Philip Brown Eyes, the community chairman from Slim Butte, is trying to get rid of them. They say the members of this family are apparently bad characters.

I had a regular session with Edgar Red Cloud and Mrs. Forshey in the latter's office from 5:00 p.m. on. Edgar had come to borrow a metal saw from Mrs. Forshey to fix Vincent's car. Mrs. Forshey says Edgar has a fulltime job fixing his car.

More bootleggers are at Kyle and in Pine Ridge. One of them used to work at the hospital here. His wife still works at the hospital. Another is a real outlaw, ever since the time Mr. Reifel at inauguration ceremonies on April 6 asked the council to state where they stand on the liquor question and then asked them to look into the innocent faces of school students. Mr. Reifel shouted and called the bootlegger's name and pointed at a former hospital employee who he knew was a bootlegger. This man also reportedly murdered an Indian woman married to a European man. Mrs. Forshey says this guy has said it is easier to murder than to bootleg.

Anyway, the bootlegger's son-in-law has two children. Their mother died in January 1954 at the Sioux Sanitarium. So the bootlegger takes the two kids, goes to the Public Welfare Office, and asks for Aid to Families with Dependent Children, stating, "Since Mr. Pistol came my whole life has been changed." I learned the bootleggers are having a tough time. They call Mr. Reifel "Mr. Pistol" and "Mr. Gunshot."

Edgar told me this and says he is helping to spread the story. Congressman E. Y. Berry was in Rapid City and had conferences with Mr. Reifel and some others from this reservation. The Indians here, especially Jake Herman, who own land in an area where the government wants to make a gunnery range, have been trying to get the money by selling off part of the reservation and the Badlands to the government. Jake and others have made innumerable trips to promote this.

Edgar says that Jake goes to Rapid City to talk to Congressman Berry about this and gets his mileage paid for by the tribe. Then, says Edgar, "He throws up an Iron Curtain." Jake had a private conference with Congressman Berry. Mrs. Forshey told me all about it. Jake told Congressman Berry that he was working for him and will continue to do so. He told him he was again elected to the tribal council. He told Congressman Berry to do something to get the bill passed for us (to get more money for those who had land in the gunnery range), and he told Congressman Berry to at least get it passed for HIM (Jake Herman).

Mrs. Forshey told me about another guy who got a lease check for $108. So she decided to take him off relief for two months. He came back with a bill for $80 for a grazing fee for his eight head of horses. He rides horseback but, of course, has no other real need for horses excepting that six of the horses were once his mother's. Then he came back with a bill for $54 for the ground gopher or ground mole extermination program on his land. These people are real corkers.

I got a letter today asking for authorization for a woman currently hospitalized in Rapid City. On checking, with the help of Mrs. Forshey,

I found the woman is the illegitimate daughter of people enrolled on the Rosebud reservation. They have lived in Rapid City for over seventeen years. Then they lived in Chadron until three months ago. They lived there long enough to be bona fide residents but left Chadron recently when that city ran off Indians who were living in a campground. Naturally, I could not authorize such care.

Mrs. Forshey brought up THE hero of the reservation as far as his World War II record. He was with Merrill's Marauders and held off the enemy while members of his group escaped.[6] He has had lots of write-ups. Anyway, he is having trouble and is much disturbed. Last August he threatened several people with a gun. He is in the hospital overnight. Mrs. Forshey is driving him up to the Veterans Hospital tomorrow.

A committee from school consisting of Miss Crescentia Gage, Miss Talcott, and Mr. Manning C. Ryder came over to talk to me. The whole thing began with Mr. Reifel in Rapid City when someone asked the condition of a relative in the hospital here. He knew nothing about it. So Mr. Reifel wrote to Pyles, Pyles to Mickelson, Mick to the committee he appointed, and the committee to me, and we met to discuss starting a hospital visitation program where high school age kids would come and help hospitalized persons write letters, bring reading materials, and play games. All okay with me. I only suggested that the kids be chaperoned by an oldster so they would actually be doing something and not wandering aimlessly. Both Mrs. Forshey and the Mickelsons are irritated by Mr. Ryder.

Ten. May 1954

Yesterday, the last Friday of the month, a community services meeting was held with Mr. Reifel. He is conducting the meetings now with each department head taking a session and presenting what he thinks a reservation program ought to consist of. Mr. Pyles, head of Education, presented what he thought a reservation program ought to be. He set up a representative community, spending considerable time telling about the kids, in and out of school, the adults, married and unmarried, the elders, those on relief, and so on. Then he set up a method of attack, a long-range and a short-range plan. What was his program, its objectives, its goals? God only knows.

May 1, 1954

Yesterday, the last Friday of the month, a community services meeting was held with Mr. Reifel. He is conducting the meetings now with each department head taking a session and presenting what he thinks a reservation program ought to consist of. Mr. Pyles, head of Education, presented what he thought a reservation program ought to be. He set up a representative community, spending considerable time telling about the kids, in and out of school, the adults, married and unmarried, the elders, those on relief, and so on. Then he explained a method of attack, a long-range and a short-range plan. What was his program, its objectives, its goals? God only knows.

Sometime ago, a couple weeks ago, the community of Slim Buttes was making great efforts to get a family into the Sioux Sanitarium. As part of that effort, those with tuberculosis and the others in the family were moved to Pine Ridge to live in a tent until the whole family was examined. In a memorandum to Mr. Reifel, I told him I'd finally gotten one member of the family to the Sioux Sanitarium, and I was impressed by the community of Slim Buttes in getting the family to medical attention since they have no car.

Then a day later, Mrs. Forshey, reading this memorandum that I wrote and that Mr. Reifel circulated, typed me a note stating the real motivations of the people from Slim Buttes. This was an excuse to get rid of the family. The community had kicked the family out once before. The family went to Chadron to live this time. Then Chadron evicted them. And they got back to Slim Buttes, which was trying to get rid of them again. They say the family stinks. Well, after I informed Mr. Reifel of the real motives of the people of Slim Buttes, I noticed that the next week in his news sheet he mentioned the fine spirit of the people of Slim Buttes to be so interested in this family and to help them get to the hospital. Along the same line, I send him reports of all people from the Sioux Sanitarium who left against medical advice. I once sent down the name of a patient who had gone to the sanitarium and left. But Dr. Carmine A. Celilla from up there wrote asking that we get back this guy, who lives in Allen. The patient returned, and after completing an examination of him, Dr. Celilla wrote back saying the boy did not have tuberculosis. So I wrote Mr. Reifel a memorandum stating that the patient went to the sanitarium and was found to be free of tuberculosis. So a couple days later this past week, Mr. Reifel wrote about the patient who had gone back and was found to be cured of tuberculosis. Mr. Reifel said it was fine that the man can live among his community, and applauded how happy his family must feel. I liked what Mr. Reifel had to say yesterday morning in conference. In dealing with people and making a program there is no place for romanticism or emotion.

The man from Oglala who was hit on the head with an ax several weeks ago and who is a peyote eater was in the clinic yesterday. He told me they were having a birthday meeting at Wounded Knee the following day. These are Half Moons; their main chief is Levi Sitting Hawk.

I wish that I could go with Wilson Brady, a Cheyenne Sioux who is going. But I have to go to the darn OCHS Junior-Senior prom. Wilson told me the altar in Half Moon is made in the shape of a half moon, the same as the Cross Fire worshipers use. Across the altar is drawn the road of life, just as in Cross Fire practice. Wilson also told me that Half Moon has a water call at midnight, whereas the Cross Fire does not have a water call until morning. Half Moon also has the water call in the morning before eating. They don't eat dog. Usually they eat a corn dish with other things. Wilson told me when he first came here from Lame Deer, Montana, he didn't understand their language. But at the first meeting he went to he could understand them along toward morning. I think this is significant in that as the "happy feeling" comes from the use of mescaline, words and objects are loved or looked at for their own being. I think it is significant that peyote eaters to whom I've talked do not have great visions of colored geometric figures. They do not have visionary minds. Instead they have a difference in perception that answers their problems since their religion is an escape for them from the discouraging earthly conditions the Indians are in.

Felix Walking told me that he once painted the agency hospital lobby and the designs or figures he used were those of the peyote cult or Native American Church, the Half Moon symbols. They were painted over several years ago.

Joe Flying Hawk raises three kinds of corn. He says he makes *wasna* [phonetic spelling by Ruby] from the squaw corn. Only the *wasna* he makes is not the old wasna (dried meat, chokeberries, and the fat of tallow and sugar) but is made by letting the corn dry on the stalks in the field, then picking, shelling, and parching the corn with heat, and finally grinding it. Sugar is then added and the fat from tallow of beef. All the ingredients are mixed and cooked. This, he says, is a delicacy.

Snow came Thursday and is still with us. It is still snowing. May first! It froze Wednesday night and froze our lilacs that are out. I have them covered with a blanket in hopes of keeping them from freezing further. It is muddy. Electrical storms last Sunday and Wednesday burned our and several other people's hot water units. They burned out our electric clock. What weather!

May 3, 1954

These people are fabulous. Nell Coker tells me sometime ago a man's son was put in jail for speeding. The father, a bootlegger, came and got him out. The new judge had some land dealings or tie-ups with the bootlegger and owed him favors. But after that they have been at such odds that they are ready to burn each other's house down, Mrs. Forshey tells me. Then not long ago the guy's kid was speeding again. He sped past Mr. Reifel's office window. Mr. Reifel lit out after him in his car. When the youth saw who it was, he sped up even faster. Mr. Reifel sent cops after him. They got him and locked him up. Mr. Reifel filed the charges. The father came and bailed his son out.

Well, this morning a man suspected of bootlegging dragged another man into Mrs. Forshey's office and said the second man had worked for him before he was injured in an altercation in Rapid City. The bootlegger told Mrs. Forshey he went to get this other guy to work for him the other day on his cattle land, but the man passed out. I just saw the guy in clinic last Friday (three days ago), and he told me no such story. Mrs. Forshey told me she knew it was a put-up deal. She says the bootlegger told her the fellow was so up against it. Apparently his business is running out on him. Mr. Reifel is making it too tough for him. Mrs. Forshey says after her interview with him this morning she is sure he is approaching an anxiety state. And what is going to happen now is that she gave the second man a grocery order. He will get groceries and trade some to the bootlegger for liquor.

Mrs. Forshey told me that when Wilson Brady gets jelly or jam he locks it up and uses it himself. She said that old George Swift Bird (father of Joe Swift Bird) locks up the food at his home. And then when he gets mad at his family he won't give them any food for awhile. I hadn't realized it, but all these people get food and lock it up. It is the only way they can keep all the relatives who pile in on them from eating them out of house and home. Mrs. Forshey once gave Mary Ann Red Cloud some jelly. She forgot where she'd hidden it, and the family ran across it. Edgar says, "She is stingy." Isn't that something! In every home you find trunks, where they hide their extra food in them from visitors. But they have to become crafty. Mrs. Forshey says some people even bury things like food, keeping it from others.

Miss Laurella Pease, one of our nurses, a white woman, is going with an Indian and wants to marry him. But Angelique High Whiteman, a nurse's aid, told Miss Pease she shouldn't marry this guy because Indian men did nothing. They let the women support them, or get drunk and won't work. We have a white nurse married to an Indian, and the situation in their home is as Angelique described it. Angelique is in her late thirties, maybe older, and isn't married.

Wilson Brady told me he is to be one of the twenty who are to dance for William Randolph Hearst Jr. when he comes through here on May 20. Charlie Yellow Boy came to the house and told me he is heading the committee to put on the dance for Hearst. He is going to pick only twenty dancers. They are going to put up two tents in the street.

The people here are noted for arguing and causing trouble. Even Mr. Reifel must have gotten his fill at some meeting lately. They apparently heckled him and annoyed him so much that in disgust he said, "I'm here to close this place down in three years time. And I'm sure going to do it."

Mr. Reifel sends out birthday letters to all employees. But I didn't get one. He found out about my birthday afterward and said doctors were the only ones whose birthdays were not listed. A letter to Mr. Reifel was received from a girl in Rapid City asking for aid with federal funds to pay for her medical expenses. Mr. Reifel sent it to me to answer with a penned note from him, "Answer a polite no."

One patient is a veteran with a brilliant war record, honors for car-

rying two wounded men to safety under fire, and other things. He received most of his elementary education off the reservation, and he
thinks like a white. He wants to work and own a home. He says his in-
laws sell everything he gets, and they get him arrested all the time. He
sure doesn't like them or their way of life. They are full-bloods, and he
says all they want to do is go from place to place and gossip. He is so
different from his relatives, who have been telling him for so long he
is crazy that he believes it. Measured on that score he is not. But Mrs.
Forshey wanted him in here for a physical examination since the Veterans Administration Hospital wouldn't take him. He came into the
hospital yesterday but left to do some business. He said he'd be right
back, but he didn't return. He is despondent.

Edgar was telling me that in Yuwipi they pray to the winds, the animals, and the rocks. When rock is put in a hole and water is poured on
it, they tell the Great Spirit, "Now we are putting on water, give us air."
If it is a treatment, as for pain in the chest for pleurisy, the medicine
man will blow that steam on the chest of the sick person.

May 4, 1954

Mrs. Forshey called me this afternoon because I saw a man in the clinic
with a leg ulcer. I wrote on the welfare application slip, "ulcer will get
well in a few weeks with care." But I doubt this guy will take care of it.
He had dirt and mud in it when seen in the clinic today. I had put a note
on the welfare slip, "Call me." She did. The patient is a Cheyenne Sioux
and a member of the Half Moon peyote sect, out by Oglala. Then Mrs.
Forshey told me that the Half Moon peyote followers are holding a big
prayer meeting this Saturday night in expectation of our visit.

They are making big plans. Edgar says they plan to have a thousand buttons and give everyone fifty. She said she was told Lawrence
Hunter was going to interpret for us during the meetings. She said besides coming in for his welfare money he was an advance party for the
peyote meeting Saturday night. Less than fifteen minutes later Char-

lie Bear Robe, a Cross Fire practitioner, came to the hospital and said he wanted to talk to me privately. He said that both groups, the Half Moon and Cross Fire, were going to meet at Porcupine and he was supposed to take me to the place.

I told that to Mrs. Forshey tonight. She knew that, of course, Cross Fire and Half Moon were feuding, and it seemed unlikely the two would meet together. But she thinks that the Cross Fire people are going to kidnap us and take us to their meeting. Charlie arranged to be at my house at 6:30 on Saturday evening. I really can't say that I've known one Indian to make such specific time arrangements. Edgar wants to go with us. Mrs. Forshey says the news is all over the reservation.

May 6, 1954

Edgar came over tonight at 9:00 p.m. I offered him a Coke. "Rather have beer," he said. I told him we haven't bought liquor since Mr. Reifel came. I had gone out to see him before 6:00 p.m. to take him some beads to use in stringing on leather, and he said he was going to Mrs. Forshey's tonight. I told him I'd take him home later. Edgar also thinks Charlie Bear Robe is trying to get us to Cross Fire service and keep us from attending the Half Moon service.

May 9, 1954

The ride out to Denby was during the nice part of the evening. We went out just after sundown. I drove Mrs. Forshey's car as she was also going to the peyote meeting with me. With us was Edgar Red Cloud, who is not a member of the peyote sect, and Wilson Brady. Brady was carrying a wooden chest, about fourteen by six by six inches. He also had a small sack. In the wooden chest Wilson had his paraphernalia that is used in the Half Moon worship service.

We turned off Highway 18 at the Denby turnoff, having gone east from Pine Ridge, and went over the rolling gravel road past the Denby store about two miles from the turn. Then we turned off the road onto a private road leading to Levi Sitting Hawk's home. It was a half mile off the road. There were other cars there when we pulled into the yard. It was about eight p.m. Levi came up. It was the first time I had met him. He said, "So you are the doctor. I've heard about you so much. I thought you would be a very big man." He said the service was not ready to begin. They were waiting for others to come. Outside there was a fire. In back of the house was a creek. It was dusk. I could hear frogs croaking. It was quiet out there. It seemed to be a nice place to come and even live, perhaps.

Levi said that the group had a tent, but it was still too cold to use the tent. Besides, the tent was in Scotts Bluff, where some of the groups were using it, so they were having the meeting indoors.

Levi told us that some who came out were eating supper. His wife was feeding them. We could wait in the car until they were ready to start. Then we could go in. He left.

Levi came for us just after 8:30. We walked into the house, through a small narrow room in which there was only a davenport and on into a longer room at the north end of the building. The room was perhaps ten feet from east to west and six feet north to south. There was no furniture in the room except two folding chairs that had been placed there for us until the meeting gets under way. We sat on them at the back of the room, which was the east end. The front of the room was the west end. There, about three and a half feet from the wall in the center, was a flat surface of packed earth about two and a half by two and a half feet. It was raised or was about three inches high. There was a curved mound of earth in the center of the room, curving and rising in height to about four inches at the center of this "moon." The convex surface was to the front side, west. At the center of the moon-shaped mound there was a small depressed square about two and a half by two and a half inches and perhaps three-fourths inches deep. There was a small thin path, or line, on top of the moon mound. On the earth behind there was a large peyote button. On both sides of the altar there was a lighted coal oil lamp. The entire service is done in light. There is not

the element of the supernatural that required darkness as is used in Yuwipi. Dick Running Bear came in. He is a past president. Levi told him
to be the leader or main chief tonight. He didn't have his paraphernalia, so he had to go after it.

While he was gone, Levi got out an old imitation leather briefcase
and pulled out the national charter for the Native American Church and
showed it to us. Then he showed us the by-laws and rules. No one is allowed to have peyote outside a meeting, to carry it, or to use it outside
a meeting. Peyote cannot be given to nonmembers, though we were invited to take it. Only the president can order peyote from the source.

Then Levi showed us an old list of members. On the list were two
medicine men and a policeman for the tribe. It just goes to show you
that one should not say anything to anyone. That policeman was at the
hospital on Friday with a prisoner, and so was Joe Swift Bird, chief of
police, who had seen our car at the Yuwipi meeting. Wilson explained
to us that long ago when a worship meeting was held all members had
to sit all night long on their knees. But it was so tiresome that now that
isn't followed. We asked if we should sit on the chairs. He thought it
would be better if we sat on cushions on the floor. So we obliged. Along
the room against each wall was canvas, old calf hides and blankets, and
on them were cushions and pillows. So they fixed extra high cushions
against the north wall apparently so we'd be comfortable enough. Edgar had warned us, or rather advised us, on three things: bring some
money, don't sign anything, and don't lean against any walls. He told
us this all before we got to the meeting.

We then each gave Levi $2. The peyote buttons for tonight cost $5
for two hundred beans, so we gave them practically enough to pay for
the peyote for the evening. We were not asked to sign anything. But we
were told we could leave at any time we wished.

Levi told Mrs. Forshey there were only forty members of this church,
whereas in the Cross Fire there were two hundred members. She detected a note of pride in having an exclusive group.

And one person in Cross Fire had done much to persuade us to come to their meeting, but that person, Edgar told me, showed up at this meeting drunk. I didn't see him, but apparently they dispensed with him promptly.

Dick Running Bear was back with his metal tool box containing his paraphernalia. Practically all men had long metal or wooden boxes in which to carry their gourds and feathers. Dick took out a silk multicolored scarf and laid it down back of the altar. On this he laid a sack of Bull Durham, feathers, and a bone whistle. He sat at the center back of the altar. He closed his box and put it behind him. Dick said he had a few words to say to us, but he asked Edgar to interpret his Sioux words for him. He welcomed us, saying it is the first time in history that white people and federal employees (Indian or non-Indian) had come to their meeting. Of course, though he didn't say this, it has caused considerable discussion, alarm, excitement, and even anticipation for the Indians all over the reservation and off, even into Nebraska. Dick told us that there were not many at the meeting because they had heard a doctor and Welfare worker were coming, and they were scared.

Dick, who is sixty-two, said he first joined when he was twenty-four years old. He said he had never been to the hospital. Peyote kept him well. His wife was there. She had had dropsy and had been cured with peyote.Dick said he had worked with white men all his life and had picked up the language that way. He said he had no education and couldn't speak too well though.

Then Levi spoke. He welcomed us. He said this was a great occasion, again stressing the first time that white men had sat in on their meetings. But then he wanted to know how long we were going to stay, that we should stay all night. I was a little uneasy. I thought it was understood before the meeting that we could leave at midnight. I didn't want to offend them. So I told Edgar, our interpreter, I had to get back to the hospital. I knew Edgar also wanted to leave at midnight. Levi speaks very good English, but he talked thru Edgar also.

Dick then asked if there was anyone else who wished to say something to us. Since we had definitely let them know we wished to leave

UNITED STATES
DEPARTMENT OF THE INTERIOR
OFFICE OF INDIAN AFFAIRS
FIELD SERVICE

This is seating and altar arrangement.   (West.)

Mrs. Running Bear · Rising Sun Drum Ch. · Dick Running Bear Main Chief · Wilson Brady Cedar Chief

Door to kitchen

16

Leo Little Boy

Levi Sitting Hawk

Mrs. Sitting Hawk

South

Nyrolf

Edgar

Mrs. Crow and Baby

Door to living room

Joe Catches Fire Chief

Joe Running Hawk

Dan Tail

Mrs. Elk Boy · Ira Elk Boy · Charles Deon · Willie Running Hawk (Brother of Joe)

EAST

1 Pot Peyote tea
2 Sack of peyote buttons
3 scarf
4 bone whistle
5 feather fan
6 staff
7 Sack of Bull Durham
8 Sack of cedar
9 Father peyote
10 Cigarette butts of worshipers
11 Cigarette butts of the chiefs.
12 Raised earth Half Moon with road of
   life imprinted on the dirt altar.
13 Coal oil lamps
14 Fire
15 Cedar pole used to light cigarettes
16 Peyote Drum

1. Native American Church meeting altar arrangement as observed and described by Robert H. Ruby on May 9, 1954. Drawing by Robert H. Ruby.

at the midnight water call, that was settled. Rising Sun got up and explained the four stations in the service. The midnight water call was the first station. The fourth was at 6:00 a.m., which ended the service. They were ready to begin the service.

The service began. Everyone was seated around the room on the floor. Joe Catches, the fire chief, went outside and with a coal scoop brought in a pile of live ashes and put them on the earth altar in front of the half moon.

Dick Running Bear, the main chief, took the peyote button from the very front of the altar and placed it in the depression at the center of the dirt half moon.

Wilson Brady, the cedar chief, took small fragments of cedar branches from a small beaded leather pouch and sprinkled them on the pile of ashes. A very pleasant aroma of cedar permeated the room as the smoke rose from the ashes.

Rising Sun, the drum chief, held the drum over the smoke for a second. Then Running Bear picked up the staff, the gourd, and feather fan and ran them through the smoke. Then he took a pack of Bull Durham and held it in the smoke. He passed the bag of Bull Durham to the drum chief. He took a paper and rolled a cigarette. He passed the bag to Running Bear. He did the same. Wilson rolled one next. And then on around the room. They each held their cigarettes.

Joe got up and went outside to the fire and brought in a cedar limb about an inch and a half across and sixteen inches long, which was not flaming but was red at the end where it had been in the fire outside. He handed it to Rising Sun who lit his cigarette. He passed it to Running Bear and on around the room. When it got to Mrs. Running Bear, who was the last to light her cigarette, Joe came forward and got it and laid it at the front of the altar with the burning end over the live coals. Joe never approached the altar and returned directly. But each time he came forward he then walked around the altar before returning to his place.

After they had all puffed a short while, Running Bear closed his eyes and prayed to Wakan Tanka.

As soon as he was through praying, Joe gathered the cigarette butts from all except the three in back of the altar. He divided them and laid half at each end of the half moon shaped altar. Those three behind Dick then sent Joe into the kitchen for the peyote "tea" and paper cups.

Dick took a calico sack from his box, which was perhaps a foot deep and seven inches wide. The sack was filled half full with peyote buttons. He took them out and placed them on the altar to his right. Wilson had placed his leather bag of cedar pieces on the altar to his left.

The pot of steaming hot tea and the cups were passed around the room. Each poured tea and drank. The sack of buttons was passed around and each took buttons.

Usually the buttons are boiled in water, so they will be soft, and are then put in a wooden bowl that is passed around the room with a spoon, one spoon that all use to put the buttons into their mouth. But because white people were there that part was altered. The dried buttons were passed around. When the tea and sack were back at the altar, they were again placed at the altar to the right of the main chief. The peyote bean is very hard when dry, and the crunching could be heard around the room.

The drum chief picked up his drum. The drum is a cast iron drum about eight inches in diameter at the top. It has three legs (which today stand for the three in one God). It has a pint of water in it. Over the top is tanned (not rawhide) calf hide. Around the top of the cast iron drum at the sides are seven projections. The leather is laced around these with a cord the thickness of clothesline rope. It is laced around each of seven knobs and, crossing the rope, is carried under the bottom of the drum to another knob. The leather continues the lacing, making a seven-point star pattern of the rope on the bottom of the drum.

The peyote drum is beaten rapidly with a regular rhythm. There is no syncopation. It is beaten with a small nonpadded stick. Before each song the drummer tilts the drum quickly so the water will dampen the leather. He holds the drum with his left hand. All fingers except the thumb are around the rim. The thumb is held down firmly on the surface and moved from the periphery to the center of the drum to alter the pitch. With the thumb near the periphery the leather is less taut and gives fewer vibrations, and the pitch is low and hollow. As the thumb is moved closer to the center, the leather is more taut and gives

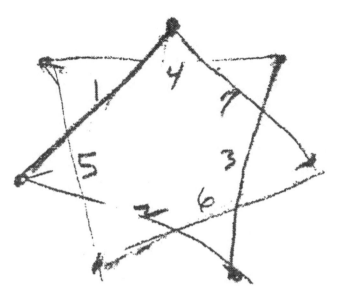

2. Lacing pattern for drum used in "peyote service" as observed and described by Robert H. Ruby on May 9, 1954. The number of spokes or projections on the drum lacing represent the number of sacraments in the service. Drawing by Robert H. Ruby.

more vibrations, and the pitch is higher with yet a hollow tone. The water gives it a dull quality.

The first one to sing four prayers was Dick Running Bear. Rising Sun beat the drum. Each singer holds the staff and feather fan in the left hand, squats, and rattles the gourd with the right hand. His eyes are closed while he sings. The singers take on an expression of pained concentration. The songs or "hymns" are scant on words. They may be no more than "Forgive us of our sins." This is repeated with a series of hums in the *eeys, ahas, oyis.*

The drum is beaten rapidly. The singer rattles the gourd in perfect "rhythm" to the drum, moving the hand up and down. At the end of a song, the gourd is rattled sideways slower. The pitch of the drum is then softened. The drummer tilts the drum again to wet it and commences again until the singer has sung four prayers. The staff, fan, and gourd is then passed to the next person. The drum is passed to the next person, the one who had just sung. This dual maneuver passes around the room.

The paraphernalia made the first round by 11:00 p.m. At that time the Two Tails family and Ada Black Crow came in. They each took the Bull Durham and made a cigarette. Joe took the cedar bow outside to burn it again and brought it back to them. Wilson sprinkled more cedar on the fire. These three women did not sing. But when the paraphernalia reached them they moved it to the left side of their body, then to the right side, and then passed it on to the person to their left. The tea and sack of buttons were passed around the room again.

The staff, which is passed around, is about three feet in length. At the top of this one were rows of beads about three inches from the top, and from the top protruded a "fuzz" of white horse hair. At the bottom was a carved point or spear in the wood. The staff is said to represent the staff that Christ carried when he herded sheep.

There was one other staff there that was not used. It was enameled in red, white, and blue, carved with a large spear at the bottom, and above this there was a series of linked chains. There were a couple of gourds with flags done in beadwork. The red, white, and blue theme is common in beadwork.

The fans are small feathers of owl and pheasant. Some are wrapped with leather, and each feather is tied into a handle so the feathers are loose and will flop to the side unless the feathers are also partially held with the handle. From the fans hang tassels or strips of leather. Ribbons hang from some.

The gourds are dried and varnished. The tops are cut off. They are filled with small pebbles and the openings attached to sticks or handles about a foot long. Some were carved. Others were beaded. Some had two-inch points at the top. Others had a fringe of white horse hair.

After a breather Joe went out and brought in another scoop of live ashes. Wilson sprinkled them on tiny cedar branches. The round of prayer songs was again done. When the drum got back to the altar, it was just about 12:00. Joe went outside and brought in a brass pail of water. He set it before the altar. He then went out and brought in more ashes and dumped them on the fireplace. He bent down and with his stick pushed them into a half-moon shape. Wilson sprinkled on more cedar. Each time he sprinkled he raised his hand in a little flourish. All paraphernalia and the drum were passed through the smoke.

Wilson stood up and said all those who have fans and gourds take them out. There were about five other sets. Those who had them took them from their "tool boxes" for fans and gourds and passed them through the smoke. Running Bear picked up the bone whistle. He blew three long blasts and then a series of several short whistles. Rising Sun beat the drum, and Running Bear led the midnight song while others joined in holding their fans and rattling their gourds.

Joe came forward again and took the pail of water and passed it to Running Bear who dipped his cup and took a drink. The water pail was passed all around the room at each drinking time. Running Bear then stood and prayed to Wakan Tanka.

Joe made a very big cigarette of tobacco from a bottle that was passed to him. He lit it with cedar limb. He was to smoke this and then pray, but he told Running Bear there was a drunk outside and he had to go out. He passed the cigarette to Wilson who smoked it then stood and prayed fervently and long. He prayed for the doctor. He prayed for Edgar and the social worker and for his tiny daughter who is ill in the agency hospital. He asked God to give him and his wife strength to raise her as she should be raised. He asked for God's help for himself and for others. He asked that we have a safe trip back into Pine Ridge. All this was done in the Cheyenne language.

Joe Catches was back in the room by now.

Running Bear then got up and went outside. Joe Running Hawk beat the drum while Joe sang the four midnight prayers. Running Bear turned to the four directions of the winds (he was outside) and made a prayer in each direction.

He came inside. The first station had been reached.

Wilson told us he was happy we had come and attended their worship meeting. Running Bear then said, "I can talk good enough English. I'll talk to you myself and not through an interpreter." He also said he was glad we'd come. He said that this was the way the Indian worshipped God long before the white man came. It was perhaps primitive. He said over at Porcupine there is another group, the Cross Fire group. "But they are smarter. They use the Bible. They can read." Why I think this is significant is that while under the influence of peyote, a person loses self-consciousness and perhaps becomes somewhat talkative. While each person sings his four prayer songs others sit usually with their eyes shut. They chew on the peyote buttons.

The whole meeting was very orderly. The only difference in individuals that I could detect was a slight crescendo to the voices in song. Talking was a little more verbose.

Levi talked to us again thru Edgar. He told what the rest of the service would be. After midnight the service was the same except that they had talks and stressed the four standards of their cult: sobriety, charity, morality, and industry.

Running Bear then talked again and thought we should come back again. He wanted us to. He said you can't understand our religion by coming once or even twice; he said he went four times or more before he understood it.

They let me take pictures of the altar. I'm afraid however that the two lamps on either side of the altar might spoil the picture. I have never seen pictures of the altar at any place. As far as I can learn, these are the first pictures allowed.

I have no doubt that there were other alterations in the service besides not boiling the buttons to soften them and passing them with a common spoon. But though I would not join and I'm very much against their belief that peyote is a cure-all, their service as I see it is not too far off from some white men's religions. It was one a.m. when we left the building.

I mentioned previously that Joe Catches made a large cigarette with tobacco taken from a little bottle. I learned later it was crushed sage brush, not tobacco. The sage is practically the same as sage grown around here, but that this sage is shipped in from Oklahoma where the peyote is grown. The large cigarette is rolled in corn husk.

May 10, 1954

Edgar Red Cloud with lots of time on his hands has been taking in some of the sessions of the current tribal council. He says all they do is argue over something superfluous and criticize someone unmercifully, especially government employees.

Saturday at the hospital Father William Fitzgerald came up to me and said one of the family members he'd been talking to from Loeffer Camp told him Doctor Ruby approved of healing in Yuwipi. That priest had been talking to them against Yuwipi. I am not surprised that they said such a thing. I am doubtful they believe I endorse it, which I don't. And I don't disapprove of it either. It is an excuse for the Indian people to practice Yuwipi, and I expect that sort of thing knowing these people as I do.

I had quite a talk then with Father Fitzgerald. He thinks the people here are too slow to change. The people are not readily accepted off the reservation in churches because they are dark skinned. That is too bad.

Father Fitzgerald is upset with the peyote cult. He said one crazy woman once came up to him shouting, pulled a piece of peyote from her mouth, and cried, "Look, the body of Christ." He says there are unknown peyote cult members who take the sacrament in the Catholic Church.

Father Fitzgerald says the peyote makes them vomit. This, they feel, is the purging of their sins. If this happens, that could well be the belief or interpretation they attach to it. According to the scientific literature it causes gastric irritation. But I saw no vomiting at the meeting we attended.

Father Fitzgerald also said their drums had the crown of thorns painted around the surface of the drum. That wasn't on the drum I saw, but I know there are so many variations to the service and the paraphernalia that this must be so in some places.

Mr. Reifel called yesterday, Saturday, and wanted me to go to some tuberculosis meeting in Rapid City for today and tomorrow. Miss Wayne is going to be there. Mr. Noralf is going to discuss their tuberculosis plan at Cheyenne, where they lock up those who will not take treatment. Because Doctors Gassman and Bragg handle most of the tuberculosis cases, I told him I'd send one of them. Dr. Gassman doesn't want to go because his daughter fell down steps and is hurt. So Dr. Bragg will go.

Mrs. Forshey gave Edgar Red Cloud a very large reprint of a painting by a popular French artist. I laughed. After the floods and wind storms of time cover this area, archeologists will uncover the picture and exclaim, "Hah, these people incorporated French culture."

Mr. Pyles is having pressure put on him by Mr. Reifel to get kids in schools. He acts in such a solicitous manner at everyone's expense but his own. He sent a girl up to the hospital with a note written by Mr. Quinn that stated the reason for referral was "Ear ailment. Should be examined thoroughly and if necessary referred elsewhere if she can't be treated here per Mr. Pyles' request." I questioned the woman. She said her girl hadn't been in school for several years because of ear trouble. The examination revealed bilateral otitis media, but she apparently told the Education people that her ear problem was the reason she'd not been in school. Said further she had come to the hospital time and time again for treatment, but nothing was ever done. A check of the record in the clinic revealed she had made TWO visits here for her ear, one in 1948 and one in 1950. She had not sought medical aid elsewhere. The fault for this girl not being in school lies with Education, and I've drafted a letter to Mr. Pyles with a statement to that fact in just those words.

May 11, 1954

Tonight Quiver, the jailor, brought a prisoner into the hospital. He is in jail on three accounts. Dr. Bragg examined him and thought the horrible pain he was complaining of in his abdomen was malingering. The prisoner asked to go to the toilet, and the jailor said "Okay." The prisoner escaped thru a hospital window. He is the guy who put up such a good story to me some time back of how the Peyote Church had reformed him. How he used to steal, fight, and get drunk but no more. Now all he wanted to do was good.

Tomorrow is National Hospital Day. We are having a program and open house. Seniors of OCHS and Holy Rosary Mission are invited to a program at ten a.m. The event has been well advertised.

Staff conferences this morning in Mr. Reifel's office. Roy Grube, Extension assistant, outlined a pretty stiff Withdrawal program. Apparently Withdrawal is in the air again, and the Indians are much disturbed by it. Mrs. Forshey said yesterday that one client of hers remarked that the sooner the white man got out of the Indians' way, the better anyway.

Eva Gap came into Mrs. Forshey's office yesterday in great anger. She wanted to know why we didn't go out to Porcupine for a peyote meeting on Saturday night. She said that everything had been set up for us. Her husband George Gap is president of the Cross Fire group out there. Mrs. Forshey thought she'd be down to see me about the same thing. Wilson Brady came into the office later. I told him about Eva going into Mrs. Forshey. He says George Gap isn't the president. You hear so many things around this place that are conflicting.

Dick Running Bear, who was main chief the other night and who goes to mass on the Sunday mornings after a peyote meeting, used to be one of the head men in Cross Fire, Wilson told me. But then he got to dabbling in the Half Moon also, and so Cross Fire kicked him out for trying to be in both groups.

May 12, 1954

A former president of the tribal council called today. His wife recently signed out of the Sioux Sanitarium. She has tuberculosis, and he wanted to get her back in the sanitarium. So I called to see if they'd take her and then went to the agency. Allan M. Adams there said the former president had tried to get a land sale for his wife. I learned her brother had some interest in it. So the probable reason for this man wanting to get his wife readmitted is so that he can spend the sale money when that happens.

Dr. Jubie Bragg, the new dentist, arrived today. His brother Robert is on our staff. I received a confidential letter today regarding a woman working as a blue girl at the hospital. She had an arrest record in 1940 that she failed to mention when she started to work in 1953. So I have to see now if it was an intentional or unintentional omission.

May 13, 1954

Last evening both Doctors Bragg were at the house for dinner when a man came in. He talked a minute and then wondered if I'd see his common-law wife because she wasn't feeling so well. I refused, not being on call. I told him to take her to the hospital. Dr. Quint was on call and would see her. That was about nine p.m. I learned later in talking to Dr. Quint that she did not go up there last night. Today the man brought his common-law wife into the hospital, where she had an upper respiratory infection treated. His ex-wife, from whom he is divorced, is the one who was in the accident near Hot Springs and was taken to Our Lady of Lourdes Hospital perhaps three or four months ago. I sent an ambulance for her, but she refused to come back here. So a couple of weeks ago she was still having some pain in one of her feet from a laceration as a result of that accident. She said, "Well Doctor, I suppose you are mad at me." She was referring to my having sent an ambulance for her and her not returning after all the expense and time.

Yesterday, Mr. Bob Reed from the state Rehabilitation Program and Johnny Artichoker, a former OCHS graduate and now with some state program, were in Pine Ridge. They are working on Mr. Pyles to start a special classroom for the thirty-six handicapped children on the reservation. They are not in school and perhaps in most all cases should be in special classes. But Mr. Pyles is reticent to start anything new.

They wanted to know if Health would examine and oversee the class. Now all of these kids should have been taken by the Education people to Rapid City to the Crippled Children's Clinic for diagnosis last week. Mr. Pyles didn't get around to it. So this made more work for us. Brother! What a day today. I called Miss Wayne, made two other long-distance calls, and performed administrative junk. I did everything except practice medicine.

Jeanne and I went down to White Clay Creek tonight and got some more wild flowers and bushes to transplant around the house. At last we have some grass coming up. The hot days and lots of moisture have brought things out and up. We have planted flower and vegetable seeds. But with no fence the horses will be walking across things soon.

May 18, 1954

The nursing situation is critical. We have only five nurses left. We can't do any surgery. Mrs. Coker and I went down to talk with Mr. Reifel last evening at 6:00 after a big clinic, so many people that some walked out, tired of waiting. I and other doctors also helped dispense medicines. I had to set up in ER. Douglas Horse was brought in all cut up about the head and face and arms. All he would say is someone did it. He has a brother-in-law, who probably is the one who did it. Then I had to admit Douglas. We simply have no help. I told Mr. Reifel I was on the way to Rosebud in the morning to operate over there because they have all their nurses. He said he would call Miss Wayne about it and about Dr. Bragg since they want him at Cheyenne for a week in June. Then Dr. Zumwalt goes on vacation.

I started out this morning. I got on the other side of Swett and had a flat and wrecked tire. The jack wouldn't work. A guy came along and jacked up my car. The spare had a big hole and boot on it. So I turned around and called Dr. Kurliecz at Rosebud from Batesland and said I'd come over on Thursday. Reported to Mr. Reifel when I got back, and he said Miss Wayne didn't want me to go over there and operate. I called her, and when I told her the story she said it would have been okay under the circumstances of having no nurses for surgery. But we decided we'd send this patient to Omaha. So Dr. Kurliecz will be burned. Miss Wayne was going to see about detailing a nurse from Rosebud and bringing her here. Dr. Kurliecz won't want that either. Miss McGill is back on duty. While Miss Holden is gone, she is acting director of nurses. She has all of our nurses in an uproar. This is the real reason nurse Stamley is off on sick leave. She is more sick in the head than elsewhere. Miss Wayne told me she didn't think Miss Valerie Pawluk, former chief of nurses here, would come back until Miss McGill was out of here.

Rosebud nurses won't come here because of her either. She says one thing and does another. A question she could answer with yes or no is answered with several hundred words of verbiage.

May 19, 1954

The CID [U.S. Army Criminal Investigation Command] got me out of bed last night. It is a fact that last night I got to bed at 10:00 p.m., the earliest since I've been here, and at 10:30 CID called to get a statement concerning a male patient. He was in the army and was drunk and fighting; then he broke into a liquor store with others and stole liquor. Miss Pease wrote a statement for me. But she put down that a fracture of the left leg was treated, and it happened to be the right leg. So the CID man came up to the hospital tonight and got another statement from me.

Had a call from Dr. Wanek in Gordon about Morris No More. I couldn't find him enrolled here. Mr. West of Extension and Mrs. Forshey of Welfare got on it. No More is an alias for Has No Horses. Mrs. Forshey told me George Has No Water is now an alias for George Bores a Hole.

I was looking over some stuff tonight about Yuwipi. Silas Yellow Boy, who was a member on the Half Moon peyote list that Levi Sitting Hawk showed us, is now practicing Yuwipi and helping Poor Thunder. I think probably what happened is that people like Silas and Willie Wounded, who know Yuwipi, probably tried peyote but are not active in the peyote services.

I have noticed something ever since I've been here. One Indian will go up to another in the hospital, usually grasp their hands, and give a few mournful sounds like wailing or crying. It is a display of sympathy. Maybe this is what Mari Sandoz calls the keening of the women in her book *Crazy Horse* when someone dies.

Miss Wayne called from Aberdeen this morning to say there was a nurse at Kyle who wanted to start work at the Sioux Sanitarium, but maybe we could get her here temporarily. I told her then instead of sending Dr. Bragg to Cheyenne Agency in June to send me for the week on temporary duty. I need to get away from this joint for awhile. She thought I was needed here and should not go, but though she wasn't definite she thought perhaps if I wanted to turn MOC [medical officer in charge] over to someone for awhile, maybe I could go.

May 21, 1954

The program planned for Mr. William Randolph Hearst Jr. was a fizzle. Mr. Quinn had asked me if I'd ride a horse, and I told him I would. They wanted some "cowboys" around. When the ten-car party passed Herd Camp they were going to have some cowboys rounding up cattle. The only good thing about the dance planned for Mr. Hearst was that photographers got some good pictures. Mr. Reifel was to drive out and meet the party at Winter or Martin or someplace, but when the party arrived Mr. Reifel was not with them.

There were to be speeches and various dances and a speech by Mr. Hearst. Nothing panned out. The speeches all were of only two sentences each and merely exchanges of greetings. I told Mr. Quinn I'd ride the horse Tiny Tim because I thought all the doings were going to take place near the Arts and Crafts shop. Actually most of the action was near Legion Hall. Mr. Hearst did visit the Arts and Crafts shop for five minutes, but I couldn't have taken pictures at Legion Hall and ride a horse at school to provide atmosphere. So I stayed and took pictures. Mr. Quinn and a couple Indians did ride the stallions.[1]

May 26, 1954

If this wouldn't cook your goose. The guy axed on the head by some woman in Rapid City a month and a half ago, who was present at the peyote meeting, caught me in the hospital. He said he was coming to the clinic Friday to see if it was okay to work because he had a chance to work at the rodeo for two days next week. I questioned him, and he said he gets dizzy occasionally. I asked him what he was to do. Ride? He said, "No." He would just "be a clown." Well, I talked on and on and told him I was sure he could do that. Then it came out. He said he was going to sue the woman who hit him with the ax. She is an Indian woman who has property here on the reservation, I guess. And he admitted he thought maybe it wouldn't be a good idea to be seen working if he were going to sue her.

The old chief came in today. He had been experiencing pain in the back, temperature elevation, and heavy breathing. On Saturday he saw Plenty Wolf, the medicine man. The Spirit told the medicine man the chief had a touch of pneumonia and should stay in bed for sixteen days. I took an X-ray. I told the chief's daughter. She said the Yuwipis were right, "But he is too darn ornery to stay in bed." It was a tussle to get him admitted. He wanted to go home. Then he finally consented to stay if he got a lot of meat to eat. He also wanted a room on the south side of the building so he could look out toward his home occasionally so he wouldn't get homesick.

Also the son-in-law of the chief came in. He had sprained his ankle last Saturday playing ball. Agnes told me she had gotten Plenty Wolf and taken Red Cloud to Plenty Wolf, and the Yuwipis said his leg was only sprained and for him to use crutches. She was at the hospital for crutches on Monday. But he wouldn't come in for me to see the leg because the Yuwipis had taken care of it. All he wanted was the crutches they had recommended. I gave them for him. But, of course, he had not been to work. So working for the school he needed a sick slip signed. So he had to come in to see me today. I X-rayed it. It was only a sprain. The patient said it had hurt badly until at the Yuwipi meeting where the Spirit pulled on his ankle and then it felt better.

I got a big kick out of reading the notes of the last tribal council meeting held the first of this month. A full day was taken to discuss Health and the Bimson Report. What these people think is that Health is being transferred to the state. They do not understand Health is being transferred to the Department of Health, Education, and Welfare. And, of course, they don't want it transferred to the state. They have been complaining about Health here, but the tune has changed. They now are pretty considerate compared to some time ago when all services might have been transferred or discontinued. I received notice not long ago that we were going to get a sanitary aid here. I then got a call from the Area Office today. We are going to now have a central pharmacy set up here for the Area.

I called Mr. Reifel yesterday about a woman with tuberculosis at Kyle. I have received complaints from her folks. She left her husband and kids and is running around spreading her microbes. There was a chance we could get her into San Haven in North Dakota. Mrs. Olinger is taking patients up there tomorrow. I called Mr. Reifel and asked if there was some way we could get her up there. "Should we try bluffing her?" he asked. "By doing what?" I wondered. "I could send John Richards out to her home to scare her." John Richards is a cop. That happened today, but I don't know what will come of it.

Mr. Reifel gets letters that he is required to answer. Some letters he refers to certain departments. He sends letters up to Health for me to answer for him. Mrs. Forshey does the same. But she is getting tired of doing it.

May 27, 1954

Mrs. Forshey told me I'd done something that had never been done before. That is to get the old chief in the hospital. Edgar was up here tonight and also said that had never been done before. The old chief is happy up there now. He felt much better today. His fever is down, and his nausea (pain) has subsided.

The superintendent here before Mr. Sande, Mr. Powers, gave a man written permission that he could rent his land himself. That is very much out of order to begin with since all renting is to be done through the agency. So this guy has been doing that, and then recently he put the land up for rent through the agency also. Ed Cocker rented to two people, and he can't get money out of one of them. He told Coker, "You can't get blood out of a turnip." They are smart. There is no way to get money from him to pay up.

The night before last Edgar knew where his son Vincent Red Cloud was. He was in a house nearby. So Edgar went over with Mary Ann to get the car. He found George Plenty Wolf had held a land sale. Someone had bought lots of liquor, and they were having quite a party. Marie Hand, who has fought with Edgar so much before, gave him lots of lip when he went after the car. It made Edgar mad, so he went down and reported it to the police. They arrested the bunch.

Yesterday, Edgar thought he'd go down and get them out of jail. Red Cloud speaks, and things happen! It wasn't so simple. Today they fined Vincent $14 but told Edgar if he'd pay $5 they'd let Vincent out. So he had $2 and got $3 from Mrs. Forshey. She lectured him about having his own son put in jail. Now he will have a police record. Edgar says he is sending Vincent out to work. That is really funny, knowing Vincent is twenty-four years old or older and has never worked before. Little Reno made it worse by telling Edgar, his dad, that he should not pay any money and leave Vincent in there a month if he wants to give him a lesson.

When I saw him, I told Red Cloud that George Plenty Wolf was in jail, and if he had such spiritual power, being a medicine man, why didn't the spirits get him out of jail. I wanted to see his reaction. He seemed concerned for a moment and then laughed and laughed. I could hear him still laughing as I was way down the hall.

May 28, 1954

Today we had a community services staff meeting in Mr. Reifel's office. Mr. Reifel is out of town. Mrs. Forshey was in charge. She presented what she thought a reservation program should be. Mr. Pyles, now acting superintendent, asked me to present the program next time, which will be June 25. Mrs. Forshey presented four problems and then a program. The problems included segregation, dependency, unemployment, and the cost to the government. Segregation is a problem especially in the schools. Dependency is a problem because of free services, and people use their incomes for pleasure only. Families go off reservation to work and return where there is no racism. Unemployment is high because the reservation can support only half of its residents if utilized. Wives frustrate husbands to get them to return to the reservation even when they have jobs. The cost to the Bureau of Indian Affairs is two million dollars a year for Pine Ridge alone, yet there seems to be no improvement in people's living standards.

Mrs. Forshey's program was directed to having the Indian find his place in society. They must do their own thinking.[2]

1. Strong public relations program. Families going off the reservation are considered only visitors to a city. We must educate the public that the Indian is a citizen and not a ward of the government.

2. Plan for Withdrawal based on actual situation. Taxation, have the state take over services only as it can. Increased emphasis on the Indian taking care of his own affairs.

3. Adult Education Program.

4. Private industry needs to enter this region.

Ben Irving, vice president of the newly elected tribal council, and Jake Herman, fifth member, were present.

Ben says there is a word for "tomorrow" now. The phonetic spelling is *Enck ee soppe* ("look out for tomorrow"). One trouble at getting to the Indians' problem is that there are no words for abstract words such as *time*, which is translated as "the moving iron" used after the first clocks they saw with the big swinging pendulums.

Alvin Zephier, head of Relocation, felt there was real segregation here, white versus Indians. No white felt that. Mr. Zephier is an Indian. All whites present admitted entertaining Indians in their homes. Then it came out that long ago bureau employees were looked upon as rulers, and Indians ran from them and took their spite out on the government, on the whites there working under rules and regulations of the government. What came out is that Indians are often invited and don't come. I presented this because we have invited Indians to our house, but they won't come. Then Jake, who does come to our house, says that it is due to the inferior feelings of the Indian because he can't then invite the whites back to his house because he has such a poor house. Okay. So part of it is economic and attitude on the part of the Indian.

Then Mr. Irving told how old concepts are carried over. And Jake said yes, and we preach these to our children. And it's wrong, he admitted. Ben Irving told a story of long ago that pointed up how Indians felt whites cheated them. An Indian was riding on a fine horse. He passed a white man who said let's trade horses. That white man was on an old nag. "How old is your horse?" asked the Indian. "He is four," answered the white man. They traded. When the Indian looked in the mouth of the horse he saw it had long teeth. The trade had already been made. Trying to pass it off, the white man said, "Yes, the horse has long teeth. They are not yet ground down." Yet the horse was really old. So now the Indians say let us tell lies and get something that way, too. So, says Ben, we do lie. Ben remembered when Indians wouldn't go to the hospital or to the agency garage. They felt doctors and mechanics were sent in here for short periods of time to do work on Indians, so as to become proficient, and then go out in private practice. However, he knows it is different. At the last I was on the phone, but Ben told Mrs. Forshey he would like to know the doctor better. At this meeting I heard the Indians admit many wrongs. I felt more accord going through the group.

At the same time, the whites admitted wrongs by whites in outlying cities of accepting Indians.

May 29, 1954

At yesterday's staff conferences in Mr. Reifel's office I remember that Ben Irving, the vice president of the tribal council, said the Indians' motto always used to be "Prepare for today. Worry not about tomorrow for tomorrow will come anyway."

Alvin Zephier was hot under the collar when he said there was discrimination by white employees against Indians. It sort of shows something. He was hot and bothered and felt that way himself. Mr. Reifel, also an Indian, was not present. Mr. Reifel can look at things objectively. The whole thing just shows why white administrators have not succeeded here in the past.

Today old Red Cloud insisted on leaving the hospital to buy some groceries and then go home. "How will you go? I asked. He made the sign language for walking. I told him to wait until tomorrow, and Agnes would pick him up and then bring him back here. He is going to Kyle where his mother is buried and some aunts. To Mission where the original chief and others of the family are buried. Then to the Episcopal cemetery where Jack is buried.

Well, I thought he said okay. Then this afternoon he was running around outside in his pajama top and his own trousers. We let him wear his own trousers in the hospital since he insisted on keeping on his wooden leg and he wanted his trousers to cover it up. An X-ray taken this morning shows practically no change in his condition, though he says he feels better. Mrs. McCrimmon was then chasing him around. She came to me and said he wouldn't come back in and he wanted his clothes, underwear, and such brought out. I told her to let him have them.

Eleven. June 1954

We ended up with different plans today than we had expected after Miss Holden and I went out there a couple weeks ago. Miss Wayne and Mrs. Jones think it would be best to use the "practice cottage" out there for a clinic. It is a log house and has no running water or electric lights. Those will have to be put in. It will be necessary to start from scratch. Then she will have to live in one of the school homes or houses. Miss Wayne asked me to talk with Mr. Reifel. I did tonight at the hospital picnic. He just told me to talk to Mr. Bertsch. So there you are. A Public Health nurse, no facilities, and no chance of getting any then. So we will be left stranded.

June 4, 1954

Aggie Iron Cloud said that James Red Cloud was Catholic, or at least he went to the Catholic Church to get something to eat, she told me. That is more likely. I know that because that guy has faith in Yuwipi.

Today I got a letter from Mrs. Forshey marked "PERSONAL AND CONFIDENTIAL." It was about someone I know well. Some weeks ago, Dr. Gassman had said that this man was okay to work and would not permit him to get Aid to Dependent Children any longer. The reservation Welfare person is working closely with the state welfare office. The man has a past record of angina. I'll have to follow through on Dr. Gassman's findings and say he is okay to work. Mrs. Forshey is concerned because the man is such a good friend of both of us. I could see why, but I don't feel I want to sacrifice principles for friendship. It must be a poor friendship if he severs it simply because he can't get welfare or relief from her.

Thursday Mr. Mickelson wondered if I'd go to school to see one of their palominos that is pregnant and received a large laceration just in back of the right front leg. It was infected. I gave him some zephrine to clean it with several times a day. Told him if it got worse we'd give the horse penicillin.

I can't be sure how I felt yesterday when Mr. Reifel showed me the rating of my performance he was sending in on me. All traits, characteristics, and work habits he checked "excellent" except two, which he checked "very good." They were "judgment" and "appearance." And under "remarks for improvement" he stated that I could do better if I used smaller words since I was working with illiterate persons.

I went out to Wanblee this morning and saw Father John Bryde out there. He is conducting Bible school. Father Bryde told me he didn't know the difference between Half Moon and Cross Fire peyote and, in fact, didn't even know there were two groups. I blurted out, "How long have you been here?" Then, when he told me four years, I was dumb-founded. Out there Mrs. Winters came up to me gloating. "You better come and see this woman. She had her baby. I had her at clinic last Tuesday, and you said she wouldn't deliver until June 26." Well, I hadn't even seen the woman. She had been to see Dr. Walters.

I drove the hundred miles to Wanblee with Miss Holden and also Mr. Charles Swallow to check on quarters for the new nurse who is to be here a week from Monday. The Health quarters out there are the doctor's house that Bruce H. Ecker, the school principal, uses. He was on pins and needles, afraid we'd take the house because it is the nicest dwelling out there. But I told Miss Holden I didn't think we'd take it. It is too big for living quarters and would cost too much rent for the new nurse, and I don't want clinic and quarters in the same building. We then looked at the old clinic building and nurses' quarters in one that is now used as a dormitory for kids in winter.

After I got back we had a conference in Mr. Reifel's office and called in Mr. Pyles. He said that if we took two of the six rooms he couldn't operate a dormitory, because it would be too costly. But Mr. Pyles suggested we use the farm agent's house. Anything not to inconvenience him! There is no running water up there. What a shyster. So I believe we'll take parts of his buildings. We decided to wait and let Mrs. Rosalie Jones, the nurse, make decisions as to where she wants her clinic and living quarters. That way, since it is so horrible out there, she won't be kicking too darn much, or as much.

June 10, 1954
Thursday

I left Tuesday for Deadwood to testify before the Federal District Court. The Black Hills were pretty as I drove north, so green and fresh. It was cold enough after I left Uncle Orrin's place to turn on the car heater. I went up through Hill City thereby bypassing Rapid City.

Little, antiquated Deadwood is plastered against the sides of a draw. The steepness of the hills is more than California's. This city lives in the past, in the era of 1876, the year Wild Bill Hickok was killed by Jack McCall and when Calamity Jane and Potato Creek Joe were popular. I found a room available at the Franklin Hotel but couldn't find a place to park. Close that is. The clerk at the hotel gave me a convention sticker that exempted me from plugging the meters. I moved in closer when a space was available.[1]

I met Dr. Michael Kurilecz, medical officer in charge (MOC) from Rosebud, who was there to testify on a manslaughter case. It involved Antoine Medicine, who killed two white men down by Martin.

Yesterday we went to court and wasted the morning hanging around the courthouse. They told us at noon to come back at four o'clock. So we drove to Spearfish and then to Lead looking for antiques. We returned at four, and they said they wouldn't need me for perhaps a week. Mike would testify the next day. So we shopped and then had dinner and then decided to go to bed. I wanted to read and rest. Mike said he would come and get me at 10:00 p.m. He wanted to go to a particular bar and see about getting two wire chairs from a fellow. But as we started out the door we met Wayne Bunch, a highway patrolman, and Dennis

LaCompt, special officer from Pine Ridge. With them was Jim Geboe, special officer from Rosebud, and Mr. Conoyer, in charge of vital statistics at Rosebud, and later three Indians. They wanted to treat us to a drink. They were all stewed already. Later, Mr. Bunch showed us the town. He grew up partially in Deadwood. We ran into Leroy Janis, an officer from Kyle, and Mathew Eagle Heart, special officer from Pine Ridge, and they also were inebriated. So there wasn't a law and order fellow in town I knew besides Joe Swift Bird and old George Iron Cloud who wasn't sloshed.

I drove on to Rapid City then home after a mission there. The hills and roadsides again today were in their prime. There are gobs of tourists on the highways. All the attractions are in full glory. Uncle Orrin told me Tuesday that Henry Standing Bear had wanted once to buy a portion of his land to put in an Indian crafts shop along the highway. Uncle Orrin says that at one time he knew James Red Cloud.

I arrived home to a voluminous amount of mail.

June 17, 1954

Jeanne came home Wednesday. The baby, Edna, was born last Saturday morning. She had so many visitors at the hospital that she didn't get much rest anyway. Having a new baby in the house changes the routine, the appearance of the house, and many other things.

I tried to put out a washing of diapers and blew out a box of 20 amp fuses and a box of 15 amp fuses this noon. For several days while doing the washing when Jeanne was in the hospital I got a shock from the water in the sink in the utility room. As Mr. Boob Janis, the garbage man, said this noon "Your house is the poorest constructed house in the town."

I drove out to see Edgar Red Cloud last night and bring him a picture I'd taken of Reno and also to take a picture of the peyote meeting to Wilson Brady. Wilson just sold a piece of land belonging to his wife. Traded it even for a "new" 1950 Chevy straight across. So he is never home now. He came to the house this noon and got his picture. He says he'll let us record some peyote songs on a tape recorder that Dr. Walters has borrowed.

I found Edgar home. He and his entire family had planned to leave yesterday for location in the Black Hills for the filming of the Crazy Horse motion picture. But they didn't get off. Reno is going to play the part of Crazy Horse as a boy. Mary Ann and Edgar are also going to be in the picture. Edgar says he will play the part of a chief. He borrowed the chief's costume. I asked him if the chief was going. Edgar said the movie people wouldn't take the chief unless he got an okay from the doctors.

Today the bus picked up some people for the movie location. Quite a number are going. But the bus ran off the road, knocked over some fence posts or something, but hurt no one. And the Trailways bus came here in town to pick up some others. I saw the old chief getting on the bus, the sly devil. They will be gone on location for about one month.

Miss Holden's last day of work was to have been at noon today. She is still here and says she'll have to work tomorrow and feels she may have to come back on Monday to finish ordering. Eldon LaCourse was over here this morning and says he thought now we'd have $4,000 left to spend as this fiscal year ends in a couple of weeks and so Miss Holden is ordering drugs and so on like fury.

Mrs. Reifel wanted a bottle of distilled water for her iron. She knows that there is so much mineral content in this water around here that it would soon fill up an iron with mineral deposits. So I gave her a bottle. She said her daughter is in need of an ophthalmological examination. She said that Mr. Reifel asked her not to bother the doctors up here, but she wondered about Dr. Quint. I assured her he was very good. She wanted to make an appointment. So I took her to see Dr. Quint. Besides, she said the money here isn't going to make any influence on what the doctor recommends. Besides, she said the personal attention is better.

The hospital is quiet. Few patients. Not too much surgery. Five operations this week, but that wasn't any real strain. Miss Wayne is coming in tomorrow with Mrs. Jones, the new Public Health nurse who will probably be assigned to Wanblee.

June 19, 1954

Pugh Young Man of Whose Horses They Are Afraid came in Friday. He goes by Pugh Afraid of Horses generally and sometimes Pugh Young Man. Pugh is legally or rightfully a chief. His father was Amos, oldest son of Chief Young Man of Whose Horses They Are Afraid. The chief died in 1912. Amos is also Afraid of Horses. Pugh told me that Frank Afraid of Horses was a son of the chief and is his uncle, but Frank is younger than Pugh's father would be and is a son of the chief's second wife. Pugh's grandfather, or the chief, had all the dealings with McGillycuddy. It is this chief's father who was the original chief of this group long ago and whose power was usurped by Red Cloud and Crazy Horse. This was simply because the last chief, the one during the McGillycuddy era, was too young to fight the white men, and the original chief was too old.

The annual Sun Dance is to be held July 28 through 31. It is open to tourists. Red Bear is giving one for his wife on July 1 that is private. His wife had an operation at the hospital and can see again. So he is going to offer thanks to the Great Spirit. Mr. Reifel told me tonight it would be as real as is possible to have a dance without the torture aspects. He said he thought it would be the last real dance, private one, that is. I plan to go and get some pictures.

Miss Wayne drove in last night and brought Mrs. Jones, our new Public Health nurse for Wanblee. I had a conference with her last night. She said if Mrs. Valeria Pawluk didn't want to come back here that she might send over Miss Glyndine F. Golden from Rosebud. She said she is going to try to get rid of Miss McGill because neither of them will come here if McGill is here. I told her that by the same token I wouldn't stay on as moc if Miss McGill stayed on as acting chief nurse. The new nurse is to transfer here from the Sioux Sanitarium.

Today I took the hospital car. Miss Wayne and Mrs. Jones followed me to Martin. We left Miss Wayne's car there, and I took them all to Wanblee. We went to show Mrs. Jones the place and also to acquaint Miss Wayne with it. Since there is no equipment and the buildings are not so hot, I thought Mrs. Jones would be discouraged, but she didn't seem to be. Mrs. Jones is colored. She doesn't need any push. I'm afraid she is going to push us to get going. She has her ideas all set in her mind. She has done much similar work among Negroes in Georgia.

We ended up with different plans today than we had expected after Miss Holden and I went out there a couple weeks ago. Miss Wayne and Mrs. Jones think it would be best to use the "practice cottage" out there for a clinic. It is a log house and has no running water or electric lights. Those will have to be put in. It will be necessary to start from scratch. Then she will have to live in one of the school homes or houses. Miss Wayne asked me to talk with Mr. Reifel. I did tonight at the hospital picnic. He just told me to talk to Mr. Bertsch. So there you are. A Public Health nurse, no facilities, and no chance of getting any. So we will be left stranded.

We had lunch with the Eckerts. He is the principal at Wanblee. Bruce H. and Mrs. Eckert both used to teach when they were at Sisseton, South Dakota. When they were at Sisseton there was a four-and-a-half-year-old half Indian and half Mexican girl in the hospital, an invalid. Her mother was full-blood Indian. The child was illegitimate. The next summer the girl needed care and rest but could have gone somewhere had she a home and someone to take her. The Eckerts said they'd take her for the summer. The second day that they had her, the girl called them mother and father. Then they started to adopt the girl, a long-winded procedure that took a full year. She said many of their friends, educated people, opposed the adoption. But they went ahead. Besides, they were told the girl would need hospital care from time to time and that she would probably be an invalid. Now the ten-year-old girl is in strong health. She lugs the Eckerts' two little boys around like small sacks of flour when it is orange juice time or time to wash a face. She is the sweetest and most well-mannered, cute little child. The girl has seen her mother only once since she became old enough to remember the encounter. The Eckerts said they have a household of kids in all the time to play with their three kids. Georgie Brown, brother of Victor Brown, comes to their home lots, especially right at meal times. Mrs. Eckert said that Georgie can stow away more food than her husband. He once drank a quart of milk at meal time.

There was a hospital picnic tonight for Miss Holden, who leaves on Wednesday. The hospital staff gave her gifts. Mr. Reifel brought a gift from the agency employees. There was a good turnout tonight for the party.

With a new baby in the house and not able to get help, it means that I must run a hospital, do so much traveling such as the two-hundred-mile trip today, and then come home and cook meals, do dishes, clean house, which I do each day, shop, and wash diapers. I blew five fuses on Thursday trying to wash a washer full of diapers. The water in the utility room rinse sink still shocks me when I put my hands in it. So there is a short somewhere. This house is a mess. I mowed our lawn. There is green in much of the area around the house. How interesting to take a picture on August 8, our anniversary for arriving at this joint, and seeing the difference from last year.

June 21, 1954

I performed two operations yesterday. I was worn out. One was a ruptured appendix case from Rosebud. Dr. Kurliecz asked me to take it. I told him I couldn't, because we have no nurses. He called Miss Wayne in Pierre. She said to send the patient over with a nurse. They did. One of our helpers was off or just didn't show up. The cops found him out on a drinking party. I called Mr. Reifel. He said that if that was so he'd can him.

Mr. Reifel called me about 7:30 this evening and asked if we'd like some strawberries. We said yes. He said he'd be over. The Reifels brought us a huge pan of strawberries. He and Alice spent some time visiting. What amazed me is that Mr. Reifel knows I went to a peyote meeting. He mentioned something about it, and I told him. Mrs. Forshey, with whom I went, said she was going to tell him she went to that and to a Yuwipi service, but she said she wouldn't mention me. I could tell him myself. So I don't know how he knew or found out. He didn't have anything to say about my going. We were simply discussing peyote and the Native American Church. He told me Poor Thunder, the medicine man, goes over into North Dakota also. Mr. Reifel says he has quite a circuit. He says he wishes he could channel those activities into something worthwhile. He looked at my beautiful picture of the battle of Wounded Knee by Andrew Standing Soldier and said Andrew should do something abstract.

I mentioned something about Jo Ann Gildersleeve from the reservation singing "Indian Love Call" for some contest. I mentioned that Ethel Merrival sang it at the inauguration and I said I thought she did a good job. Then Ethel was the subject. "That's right. She was one of the first persons you talked to me about right after you came." I told him that since then, I hadn't heard a word out of her or by her. He just beamed. But he really has done a remarkable job of shutting that woman up.

Mrs. Reifel says her daughter Louise and Jo Ann Gildersleeve are leaving today for Custer State Park to be in the movie "Crazy Horse." Jo Ann's folks are the Gildersleeves from Wounded Knee who run that store out there. Mr. Reifel was going to call Father Harold Fuller today to borrow women's buckskin costumes for the girls. He showed us on the map where the film is being made. He said if we go up there, we should look up Dave Miller and tell him where we were from, and he would supply us with dinner, with the stars, no less. Mr. Reifel has read the script and told us about it. It is going to be a boy-girl-boy movie. In the end, Crazy Horse is shot by the boyfriend of his wife, or something like that. A love story.

A month ago we were watering our ground about the house constantly to keep it moist and soft so grass would grow. Now we have quite a bit of grass with bare spots mostly where Captain runs, and we don't have to water it so often.

Dr. Gassman is back from vacation. Miss Holden leaves in the morning for her home on her retirement. I bid her goodbye tonight. I do hate to see her leave. Mrs. Coker in is charge now while McGill is on leave. Mrs. Coker is good but has not had the experience. Miss McGill has had the experience and is awful.

June 23, 1954

I left the hospital at 7:00 this morning for Rapid City by a new route for me. I went up to Red Shirt Table and then on up to Rapid City. It is much shorter, but much of the route is gravel. I still made better time than the usual way. I took Willard Under Baggage with me on business. He is the grandson of the previous president of the Sioux tribal council. His grandmother, Nancy, and his father, Russell, are both ill.

Today was the hottest day so far. It was 104 in Chadron. I stopped a moment in Rapid City and then went to Hermosa where I had lunch. I then went on down to Custer State Park where Universal-International is filming the picture *Chief Crazy Horse*. I was able to get inside the ropes. There were gobs of spectators. It was so out of the way that I don't see how so many tourists knew about it and found it. Just as I drove in the area where they were filming, I saw and talked to Mr. Reifel. He had with him Miss Theisz, whom he'd picked up in Rapid City. She is from New York and is interested in Indian affairs.

I went on over to the place where they were filming. The first person I saw that I knew was Edgar Red Cloud. Edgar had on a wig of long braided hair and extra brown for makeup. He looked like an Indian for sure. He took me in to meet Dave Miller. Dave is in charge of the Indians. Then he introduced me to the company doctor, John Tracey. John told me he was a registered nurse rather than a doctor, but he'd been with the navy as a hospital corpsman for over twenty years. John was handing out salve for sunburns, headache pills, eye ointments, and so on. He ran out of salt tablets, and everyone was giving him a hard time.

The setting was one of numerous Indian tepees. I saw Andrew Fools Crow. He sent Dave for me knowing I was here. Andrew said he had a loose tooth. He wiggled it. I told him we'd just pull it. We went over to the "docs" tent, but then when we started to do so, he backed down and showed us that several more were loose. He said he just wanted something for pain.

Edgar told me that white men fixed up to look like Indians looked more like Indians than the Indians themselves. That was partly true. Ben Chief from Pine Ridge was there. He doesn't look any more like an Indian than I do.

John Tracey spent most of the three hours I was there telling me about his past experiences, the company medical advantages, and so on. He introduced me to practically everyone, from the lowest flunky to the director, Mr. Sherman, who had been out here four years ago to film *Tomahawk*. He introduced me to John Lund, the actor who Tracey says is tops.[2] He introduced me to Robert Warwick, acting the part of a chief. Robert is an idol of the old silent film days.[3]

The stars are Victor Mature, Suzan Ball, and John Lund. Victor Mature is playing the part of Crazy Horse. I caught him during a lull drinking a can of beer.[4] Suzan Ball had one of her legs removed last January because of a melanoma. She recently married. John Tracey told me the studio bought her wedding dress and paid for her honeymoon.[5] Her husband is a bit player. Her nurse called me aside once and said that Susan was having a lot of trouble with her stump. She had first gotten a stump to fit high heels. Now, just before coming here, she got a new stump for low heels, since she has to wear moccasins. The nurse said she was having so much trouble. I told her that that was to be expected with a new stump.

Mr. Sherman said he liked to work with the Oglala Sioux. They were quick and had a good sense of humor. I saw many of our Indians, many who knew me but whom I didn't recognize because I couldn't tell who they were with makeup on. I saw Ben American Horse—who lives near Oglala, is ninety years of age, was in the Custer battle and has a wound in his leg to prove it—playing Sitting Bull in the movie. I also saw Matthew Two Bulls, who applied for a sanitary aid job at the agency but didn't have enough education to get it.

I was interested in the rock fires, the make-believe clay bowls and dishes, and the racks with strips of imitation meat drying. I enjoyed talking with the special effects man, who told me how he made arrows "go into" a person's chest. How he made the "bullets" hit rocks or wood, and how he made machine gun effects. He puts numerous little capsules of a powder where the bullet is to hit and each one is wired to a gadget to set them off. Thus he can rapidly produce noise and smoke of bullets hitting in dirt or a building.

They are to move next week to Red Shirt Table on the reservation for more filming. Afterward they are going to take some shots down around Crawford, Nebraska. I had to laugh. Universal Studios is complaining because they wanted to hire and feed 85 Indians. But there were 250 who came, and so they are having a hell of a time feeding that many. If they knew these people, they would have planned on more food.

I got home tonight after first stopping at Hot Springs to check on a man who was taken to the hospital while I was in Deadwood. He'd been shot in the leg by police for stealing and running from John Richards. He was doing fine.

When I got home I checked my mail. Among notes was a note from Weldon Rolfe to get me to sign an authorization to purchase stamps, saying Miss Holden had done so before she left. I'd be willing to bet my bottom dollar that is not so. I'll sign it, but I'm going to write and ask Miss Holden if that is so. I'll bet it isn't. I also found a copy of HR 303, 83d Congress second session, Calendar #1541, a bill for the transfer of Indian Health to the Department of Health, Education, and Welfare.[6]

Mrs. Jones, the new Public Health nurse, made a trip with Mr. Pyles to Wanblee to settle the issue as to what house she'd get. Mr. Bertsch of Maintenance went along. Tonight she told me that Mr. Pyles takes the path of least resistance when it comes to Education. Amen. She has found him out perfectly. He is a stinker. But she stuck to her guns and got a desirable building.

June 26, 1954

It never fails to happen. I thought it being Saturday I'd get to sleep in. I get that feeling of happy wishes every Saturday. So I read the *New York Times* until 1:00 a.m. and then had fitful periods of rest. Baby Edna was wakeful through last night. This morning I was sound asleep at 8:30 when John Richards, a cop, called and said there was a child lying in a yard on the east end of town, dead. He came after me and took me over. It was Taylor Palmier's kid. He was apparently electrocuted in last night's storm. The lightening was flashing right close. There were two wires lying across his neck.

I really had a conference with Mr. Pyles. Old Albert is trying desperately to retain his control of houses that belong to the Health department at Wanblee. He does not want to inconvenience himself in having Mrs. Jones, our nurse, move out there. He made some statement to Mr. LaCourse and Mr. Bertsch and me that he would give up one of Education's houses to her. I made it plain to him that I didn't like his attitude because he wasn't giving us a thing. Health has a huge four-bedroom house out there that the principal Mr. Eckert is using and wishes to keep. So in return for that a smaller house was no gift from Education.

Dr. Walters really blew up the other day. We are now having very hot weather, up to 104 degrees. Not sultry like St. Louis and not noticed as much. But it is ice tea time. The old clunky old refrigerator given Joe Walters wouldn't make ice cubes. So he was really blowing his stack. I don't blame him. But it is Maintenance's job to get him a new one since his original one blew out. Well, I ordered one for him, but it isn't here. Then I told Mrs. Coker to put the good one from the emergency room in his house. I guess he didn't know I'd done that so he was even lighting into me.

The medicine man who conducts the Yuwipi meetings in English is Mark Big Road from Manderson. Wilson Brady was just in. Wilson told me he is going to Scottsbluff to be main chief tonight in a peyote prayer meeting. There is always a lot of activity around Scottsbluff. The peyote users there have a tent for their meetings. Now that the Indians know me and know that I have no designs to stop their meetings, they don't hesitate to tell me a thing about where they are going or who belongs to their church. Levi Sitting Hawk told me about the early days when the law was after them all the time. He says at the present time they are getting their supply of peyote from Texas, without any trouble.

Levi tells this story. There was once a Comanche Indian who got lost from his band. He wandered around the hills for days with no food. He became very tired and famished. Finally he couldn't go on any further. He'd been wandering around trying to find his band. When he lay down he heard the steady beat like a drum. It was a rapid continual beating. He looked around but couldn't see anyone. He looked across the ravine to a hill on the other side from where he thought the noise came. But he couldn't see anyone. He got up and started to where he thought the noise came from. He couldn't see a thing. But the beating noise sounded louder as he approached the side of the hill. Presently he came to the spot where it sounded as if the noise was originating there. There wasn't a thing unusual in sight. The noise was coming from down at the ground. Still he couldn't see a thing. He bent down. The noise was coming from the inside of a plant, the peyote. He broke off the plant. He ate it. It was bitter, but soon he felt refreshed after eating the succulent plant. And so developed the peyote cult, eating the "button" as a sacrament in worship of the Great Spirit who provides for all needs.

June 28, 1954

Saturday was quite a day. First I was called for a conference about the electrocution of Buster Palmier. Then the school found another injured horse, a palomino yearling that had torn an eight-inch strip of hide off its chest. I went over and sewed it up, hoping the torn hide will live and grow. Then Dr. Gassman's dog, Penny, got hit by a car. They were all upset and thought it had a large laceration, and so they called me to come sew it, but it was just an abrasion. And I found a large dent in

217

the right rear side of my government Pontiac. I don't know when that was done, but certainly not when I was in it.

Jeanne and I were honored. Charlie Yellow Boy told me that the Indians had named our little girl Oglala Wi, which means Oglala Woman.

I talked to Miss Wayne last weekend. She said Miss Golden from Rosebud would be released if it was okay with the superintendent over there. She would probably be here until November when Miss Pawluk will be back.

I had quite an enjoyable ride Sunday. I went to Oglala. I went out to Willie Wounded's and talked with him. He is probably one of the most popular medicine men around here. Willie came out of his house wearing glasses. He is a thin, stooped, frail-looking sort of person. Remembering the story that he had tuberculosis and was sent home from the agency hospital to die and then he became a medicine man, I thought he had something now. He was breathing hard, I noticed, like an asthmatic. Then Willie told me he had asthma. His hair was short. I thought he'd have long braided hair. In the yard was a cooler. His wife was boiling water over a fire. Downhill a ways was the sweathouse. I told Willie if he would come to the hospital I would give him some medicine. I asked Willie if I could come and take a picture of his altar. Then he told me, and repeated it twice again before I left, that he just doesn't go out, but his services are "by the people, for the people, and of the people" and that he is asked to go somewhere.

Willie told me he became a medicine man about fifteen years ago. But his own story is different. He was driving a Packard late one night. Just after turning off Highway 18, coming up the hills, and reaching his place, he rolled his car over after he passed Number Four Day School and crossed the bridge. He wasn't found until the next morning. He was paralyzed on the right side of his body. But he worked his hands and feet and showed me he was all right now. It was then that he went to the mountain to become a medicine man.

He treated his wife once for four days when she had a serious ailment. She got no better. So he then sent her to the hospital here, and she was sent to Omaha for surgery. He has been working on a guy with a stroke at Rosebud. Willie told me he got the guy's mouth to come back some. Then he said he got one of his legs to come back some. Willie tells me he doesn't have a license from the tribe. Joe One Feather told me Willie did have a license. Willie says the medicine men at Rosebud are licensed. I told him I'd been in one of Poor Thunder's meetings. Willie says, "Those old guys are awful slow." It was Willie who tended Red Cloud for his pneumonia and also Dick Elk Boy for his sprained ankle. Dick said the spirits pulled his foot, and it felt better afterward. Willie, in telling me about it, said he was the one who pulled Dick's leg.

Ira Elk Boy just came in tonight and picked up the picture that I took of him one time. He was quite pleased with it. He had seen Wilson Brady's picture of the peyote meeting and the altar, and he says that once he tried to take some pictures with black-and-white film, but they didn't come out. He says that on July 24 he is going to have one of the fellows who has a tepee bring it over from Scottsbluff and hold a meeting at his place. He wants me to come out and take some pictures for him. I'll be very glad to oblige.

I saw Levi Sitting Hawk in the clinic today and asked him if he went to the meeting in Scottsbluff last Saturday night, the one Wilson went to. He said no, he went to a peyote meeting at Porcupine on Saturday. Father's Day was recently. They had a big meeting in the tepee that day in Scottsbluff.

Twelve. July 1954

Nell Coker was telling me the other day that Ben Reifel told her husband that he now chooses the places where he stops his car. This was prompted by a story that one of the agency workers stopped his car out someplace, and those who had it in for him slugged him. So even old Ben has some fear of his own people, just for trying to help them.

July 1, 1954

Joe Red Bear of Oglala is giving a Sun Dance as a vow he made to the Great Spirit if his wife could again see. She had an operation for cataracts and can now see. So today was to be the beginning. John Means of Wounded Knee got a half a buffalo from the state park for the deal.

Dr. Walters and I went out today to take pictures. When we got to Oglala and saw the camp groups, there were perhaps not more than a dozen or so tents. We went up to one where there was a cooler and some Indians, half a dozen women and three old men sitting around.[1] Mrs. Red Bear was in a tent nearby on the bed. She is ill yet with various ailments. We talked awhile with the Indians there. They said the religious part of the Sun Dance probably won't begin until tomorrow or the next day. There would be some sort of dance tonight, but not the regular part.

In a couple of tents down, the grandma brought over the two Swimmer twins. She asked us if we wanted to take a picture of them. We had our camera equipment with us and did want their picture. We went back to the first place and then went out and took a picture of a regular tepee. We don't see tepees much anymore, just tents.

Finally Mr. Means asked who we were. We introduced ourselves. There were some ohs and ahs, as there usually is, when they said, "Aren't you the head doctor?" When I told them yes, Mr. Means said how about fixing us up to get some of the relief money. These people have the idea that I dole out the money. I told him that relief funds are not mine to disburse and that I have no jurisdiction over them. They had to see Mrs. Forshey for those. Finally, Mr. Means said to me, "Do you know who this is?" He pointed to an old man sitting on a chair. He had on a dirty black felt hat, a blue and red flannel shirt, a pair of old navy blue trousers, no socks, and a pair of beaded moccasins. I said, no, that I didn't know him. "That is Dewey Beard," Mr. Means said.

I can remember once when compiling some stuff on the battle of Wounded Knee that Dewey Beard was mentioned and that I almost drove to Cedar Pass, which is up near the Badlands National Monument, to talk with him. What an opportunity today. No Sun Dance, but this would suffice for this trip out. I asked Dewey to pose for me. He did that gladly. Then he asked for money. We gave him money. Dr. Walters took pictures too. Dewey had stood by a horse belonging to another fellow so Dewey handed half the money to that guy.

Dewey doesn't speak English. He showed us the card he carries that reads, "This is to introduce you to Dewey Beard (Iron Nail). He is a full blooded Sioux." Mr. Beard is ninety-two years old. He is a survivor of the battle of the Little Bighorn and of Wounded Knee. Dewey said he knew Crazy Horse well. He said he had been in four battles with him. What I was most interested in asking Dewey Beard was, "Who fired the first shot at the battle of Wounded Knee?" He said, "The army men took all the bows and arrows, guns, and other weapons from the Indians. There was one Indian who had a gun and wouldn't give it up. Two soldiers went out to take it away from him and in the scuffle the Indian fired his gun."

Then Dewey asked, "That is a big murder. Do you know it?"

I replied, "Yes."

Dewey said they tried to get him to go where they are filming the movie on Red Shirt Table, but they wouldn't pay him enough. He gets lots of money for personal appearances all over.

I shook hands with Dewey, and he left. His wife was nearby. She offered me her stool to sit on. Then Mr. Means said the Indians don't make a fuss over Dewey like the white people do.

Dewey showed me wounds on his chest, his back, and his left thigh that he got in the Wounded Knee battle. I checked in the agency enrollment book, which lists Dewey Beard's birth date as 1862. Dewey had said this morning that he was fifteen at the time of the Custer battle of 1876.

Here at the hospital Mrs. Olinger, who is the Public Health nurse at Kyle where Dewey's home is, says that Dewey was married, and his wife was killed in the Wounded Knee battle. They had a tiny baby, and Dewey has always had the feeling that it was his baby who was adopted by one of the white army officers.

Edgar had told me that Reno was going to play the part of little Crazy Horse. But I see in today's Rapid City paper that Todd Fast Wolf of Red Shirt Table is to be the young chief.

July 6, 1854

Nell Coker was telling me the other day that Ben Reifel told her husband that he now chooses the places where he stops his car. This was prompted by a story that one of the agency workers stopped his car out someplace, and those who had it in for him slugged him. So even Mr. Reifel has some fear of his own people, just for trying to help them.

We have a janitor's job open, and all applicants so far are not worth a darn. So when I saw Chief Pugh Afraid of Horses, I asked him if he wanted a job at the hospital. Pugh said he was interested. He said he would come in this week to see me.

Amen! I heard from the American College of Surgeons. I made the grade. I have to go to Atlantic City on November 15, I believe it is, in cap and gown for my fellowship. And, of course, send them money.[2]

We have a house full of guests: mother-in-law [Mrs. Henderson], Mrs. Ella Scott, and her son, Dick Scott, all of Chelan.

July 8, 1954

Mr. Reifel sent up an envelope marked "To be opened by Dr. Ruby only." In it was a letter to Pierre LeGrande, the hospital orderly, concerning his AWOL of a couple Sundays ago. Mr. Reifel was going to fire him, but Mrs. Coker let him make up the day later in that week. So Mr. Reifel didn't think the charges against him would be severe enough. Pierre was intoxicated the day he was off. He has so many past records of having been drunk and off duty that it is high time to get rid of him. Mr. Reifel's letter was a warning. No definite action is to be taken until Pierre writes Mr. Reifel a letter explaining his actions on that day. Pierre told me he was going to get a lawyer to write that letter for him.

July 8, 1954

You'd die if you knew what I was doing. There are times when I get so disgusted with Indians. One kid, who is eighteen years old, is only in third grade. I handed him a box of ACPS [acetaminophen, such as Tylenol] with directions, and asked if he could read it. He said, "Yes." He started to dash out. So I said, "Wait, read it to me." Then he said he couldn't. So I spelled it out, and he still couldn't read it. So I told him what it said. Next patient was a fourteen-year-old girl with a bloody nose. I asked if she'd ever had a bloody nose before. "Yes." How long ago? She didn't know. Well, ten years? "No." Then how long? She knew it wasn't ten years ago, but she couldn't give me an idea of how long ago. So I walked off and left her there to think about it. While she thought, I told her I'd come back and then finish examining her. It was 9:00 p.m.

Well, something more pleasant. The baby is growing by leaps and bounds. Edna will be four weeks Saturday. She can turn on either side from her back or from her stomach. Can't hold her head up completely yet but she can sure turn it around, and she looks at things. She is having a little bowel trouble. Not enough water in her diet. So now we are giving her water and orange juice mixed.

Mrs. Henderson (Jeanne's mother) and the Scotts are here yet, will be a week Saturday. Today they went up around to Kadoka and through the Badlands National Monument. They also went to Wounded Knee today. They went by themselves because I was working and Jeanne couldn't leave with the baby. I'm going to take Saturday off, though I'm on, and take them out on the reservation and look for fossils, if it is not too hot. I'm honestly afraid of rattlesnakes.

Got a nice card from Aunt Mildred with two new shiny crisp dollar bills for Edna Phyllis, her first money. We'll start a savings account for her. Do you still have savings accounts for the boys?

Saturday—

Put a cast on Homer Stands from Oglala today. He told me that last year he had a bloody nose. He had come to the Pine Ridge Hospital. It was treated with a plug, but it didn't stop bleeding. He went to a couple of other doctors who did the same, but still it continued to drip a little around the plugs. So he finally called in Willie Wounded to treat it. He said after the flashes of the sparks and the noises he felt a furry feeling on his face and then Willie or the spirits pulled out the plugs, rubbed over his nose, and even told Homer to blow his nose. Homer said he was skeptical, but did it and sure enough, his nose didn't bleed anymore.

Both Nancy Under Baggage and Vera Mae Brown Bull, both tuberculosis patients who left the Sioux Sanitarium AMA and who are now receiving care at San Haven near the Canadian border, have both written asking to be transferred to a facility where they would be closer to home and no doubt could escape again. Since I told them there were no beds available, they are now raising complaints that they were picked up on one hour's notice and taken to their present facility without having time to pick up supplies, which they were told anyway they wouldn't need. All wrong. Mr. Reifel wrote me the note about this. Well, what happened, and it has sure escaped Mr. Reifel's memory, is that they were both notified one week in advance. Brown Bull refused to go to the sanitarium, so Mr. Reifel sent Mr. Richards out after her to warn her to get up there. And Mrs. Olinger did not tell them they would not need any supplies. Those two are agitating just to get out of there.

July 9, 1954

Mr. Reifel sends me the congressional bulletins of bills referable to the Indian service. The Health Service is to be transferred to the Department of Health, Education, and Welfare, as part of the Public Health Service. The Indians here are much upset about it and are asking questions. A portion of the bill states that health services may be transferred to public or private hospitals where they are available, but only with the consent of the tribal council where concerned. That worries them.

He sent the weekly printed sheet sent out by Senator Karl Mundt, who recently completed the Army-McCarthy hearings as its chairman. He reflects on the hearings and believes it is a great thing to have a government such as ours where such things and personal feelings and arguments can be expressed for the reflection of the minds of men.[3]

July 10, 1954

We went out today hunting for fossils. We went to the place where Jake Herman took me one time, north of Manderson on the Rosebud range. It was very hot. Captain got the hottest. We ate our lunch under a pine tree. We found a few fossils. Coming back we decided to go to the Manderson school to get a drink of cold water from the Bowmans, the teachers there. They were gone, but we found Elizabeth MacDonald there. Her husband, a professor of paleontology at the School of Mines in Rapid City, is camped there until the middle of August. They were out looking for fossils. She gave us some good cold water and was quite entertaining. She also gave us some fossils from their "junk" pile.

Mr. Reifel called yesterday. He thinks the jail should be inspected once a week to help morale. He believes above all that mattress covers

should be ordered and cleaned by a departing "guest" for the next occupant. We start next Tuesday morning.

July 17, 1954

One of the most peculiar things happened, beginning on Thursday
morning. Mr. LaCourse, the administrative officer, called me to tell
me that chairs, a table, and a chest of drawers had been stolen from
the nurses' home. Mr. Reifel left him a note telling him to check with
me. Mr. LaCourse did not know who had reported stolen furniture
from the nurses' home. So I checked with Mrs. Coker, who is the acting director of nurses, and she knew nothing about it. I checked with
those nurses and others who live in the nurses' home. Only one nurse
said she had thought a chest of drawers had been missing. But that was
all she knew. So I checked several times with Mr. Reifel's office, but I
could not get a hold of him. I even called him on Thursday night, but
he wasn't home.

So I checked with Mrs. Mathews of Property and Supply, and she has
no inventory of furniture over there. Thus she had no way of checking for us what pieces were gone. I was to leave early Friday morning
for Rosebud for one week duty. When I called Mr. Reifel shortly after
8:00, Friday, yesterday, I asked him who had reported stolen furniture
from the nurses' homes, that no one, particularly the acting director of
nurses or myself, had had any word about it. What happened is that he
would not tell me who had called other than that "Someone had called
yesterday morning from up there stating that the furniture was gone."
Then he hemmed and hawed and said that he wasn't too concerned,
that I was in charge of the furniture, or rather, that it was under my jurisdiction and that we could forget about it and just let it go.

When Mr. Reifel came here he was adamant on four points: no drinking, care of government property, no clock watchers, and a channel of
command. As far as I'm concerned, without further explanation he is
violating one, even two, of his own rules. It is a flagrant violation of care

of government furniture not to investigate and find out where it may be, and I think also it is a violation of the channel of command.

He should tell us who reported it to him so that we could investigate the matter because we are unable to find anyone up there so far who knows about stolen furniture from the nurses' home. My estimation of Mr. Reifel, which has always been as high as the moon, has just taken a solo dive.

Last Tuesday I went with Mr. Reifel to inspect the jail. He had made an appointment with me the week before to meet him on Tuesday of this week. I didn't know where he wanted me to meet him at 8:00 a.m., at the jail or at the office. I went to the office, and when he walked in I said, "I didn't know whether to come here or go to the jail." He laughed. He thought I was being facetious. Then he remembered our appointment. We walked through the jail. He found it cleaner than he had expected to find it.

I started out yesterday shortly after 8:30 for Rosebud. I took two patients from Rosebud back with me. I took a detour to Wanblee to see Mrs. Jones since she had requested that I come and see her setup. She is quite happy now. No work done yet on the clinic or house, but she is set up for business. Things in the clinic are arranged nicely. The kids out there have been bringing her live fish, snakes, and birds for gifts. I went on to Rosebud where I am to spend a week of temporary duty. Miss Wayne wanted to send one of our doctors here for a four-week tour. She said we could divide the time some.

There just seemed to be no one who wanted to go there and spend more than one week. That meant we would have to rotate. Well, I for one wanted to get away from the mad scramble at Pine Ridge. Dr. Walters spent last week at Rosebud. This really is a vacation. Held clinic yesterday afternoon with Dr. Stephen A. Parks. We had fourteen patients to divide. That is all the patients they usually average. The rest of the afternoon and evening we were left to relax. I started to read a book on plastic surgery. I then spent the evening talking with Dr. Parks and his wife on their lawn, telling them Indian lore and talking stamps. He is a collector. The Parks are from St. Louis.

Today, Saturday, I'm on call. But I spent the entire morning until noon with the Parks going to Valentine, in Nebraska. We went through Crookston, a small town that looks like Mabton.[4] We then went on to Valentine. What a clean, prosperous little berg.

Eating is good here. In one day I've gained weight. We had T-bone steaks last night. Today at noon roast pork and chicken. Tonight sausages and hard-boiled eggs.

The chief nurse here is Miss Glyadine Golden, the one who is supposed to come to Pine Ridge in about a month.

Cities and towns around this part of South Dakota say that Monday of the past week the temperature was the highest ever recorded around here. I'm staying in the house formerly occupied by Dr. Kurliecz. I have the whole house to myself.

The Rosebud Indians seem much nicer than ours. They all are pleasant, and all say "thank you" after receiving service. The scuttlebutt here is that after Mr. Will J. Pitner, the superintendent, leaves Rosebud, it will be made a sub-agency of Pine Ridge, and Mr. Reifel will also be superintendent of this agency. Mr. Reifel's daughter, who had a couple dates with Dick Scott, our house guest of the past two weeks, is engaged to the son of the second cook at the hospital here.

July 18, 1954
Sunday

Steve Parks woke me at 4:00 a.m. We went over to Oliver Russell's and had coffee and were off to Burning Breast Lake. There we did some casting for bass. Oliver got one, Parks got two, and I got none. We were there for only one hour when it started to rain, so we came back. The roads are gumbo when they get wet. While dry they are all right. Some grouse flew up. Wish we had a gun with us. I had breakfast and then slept until noon. After dinner I went over to St. Francis to talk with Father Eugene Buechel. After returning, Steve, Oliver, and I went to dig worms. Then I read an article on Dupuytren's Contracture. By then it was time for supper. After that we went out to Heffer Lake. I caught twelve small bass and one perch. I brought those home and cleaned them tonight. After that we went to the hospital for a night snack. I had chicken, ham, steak, pork sausage, and roast. Sounds ghastly, but tasted good.

I get such a kick out of Oliver Russell. He is half Cheyenne and Sioux and has no use for these Indians down here. Steve Parks remarked that some algae should be thrown into one lake to clear it because it is so soupy. Oliver said, "Throw in a couple of dead Indians."

This being rodeo week, he says all the darn Indians here go to Mission with nothing on their minds and come home with knots on their heads. Some of the nurses said they went to the rodeo, and even Indian women were lying around dead drunk. Catherine, a hospital attendant, says that at Mission they had to build a jail for women and enlarge the one for men.

I think of the book *Speaking of Indians* by Deloria.[5] Catherine said that during World War II a bomber crashed on the reservation, and the Indians near where the crash happened went into the church to pray. Oliver says that near here a bomber crashed during the war, and the Indian boys went out, and the first thing they did was go through the pockets of the dead soldiers to get their money. He says that if the Indians get money they'll do it all the time to get it for doing nothing. Oliver is a well-integrated person. His wife is very nice, and their home is neat as a pin.

The most primitive place around here is Soldier Creek. There the Indians still jerk meat. That is the traditional way of curing buffalo and later beef. Small thin pieces are "jerked" or stripped from the animal and hung up to dry and cure in the sun. The village is the main peyote worshipers' point for the reservation.

Visiting with Father Buechel, he told me an Indian man's wealth was determined by the number of horses he owned. Father Buechel first went to Pine Ridge from 1907 to 1914, I believe it was. The agent then was Brennan. Brennan used to send Father Buechel cigars and cards at Christmas, and Father Buechel sent him some wine.

Father Buechel has three mats made long ago by the Indians. They are narrow small willow sticks held together by sinew threaded through holes in the sticks. These then were rolled up and probably unrolled and used when the ground was wet, Father Buechel figured.

Especially interesting to me was the large root of the bush Morning Glory. The large bulbous roots extend down several feet into the soil. This root, when dried and ignited at one end, burns up through the center. The Indians, long ago before matches, had to keep fire starters, so they packed these roots with them. Father Buechel said they would burn inside for three to six weeks. They would be on the order of "punk" used by kids to shoot off firecrackers. To get sparks from the inside, the root was swung round and round, and the sparks would come out to ignite dried rotten wood.

Father Buechel had two sets of paraphernalia used in the adoption ceremony of long ago. He could not tell me who was adopted, that is, what children. In their old relationships a child was hardly ever without parents, so under their code the few who were without parents or relatives were children who had been lost and then found or, as Dr. Parks suggested, children taken from other tribes. An adoption ceremony lasted three days. The man who was to adopt a child would carry it around on his shoulder. During this ceremony was the only time a Lakota woman wore a feather in her hair. The ceremony consisted of songs, dancing, and special incantations using two sets of rattles, two "pipes," and a stick of corn. The ear of corn stuck on a long willow signified fertility. The rattles were about two feet long (cans filled with rocks were used after the advent of the *wascui*). The "pipes" were not smoking pipes, but two long sticks, each two feet long, decorated with a spread of eagle feathers, cloth tied at the bottom, and wrappings along the stick.

The Parks and Oliver Russell visited with me tonight. The talk was mostly food. An interesting day, almost a vacation over here.

July 21, 1954

I am still at Rosebud. I just saw Oliver Turkey. His folks live at Soldier Creek. Oliver was a patient earlier but looks fine now. He is big for his age, nine months. Soldier Creek is the Skid Road or Hell Hole of this reservation. As Dr. Parks says, it is all filled with disease and should be plowed under, every bit of it, and then salted down.

I just got back from fishing at White Lake, where I didn't get a thing. The only one who got something was Oliver Russell. He got two big bullheads and gave them to me.

Dr. Bragg called me this afternoon to tell me that Mr. Kessis had called from Aberdeen and wanted someone to go to the Sioux Sanitarium for three days or so. Something happened in Dr. Celellia's family. Dr. Bragg said that Dr. Gassman wanted to go. He was to come over here to Rosebud for a week beginning Friday. So Dr. Bragg will come here and Dr. Gassman will go to Rapid City to the Sioux Sanitarium.

The food here is wonderful. I'm the only male with five females at meals. The chatter runs to something about pregnancies and deliveries. Then they talk about all the illegitimate kids. There is so much of that here. Just like Pine Ridge. The chief of police brought his pregnant daughter in the other day to have her baby. She has no husband. In clinic we saw a mother with three kids. She's never been married. All the kids are registered in files by their first name and her last name and also all are registered by their first names and the last name of the alleged fathers, so they all have different last names.

I learned that Mrs. Fairburn cooks for the jail here. Last weekend was the rodeo at Martin. All three of Mrs. Fairburn's boys were drunk, and she reported them and got them put in jail. "She wanted to get them fed well," someone added.

I will leave here sometime on Friday morning, just in time to get to

Pine Ridge and help Dr. Walters in the clinic since the other two men, Drs. Bragg and Gassman, will be gone. I've enjoyed it here, but I will be most anxious to get home to my wife and little baby.

July 22, 1954
Rosebud

One of the fellows in the hospital here in Rosebud is Daniel Small. He is eighty-four years old and from Chamberlain, South Dakota, from Fort Thompson, I believe. Anyway, since he was a kid he has had two holes in each ear lobe. He doesn't know why he has them or how he got them, but it could be a safe bet that he went through the traditional ear splitting ceremony that was done on kids.

Dr. Parks is sick of the common service that his department supplies for the rest of the agency. I told him not to worry about it, that we paid salaries and car expenses for two people at Pine Ridge we never see, besides many other things we pay for out of our funds.

One of the kitchen help here, Sophie Bordeaux, loaned me a picture of Spotted Tail to copy. The picture is one printed from some old image and handed out by C. B. Weston, who owned a store at St. Francis. He married a relative of Sophie's. He was a white man and was reportedly once a senator from Illinois.[6] He came here early and took Spotted Tail to Washington DC on one occasion. Sophie said it was his first trip, but she must have meant that is was his first trip after the agency was established here. She said that every place they stopped people gave him flowers and were eager to see Spotted Tail. She was telling me about the two-story house built by the government for Spotted Tail. He didn't live in it but lived instead in a tepee pitched just outside the house since he was used to living outdoors.

I don't think that at Rosebud you find the feeling so much as we do at Pine Ridge that before the white man came our Indians at Pine Ridge believe the people lived longer before we introduced them to our way of life and medicine.

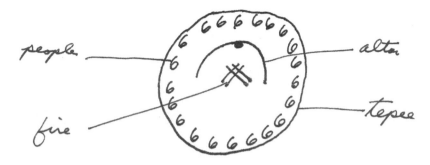

3. Native American Church meeting altar arrangement, as observed and described by Robert H Ruby on July 25, 1954. Drawing by Robert H Ruby.

July 25, 1954

All day long Louise Elk Boy had prepared for the meeting that was held beginning at 9:00 last night out near the Holy Rosary Mission. She hitched up a team of horses and drove over on White Clay Creek above the mission for wood. White Wolf, a Cheyenne from Montana, made a large clearing in the dirt, cleaning away weeds so the tepee could be erected. In the evening, Wilson Brady took the team and went for water at Holy Rosary Mission. I wonder if the fathers would have let him fill his barrel had they known the purpose was for a peyote meeting.

In the evening I went out, and I took our head nurse and acting director, Mrs. Nell Coker. We saw Agnes (Red Cloud) Elk Boy and her husband and Dick and Vincent Red Cloud. Agnes said they were coming just to see what the meetings were like. They're strictly Yuwipi practitioners, so they've never been to see a peyote meeting before. There were so many there for the meeting that since only about thirty-five could get in the tepee they held a meeting in the house for as many more. The tepee was about twenty feet in diameter and about twenty feet high. The altar occupied most of the center. The altar was about ten feet in length and curved to include half the circumference of the center of the tepee. The fire was built inside the altar's half moon.

It was not one bit smoky in the tepee in spite of a big fire. The smoke rose straight up and out the top opening. The sparks rose straight up. The fire was kept going by crisscrossing small chunks of poles at an apex. The mud altar was as usual. The Road of Life and the Fetish Peyote were at the center of the altar.

The drum chief, the main chief, and the cedar chief sat at the front against the west end of the tepee and facing the opening at the east. The opening was guarded by the fire chief and his helper. The fire chief showed us some green peyote plants and buttons.

The entire circumference of the tepee was lined by Indians. The Bradys had a small child sleeping back of them. There was a family of Winnebagos, and they had a small baby in the tepee with them. Nell sat next to the fire chief, then me, then another, and next was the interpreter.

The meeting began with everyone rolling a cigarette from Bull Durham. We tried it. Mine looked like a hunk of sausage. But then the fire chief passed the burning stick for lighting the cigarettes. I lit mine. Mrs. Coker puffed and puffed on hers, but it didn't burn. She asked to light hers from mine. Still it wouldn't burn. I puffed on mine, but the bottom fell through. So we saved our butts for the Fire Chief to collect. One must smoke before he can pray.

The main chief then offered the beginning prayer. Ira Elk Boy and his wife were sitting next to the cedar chief. Ira was sponsoring the meeting and gave the purpose of the meeting. This was a memorial service. It was for his aunt who died July 21 one year ago.

After Ira's remarks in Sioux, the interpreter explained what he had said: "Ira's mother's sister had died. Before she died she said, 'Remember me.' So all year long Ira and his wife have lived a good life free from sin. They didn't lie, didn't drink, and thought of the lady who died and asked to be remembered. So this meeting is so we may think of her and our thoughts may be with her. We want to think good thoughts. This is our old Indian way of worshipping. Long time ago the government tried to stop us, but lately President Eisenhower fixed it so we could worship as we please in our own way and not be bothered. We have lots of people here tonight. Some are Winnebagos. Some are Cheyennes. In the old days we scalped other tribes, but nowadays they say the white man skins another white man alive. So I'm going to interpret for you and for some others here who can't understand our language."

White Wolf, a Cheyenne from Montana here mainly for the upcoming Sun Dance, was at the meeting. He told me earlier in the day, when I dropped out to check on the meeting, that he figures the reason people have tried to stop the peyote use in services is because they want the Indians to join the other churches. He says they all belong to Christian churches.

The cedar chief sprinkled cedar on the fire. Then a bundle of sage was passed around. This is a part of the old custom. We all broke off tiny pieces, rubbed it in our hands, and then rubbed the hands over the body and head.

Then tonight, instead of the singing with a fan, the bunch of sage was used with the staff and the gourd. Different tonight also is the fact that the main chief blew the whistle at this time. He gave four long blasts and two blasts of a series of about six each.

The peyote was passed. Tonight they did it in traditional style. They had no peyote tea. The peyote was in an aluminum pan. It had been cooked and apparently ground or smashed into a thick paste. In the light of the tepee or altar fire it looked like the chocolate syrup put on ice cream sundaes. But let me tell you, it was the bitterest stuff. A common spoon was passed with it. The pan made the rounds about three times up to midnight. The meeting was sort of drawn out. The serial singing moved around the tepee only one time before midnight, reaching around to the main chief at that time. Each person sings four songs while the one next to him drums for the accompaniment.

The drum appeared to be made of brass this time with the three legs and knobs for tying the rope that holds down the hide. White Wolf told me the hide used is deer hide. He said the wetting is done for tone.

At midnight, the main chief blew the whistle with the same sequence of whistles as at the beginning. The fire chief rolled a large Bull Durham cigarette and smoked part of it so he could pray. Then he prayed fervently, some in Sioux and some in English. Soon tears came, and he could hardly pray for awhile. "Help us. Guide us. I've had no education, and in my own humble way hear me. We pray for those who are on the highways. Maybe right this moment someone is in an accident. There will be sorrow. Help them. We pray for their relatives and loved ones. We pray for the white people. We want peace with them. We want to live peaceful. Help us. We pray for colored people. We want to get along with them. We pray for all colors and races. We pray for the Mexicans. Help us. Guide us. We ask for good health."

This main chief did not go outside to face four directions to pray. The Midnight Song was sung. Everyone took out their feather fans now. The cedar chief put cedar on fire. It sure smelled good. The main chief had smoked another rolled Bull Durham. Then he prayed. There were prayers for the doctor and the nurse.

Next the main chief made a speech of how thankful he was we came. He said it was nice of us to come and so on. It was hard to hear him, but the interpreter repeated it. Then he ended that translation with, "It is hard to hear way up there so I repeat what they say and repeat what you say for them, but if I said you had lots of money back here they would all hear that," after telling them up there what I had said. I thanked them for their prayers and kind thoughts and thanked Ira and all of them for letting us come.

Then came the water bucket with a common cup. This was passed all the way around the room. While it was going around a Winnebago got up and said, "This young girl here is my daughter. She was twenty-two years old yesterday. She has two little children. Her husband is a Mexican. We are so happy to be here with you. We thank you for letting us come here and sit with you. My daughter has never been in these places before. I hope she comes to like this way of life and will join with us when we go back home. We came here for food and for clothes. In the morning we will eat. This is fine. We are happy. We have been treated nice up here." Then repetition. Then "I have another daughter older than this one. She has been in the sanitarium for two years. Will you pray for her so that when I go home I will find her in good health? We thank you."

There were numerous grunts and "Hows."

At about 11:00 Mrs. Coker kind of flinched but then looked around, and I figured she was looking for something. It was shortly after she had tasted the thick peyote. Then she nudged me and said, "Look at the toad back there." I thought sure she was hallucinating. But sure enough, there it was. It hopped up to the fire and actually jumped in. Then it jumped off the coals, and the interpreter said, "Get that toad and throw it out." Later, Mrs. Coker told me something hit her back, and she figured it was a hand from the outside, reaching up under the tepee, and she decided to let it go. She felt it again and knew it was some sort of animal, and then a toad hopped out past her and she knew what it was.

We took our leave after the water at 1:00 a.m. It always takes an hour to dispense with midnight ceremonies. On the way out we looked into the nearby house. In there the people inside were all sprawled out, reclining instead of sitting against the wall. "They must have eaten a lot more of that stuff than was eaten in the tepee." One thing that I noticed about those in the house was that they didn't take out much time for midnight ceremonies, if any, because they didn't have all the stillness that we did. So they couldn't have done too much praying or even have taken long to drink their water. Charles Bear Robe was in there. He is the one that tried to kidnap me and Mrs. Forshey the other time. I was afraid he was coming in the tepee, but he went to the house meeting. He is such a crook according to Mrs. Forshey. Now he will probably spread a lot of malicious stuff about how peyoted-up Mrs. Coker and I were.

July 26, 1954

I saw Jake Herman at noon. I took him by his house, and he gave me a souvenir program for the Sun Dance that is being held this week.

Mr. LaCourse called and wanted me to get a work order in by the morning. Someone suggested an electric stove for Miss Janis, nurse's aide, for her home.[7] Joe Walters now holds me personally responsible for the fact that he didn't get an electric refrigerator in his home for a long time. Now that one has recently arrived it is in his home. I may just as well order an electric stove for Miss Janis. As soon as it gets in, she will be moved out. Then they won't let me take the electric stove out so someone else from a different department can move in and use it. When we hire another nurse's aide and when she gets into another house with practically no equipment, then Health can furnish that house as well, as they have used hospital funds for so many houses around here.

Mrs. Forshey told me Saturday that Edgar Red Cloud is back from his movie work. He spent three days walking up and down the street shaking hands with everyone. He finally told Mrs. Forshey he was terribly tired of shaking hands.

She told me she had written a sassy letter to Area Office about her boss, Mrs. Heineman, who kept postponing the Area Office meeting for the department for so long and so many times until it ran into her leave time, and she flatly refused to go. She cited the Health Department that made plans for meetings and then didn't hold them.

We have a new water heater in our house. Rents have been slashed 53 percent. We went from $22 for every two weeks to $9.50. That's the same as a jump in pay grade.

The staffing situation is about to erupt here. Now nurse Mrs. Nierenhauser, who said she wanted to come here as a transfer from Sioux Sanitarium about two weeks ago, did so, but only to escape relative problems in Rapid City. Now she will leave us in about two weeks. Two other nurses are leaving, too. Dr. Bragg handed in his resignation to be effective on August 31.

July 27, 1954

Edgar Red Cloud came over to see me at noon. He was telling me that he and Andrew Fools Crow were the only two old guys at the movie to ride a horse for the Custer battle scene. No, it was he and Iron Crow. Old

Andrew got married while he was up there. His wife died a few months ago, so he got remarried when he was working on the movie. When he came home his daughter wouldn't let the other woman around the place and didn't want to see this woman wearing her deceased mother's clothing and such, and so Andrew and she separated and will be getting a divorce. Andrew is in charge of the Sun Dance.

Edgar told me about the white boy from Pennsylvania who is living with him. Wants to live here with the Indians and get a job, but Edgar says he is too slow to work, and Edgar doesn't want him around much anymore to feed. Vincent took the boy to the Peyote meeting at Ira's the other night. I saw him with Vincent, but it was too dark to see his face. Edgar says in the Cross Fire group that was held in the house, the one we didn't go to, that they all ate too much peyote, and the kid didn't get back to Edgar's home until Monday. Then he told Edgar he looked out and saw the blue hills and a man, all red with wings, come flying down. Then he saw himself with hair or fur all over his body.[8] Edgar told him he was going to become a monkey. So that group of Cross Fire is quite a peyote-eating bunch. Charles Bear Robe was at that meeting. He came to the house Monday, Bear Robe did, and asked Jeanne for something to eat for his kids. She fixed him a stack of sandwiches.

Incidentally, it was like Grand Central Terminal at the hospital. It looks like a camp city has sprung up overnight east of the hospital, with tribes here from all over the central, west, and southwest for the Sun Dance, which began this morning actually. Charlie Poor Thunder is to be the medicine man leading the dancers. This morning before sunup a sacred pole or tree was cut after offering up the peace pipe. It was hauled to the Sun Dance grounds, and tomorrow morning four men who have led a good virtuous life this past year are to carry the pole in. Edgar told me this noon, "I don't know who they could get. There hasn't been anybody who lived a good life this past year." Mrs. Forshey told me later that Edgar sure didn't think for one minute, did he, that he could be asked. Edgar did do that one year. He is going to drum and sing this year. Tonight they are practicing their songs.

The pole raising and dancing begins tomorrow just before sunup. So that probably means at 4:00 a.m. I'll go out, but not that early.

July 28, 1954

They opened the Sun Dance today. Last night those four dancers took a sweat bath and got their instructions from George Poor Thunder, the medicine man. George is the one who conducted the Yuwipi ceremony I attended.

This morning the four virtuous men planted the pole after the medicine man had tied at the top the symbol of the buffalo and the man cut from cow hide.

At 9:00 this morning the four dancers came from the tepee followed by Andrew Fools Crow, who carried the sage and buffalo skull. Each dancer carried a wreath of sage to which was attached eagle feathers. On their heads was a wreath of sage. Around their arms and ankles was a wreath of sage. They led the process, with singers and drummers following.

The peace pipe was offered up by Poor Thunder. Then he led the dancers from where they sat to the arena. They faced the sun. Their faces and bodies were painted with bright yellow suns. They wore only scarf blankets around their waists. Around their necks were bone whistles. They faced the sun and danced, taking several steps forward and several steps backward while bobbing up and down and continuously blowing the bone whistles. There were three from Lame Deer, Montana, two of whom were Korean War veterans. They were the three who are visiting Wilson Brady and attended the peyote meeting in the tepee Saturday night at Ira's. One of them on crutches was still on crutches. These men fasted all yesterday and will today.

At intervals of about eight to ten minutes Poor Thunder led them each, not by touching but by putting sage leaves around their arms and leading them a quarter of the way around the arena, a circular enclosure. At each time around one (they took turns) would offer the peace pipe to the drummers, and then they would sit for fifteen minutes in the shade before starting again. This kept up until about 1:30 today. Then Andrew Fools Crow led the dancers out of the arena. At the tepee Poor Thunder talked to them again, and then they took a sweat bath again.

Attention was distracted from the dancers for a while this morning when two tepees close together and a cooler went up in flames and burned down in about ten minutes. A Pueblo Indian living here and a Sioux living in New Mexico brought up several Pueblo people who put on the Eagle Dance later in the afternoon. Their costumes are impressive.

Ben Irving, vice president of the tribal council, gave me an official sticker so I can get in the Sun Dance grounds any time. Aggie Iron Cloud, the hospital cook, is there and selling pop. Her husband is a Sun Dance big wheel. This afternoon Andrew Fools Crow gave me a silk official badge.

Mr. Reifel with Eddie Coker showed Hal Boyle around.[9] Mr. Boyle is the columnist famous mostly for his Korean dispatches. Warren Morrell, editor of the *Rapid City Journal*, and Earl Buckingham, owner of the Buckingham transport outfit, were also in that party. The whole bunch will leave here tomorrow in their private plane, fly to a ranch in Wyoming, and spend the weekend with some friend of Mr. Morrell's.

Mr. Morrell asked me the bluntest questions anyone has. He had quite a few questions to ask me concerning Health for an interview for his paper, but he somewhat startled me with one of his questions.[10]

Hal Boyle was introduced. His Indian name given some time ago is Leading Eagle Jr. Since there are no words for *junior* and *senior* in the Indian language, it is "first" for *senior* and "last" for *junior*. He was given the name some time ago when Henry Standing Bear was present. Henry protested violently, saying that President Coolidge was given that name, so then someone said he could keep the name and be called *junior*.

The fourth Sun Dancer this morning was William Brave, in his early eighties. Today I talked at length with John Nelson, who is ninety-eight years old. He traveled with Buffalo Bill along with American Horse, the father of the present American Horse, the chief.

This afternoon about 2:30 two jets made three flights right over the Sun Dance grounds. This was done by the commanding officer in charge of Ellsworth Air Force Base near Rapid City in honor of those who danced in the Sun Dance. This occurred right after the flag-raising ceremonies. There were several veterans including Eugene Rowland, who had been a prisoner of war in North Korea and who raised one of the two flags. One flag raised belongs to the Iron Cloud family. It was for a son of James Iron Cloud who died after returning from the Korean War. The other flag is in the Woman Dress family. When the flags were raised, there were several women who made keening cries. It was sort of eerie.

This morning when I went around to where Poor Thunder was relaxing during a brief rest period with the dancers, I first went up to him and asked, "George, can I take a picture?" He turned around quickly and said, "Oh, I thought you wanted to give me something." Then he recognized who I was. Finally, after pictures, he asked if I'd buy a package of Camels for the dancers to smoke between dances. So I went over and got them some Camels. Tonight Dr. Gassman and I went out to the Sun Dance grounds. I took some medicine to Charlie Yellow Boy, one of the drummers.

Thirteen. August 1954

I had heard from several sources that Mr. Reifel really gave a good talk at the dedication of Number Five Day School at Oglala the other day. Tonight Mrs. Mickelson told me what he had said. First Mr. Sande, now in the Area Education Office, gave an opening talk. He told how he had personally had a hand in seeing the project develop. He talked about how the funds were asked for and appropriated. He then turned the forum over to Mr. Reifel, who got up and said thank you for the key to the school, but he wasn't sure he ought to give it to the people of Oglala. He wasn't sure how they would treat it. He said that everywhere he went he saw initials carved in school desks and seats and in church pews even. He said he wasn't sure the people deserved the school. He said they acted like POLLYWOGS. Parents just didn't seem to get their kids in school. Lillian Mickelson said he really poured it on the Indians at Oglala.

August 1, 1954

The Sun Dance festivities are over, but I noticed this morning at about 4:00 when I had to go to the hospital to take care of the big wheel for part of the celebration that most of the tents are still there. They will most likely be pulled out today. Jake Herman drank two beers and two cocktails last night, he said. He was horribly tired and wanted to stay in the hospital for two days and rest. So I kept him in. But on Friday when Jeanne and I were at the Sun Dance, he told me then he was very tired. Jake was instrumental in getting Hal Boyle, the Associated Press columnist, to come here for the celebration.

Ben Irving, the vice president of the tribe, was unusually nice, and he is a real gentleman. He extended to me a personal welcome to do as I pleased and enjoy myself and call on him at any moment I might want help at the celebration.

There were a lot of horses and kids particularly riding them. Many had wool Navajo blankets for saddle blankets. The most popular dancers were the Bacas from Albuquerque. They are Pueblo Indians who came up with Mrs. Hendricks, who is a sister of Sarah Looks Twice. Mrs. Hendricks lives down there, but is Sioux. The costumes for dances were pretty. The *waiscu* (white man) who lives with Edgar had a very nice costume, but he looked like a *waiscu* dancing. He tried too hard at times to be an Indian dancer.

Friday there was a parade. They wound up by the hospital. Mr. Reifel was in full chief's costume. Wilson Brady was on the front of one of the cars all in warrior costume and was with his little girl.

Yesterday I went out all day with Mr. Carr and Mr. Hockenberry to hunt agates. I found a very fine specimen. I found a couple that weren't so hot—in fact, that don't even count. We planned on going to the Badlands with Reverend Obert of the Oglala Presbyterian Church, but he had too much to do and couldn't go. If he was driving his jeep we would have gone to the Badlands, but we had to settle on an easier road and went to Slim Buttes.

We are in a dilemma. I bought two pair of children's moccasins at the arts and crafts store at Rosebud. When I got them home I noticed they were dirty. So Jeanne washed them. Now they are hard as rocks. I must find Edgar or Wilson to see how to soften them. I unsuccessfully tried mineral oil last night.

Joe Running Hawk came to the hospital on Friday night and asked Mrs. Coker to call me to tell me his brother was having a peyote meeting at Porcupine and that he'd like me to go to it.

August 4, 1954

I thought my car was going to explode yesterday. Monday night Edgar Red Cloud helped me load the garbage can from the house into the trunk of my government Pontiac because it was getting so rotten. It had not been picked up for over a week. We couldn't get the key out of the lock then. We finally broke the key. After the key was broken, Edgar let the trunk slam, and there it was locked, no key, and with the garbage in the back. The garage finally got it opened yesterday and put a new lock in. So I got the car and merrily drove out to the dump grounds near Edgar's place. I opened the trunk, and someone had already disposed of the garbage.

Edgar has a petition he is passing around. He is trying to collect money to send Reno to Sheridan, Wyoming, to dance in the Indian celebration up there. I was the third one to donate a dollar. Ben Irving was before me and Harry Tylee. Edgar said he would let the old chief take the request or petition around, except that he was afraid the old chief would keep some of the donations.

I ran into Adolph Red Cherries and Calvin White Wolf down at the telephone office yesterday at noon when I went to pay a telephone bill for the time I called Jeanne from Deadwood. Those two were there trying to get money to return to Montana. Calvin White Wolf is quite a very nice person, talks well, and must have a high school education. He is interested in agates. He hunts them frequently for a shop in Montana that pays his expenses around to find them. I told him about the beauty I found Saturday. He wanted to see it. So last evening I took it out to Wilson Brady's where he is staying and took Wilson some jam.

I enjoyed talking with them about this Sun Dance. These are some of their comments. They wore the same sage head halos, arms bands, and leg bands both days out here. At the Sun Dances in Lame Deer, Montana, they never wear the same sage bands for more than one day. White Wolf and White Man had been given bone whistles, but Red Cherries didn't have one. He asked George Poor Thunder for one. George found a bamboo whistle for him. It was so big, and since he had to hold it in his mouth with his teeth, his jaws ached very much that night.

They took three sweat baths out there. It was the first time White Wolf had ever taken a sweat bath. He said he nearly roasted to death before they let him out.

They ate all the meals and drank water. They were well fed, they said. They ate buffalo meat and also one day dog meat. White Wolf doesn't like dog meat. Too fat and too rich, he said. Up at Lame Deer they fast two days and two nights and then fast during the dancing. They couldn't understand the fasting that is done up there.

The effigy at Lame Deer is only that of a man. No buffalo, in addition, as is used here. Up there they had a whole buffalo hide at the base of the main pole.

Up there they do not have a circular enclosure in which people sit and kids can run across the grounds. The Sun Dancers stay in a small enclosure by themselves at the base of the main pole. And they stay right there day and night until the Sun Dance is over. They don't go to the main tent until after all the dancing is over. The tents of Indians here are placed north and south in a horseshoe pattern with all openings to the east. And the main Sun Dancers' tent is open to the east. Here the main tepee was open to the west.

In Lame Deer they use real Indian soil paints.

They said that Poor Thunder used white shoe polish and lipstick, mixed them, and painted them, and not all alike. It burned their skin.

When all was said and done, they volunteered this information. "The Sioux don't believe in it," they said, meaning the Sun Dance. They do it for effect or for show. They don't seem to be serious. Red Cherries said he really believed in it. He has danced before at Lame Deer. He showed me a picture of him dancing up there and their enclosure.

So I asked him then if he'd lived a year as a good person. He said yes.

Then I asked him his purpose for dancing, and he said his mother had been ill and then got better. So he danced to thank the Great Spirit through the Sun God. Wilson told me today that Edgar and his family left for Sheridan, Wyoming, for the Indian celebration to be held there this week.

246

August 6, 1954

Mr. Reifel got back last night after nearly a week in Aberdeen at the Area Office, where he discussed many things in a conference of superintendents from the Area. So he called a meeting of all branch heads to let them toss around the ideas he'd picked up. There was nothing on Health except that the transfer of health services to the Department of Health, Education, and Welfare has taken a setback with so many objections now from representatives of different Indian tribes.

There has been a major reorganization of particularly the Resources group of the BIA from the Washington Office on down. Many things will be cut out and put into one unit, such as SMCO [Soil and Moisture Conservation Operations], Forestry, Grazing, Irrigation (of which we do not have a branch here), and so on.

Mr. Reifel left to take a call from California. The banter that went around was chiefly from those who now head those departments. The comments were certainly off the cuff. It seems there have been increases in pay grades at the Area level and on up that will absorb much of the money allotted by Congress for those departments that are already so short of money that Mr. A. M. Adams, head of Realty here, says they have only enough money to operate for six months this fiscal year. And as someone mentioned, the Area Office says, "Don't worry about your salary. Let us worry about that." "There are too many generals and not enough privates," said Mrs. Coker.

Mr. Reifel read an article from some magazine written by an Indian about the cunning white man and broken treaties. The idea is played up for young Indians growing up that the white man stands behind them with a knife. This is a detriment to the kids. What has to be done is to work with the situation at hand. The Indians had nothing at one time, said Mr. Reifel, excepting some food and clothes on their back. Now the Indians have so much more, Social Security, opportunity galore to work and make money, all the federal programs for health, welfare, and education, federal benefits, aid to the blind, and so on. And the Indians complain about some white men who use their land or any land and make lots of money.

There is Earl Buckingham, who visited Pine Ridge last week. He and his brother graduated from some place near here in Nebraska. They could have sat around and figured the world owed them a living. Instead they started a trucking business that grew to such proportions that it grossed five million dollars last year. And they started a lumber business that grossed five million dollars last year also. They employ hundreds of people. And, of course, that is the sort of society in which we live, a capitalistic one that is competitive. The Indian has the opportunity also to form a business.

One of the problems discussed at the Area meeting of superintendents was the heirship problem. There are over five hundred unprobated estates on this reservation. In some instances there are now thirty heirs. Several may want to sell the land, and others may not want to sell. What to do? The estates could be turned over to state courts. In such a case a piece of land could be sold without unanimous agreement to sell. But much more land would be sold. Someone suggested that the tribe buy up the land. Mr. Reifel said that is not the policy. The tribe could if it became a private corporation and was no longer under federal control. Some tribes do this.

In all the discussion Mr. Reifel used the word TERMINATION whereas it used to be WITHDRAWAL before. Mr. Reifel seemed to think termination ought to be done by individuals and not tribes. One bill now before Congress would eliminate anyone from federal help and control who possesses less than 50 percent Indian blood.

Thus this would give more time to the full-bloods, who certainly as a group do need more attention than persons of mixed ancestry. A dentist in Rapid City, who is less than half Indian, came down for help the other day. Mr. Reifel said they had to help him because by law he is entitled to it, but he is fully competent and should not ask for so much help.

Mr. Reifel said an inquiry is coming through to all Indians employed by the government asking them why they had not gotten a patent fee on their land. Mr. Reifel said he would frankly put down, "Because I do not wish to pay taxes on the land."

Mr. Reifel went through the TIME business again. He said he wasn't so concerned about the land and material resources of the Indians as he was the mental attitudes. If the Indians learned to value time, they would then take care of or be interested in saving material things and providing for themselves. He saw a family fixing a flat tire the other day on Red Shirt Table when he was on his way to Rapid City. Mr. Reifel was biting his teeth for fear he'd be late for his appointment in Rapid City. The Indian family fixing their flat was in no hurry. If they were not there, they'd be someplace else. What difference did it make where you were just so you were?

Mr. Reifel talked about the transition of the Sioux. The Sioux are thought of as "the" Indians of the United States because of the Custer battle and because Buffalo Bill toured them through Europe. But, says Mr. Reifel, they are a fairly recent tribe that is an admixture of cultures of many other tribes. They picked up the culture of other tribes very quickly, so he was in hopes they could make the transition to a white man's society fairly quickly. I don't agree with Mr. Reifel. I always get the impression that he means in a matter of two or three years, but I think he is counting on too much change too rapidly.

But on the other hand several things came out of the conference that I think mean progress. Mr. Reifel has stated that at the Sun Dance last week he counted about 150 cars and 3 wagons. Twenty-five years ago the numbers would have been reversed.

The National Congress of American Indians is now taking Indians from various tribes all over the United States to Congress to fight the legislation concerning termination of Indians' relationship with the federal government. In some instances Indians are being asked what they think of certain legislation. Before the legislation was even read, the Indians said, "NO." They are being prompted by this organization to not accept new legislation for Indians that would dissolve their reservations.

The weather the last few days has been marvelous. Just like fall. Cool. We even had the furnace on a few moments last night to take the chill off the house. I actually like to can vegetables and fruits and preserve other things for winter's use. We have already gotten cabbage and cucumbers from the mission and made sauerkraut and pickles and canned some beans from our own patch. Mr. W. E. West, head of Extension, put in a large patch of corn. Mrs. West and he went out one evening and found their corn ripe and ready for picking. They decided the next morning to get up early and pick the corn and can it. The next morning two-thirds of their patch had been stripped. That happens constantly around here. The Indians strip gardens.

August 14, 1954

I did some high-class politicking, or so I thought. Mr. Kessis called and wanted Dr. Bragg to go to the Yankton hospital in Wagner, South Dakota, until he leaves here. He is getting out of the service on August 31. Then he said no, we'll send him to Rosebud. Practically everyone around here rebelled, particularly me. They do not need that much help at Rosebud. Mr. Keesis said skip it this week then. But in Rapid City the other day he told Dr. Bragg to go for one week only. Thank heavens. Only one week.

I thought I was going to get rid of Miss McGill. Sure want to. Miss Wayne said I could put it up to her to see if she wanted to go to the Sioux Sanitarium on a transfer. Miss McGill got terribly indignant. She said she'd think it over, and four days later said no. So now Area Office is going to try to get her to go to Alaska.

At a meeting in Rapid City, Mary E. Simms, an anesthetist and the new hospital administrator for the Area, said she thought she knew Miss McGill. Then Miss Simms realized she was sure she did. She knew her as a student. And she says that Miss McGill has always been like she is now. Miss Simms said the director of nurses, wherever it was that they were in training, thought Miss McGill would drive her nuts.

I've advertised the janitor's job three times now because we can't seem to attract anyone who is desirable, someone who will work and do a job. Indians are funny. They demand so much service, yet those Indians working in jobs don't put forth the same service that the people demand of government. So I went out to recruit Pugh Young Man Afraid of His Horses, and now there is a big stink because he is a cattle man in addition. They'd have you hire anyone who can loaf. So I guess we'll be forced to take a transfer of Bill Goings, a man who now works in an agency elsewhere. He wants to come up here, but he is no hotrod at work. But better than what we have for applications. Pierre LeGrande's son applied and gave a big letter on his federal offense of altering a check from $45 to $245.

I went up to Rapid City on Wednesday for the Area dental medical meeting and the election of officers. I nominated Dr. Walter R. Carey of Standing Rock for president again. He loves it. I nominated Dr. Walters for vice president, and he was elected. Dr. Quint and Dr. Bragg I nominated for two of the three directors' positions. So Pine Ridge will be well represented.

We had a fairly good conference. There was lots of discussion of the tuberculosis patients. It all centered on what to do with the patients who check themselves out against medical advice [AMA]. The most important thing to come out of the meeting was that the doctor should not impose prison existence or sentences, otherwise the doctor-patient relationship is ruined.

Mr. Allan J. Brands from the Washington Office, a pharmacist, was there. With all the pharmacy stuff coming in here, we are receiving too much material for us to store. Now he tells me that because of money we won't get a pharmacist here at Pine Ridge until July 1955. I'll be gone then and won't have to worry about getting him space.

Mr. Kessis took up some time to go over the budgets with those present. It really was a disturbing thing to sit there in the conference this year. I remembered the conference one year ago in Aberdeen. The only hope I could seem to see was the announcement read by Mr. Brands that Public Health definitely would take over the Indian Service hospitals next July. But this year there were so few there compared to one year ago. And it looks as if the doctor situation is going to become so short as the fellows leave, and there just are not replacements for them. Right now the Area is short five doctors. Soon they will be short seven when Dr. Bragg and Dr. Gassman leave. There are no replacements. And more tragic is the cut in funds and budget with absolutely no additional allocation from Washington later in the year.

We are to get a new Area medical director in September. A Dr. Herbert A. Hudgins, Area medical officer, who is coming from seven years out of the States. Maybe he can take some of the problems of money and personnel off of Mr. Kessis and Miss Wayne that seem to be looming.

It just seems to me that cuts in our program are going to have to be made. I think glasses should be first. The copy of our new budget for Pine Ridge that I have here says, "This is to inform you that no funds are provided for outside hospitalization where a government hospital is operated within your jurisdiction."

But a review of our budget shows that last year we were allocated $193,000. We spent $204,000. Our budget calls for $193,000 this year. So while all other places are screaming about their cuts, we have again all we were allocated last year. But I am going to cut down on eye glasses.

August 17, 1954

I saw a lady in the clinic yesterday who brought back a whole train of events. I remember the woman well now. She has been in the clinic on any number of occasions. She is of a nervous disposition. She is in menopause (surgically) and has hyperthyroidism. She has many nervous complaints. Reassurance helps her only for the short term. Then suddenly I remembered her as the latecomer to the peyote meeting at Ira Elk Boy's about a month ago (July 24). I remember that I saw this lady come in late that night. She seemed a bit out of place and appeared a bit apprehensive as she sat down and surveyed the situation. She told me about it yesterday. She had never been to a peyote meeting before. But in the course of all her nervous ailments the peyoters had told her the medicine would cure her, so she went.

The woman told me she felt worse than she had ever felt for two days after that. The peyote made her sick and also sleepy. She said her husband came and went to the Cross Fire meeting in the house. She told me the meeting was for Lena Smoke. All those Indians have been having meetings for Lena for so long for her illness with no avail. We at the hospital tried to send her away for specialized treatment twice. Each time elaborate arrangements were made and then the family, as would be typical, just didn't carry through. About three weeks ago they wanted very much to take her, but then the Area Office put a crimp in things and said to get her in St. Elizabeth's in Washington DC. That entails correspondence and much red tape. But a letter came through just yesterday. The Washington Office said to send her to a state institution. A brother-in-law of Lena's is one of the tribal police, Mathew Eagle Heart. One man who is a member of Half Moon, Roy Martin, quit the tribal police force and went back to his ranch.

Joe Running Hawk brought in his daughter Dorothy. She is the one who was with Russell Sitting Holy, the driver, and Rebecca Hump when they ran into two whites and killed a woman. Rebecca is out of jail today for disorderly conduct as of a couple days ago. She is ill. Joe had his peyote meeting for Dorothy last weekend and came to invite me, but I was in Rapid City when he came to ask me to come. Dorothy is doing fine after treatment.

This morning I grabbed a couple pieces of toast and bacon. Didn't get it all eaten before I got to the agency at 8:00 a.m. So I left the bacon in the glove compartment. Then I forgot it. Leroy took that station wagon to Rapid City to take a patient to the Sioux Sanitarium. My breakfast was gone when he got back. So they must have gotten hungry on the way up. Mr. Reifel had forgotten today that Tuesday is jail inspection day. On the way over we picked up perhaps twenty-five nails apiece on the road from the commissary to the jail. I saw Boob Janis and told him to come empty my garage.[1] It was overflowing with refuse from all the canning we did last week. He must have come pronto. But he is missing days at work now. Mr. Reifel said, "You have Miss Golden now. She is supposed to be a good administrator. Miss McGill, I understand, has her heart in the right place, but she is rather annoying." I wonder who told him. Must have been someone in Area.

When we got to the jail (they expect us on Tuesdays now) it was clean except for refuse on the windows. Several people were there to look at a brand-new Buick in the backyard of the jail. It had belonged to Lewis Hawk, who died in the jail one and a half weeks ago. That new Buick was there last week.

I remember one week ago today I had jail inspection. Mr. Reifel forgot today; I had forgotten last week. Emmaline Sauser, his secretary, called to remind me. A week ago I had gotten only one bite of cereal down and left. That new Buick was standing in the jail yard then. I asked Mr. Reifel whose it was. "That is Lewis Hawk's, who died Saturday in the hospital. There is his brand-new car, and he had no money. It took me two hours to scout around and find enough money to bury the bastard."

Today, on the way back from jail, we stopped back at his house for a cup of coffee. Alice was just getting breakfast for guests of theirs from Texas, so he had breakfast also. He invited me, but I drank my coffee and got back to the hospital for surgery.

Miss Golden scrubbed for the thyroid operation we were going to do today, but the patient developed tachycardia and so we had to postpone it. Right after that her heart rate went down to normal. Dr. Gassman took an EKG, and it was normal. To get away from things, I went over to visit Mr. Mickelson in his office about 4:00 p.m. I was talking none too well of Albert Pyles and soon in he walked. I kidded him about Ethel Merrival trying to get the school herd of horses and the Herd Camp away from Education. He said he had answered the resolutions on that and wondered how I knew. I told him I read the tribal notes. Mickelson and Pyles wondered where and how I got them. I told them I just went in and took copies from Emmaline. I told them I used to keep an eye on the comments on Health and their complaints and fussing about Health. But I said they don't run us in the ground now, especially now that they are afraid of losing Health. I've had quite a few questions about the transfer of Health to the Department of Health, Education, and Welfare under Public Health. It is to go into effect now in July 1955. Yesterday Mr. Reifel made the announcement in the daily "poopsheet," as Mr. Reifel calls it himself.

I am sure glad to have Miss Golden here. She said tonight she wanted to call Aberdeen tomorrow and try to get some of Rosebud's nurses over here. I called her over and talked to her at the hospital last night.

George Swift Bird just came here to the house. He was in the hospital about a week ago for a week. He signed out against medical advice. He told me tonight his wife is claiming nonsupport now during that time, and he wants me to write a letter to the tribal judge supporting the fact that he was in the hospital.

Jeanne and I were not unmindful of the fact that last week and a half ago was our anniversary of arriving at Pine Ridge. The old place looks a lot different than it did a year ago. We have the pictures to prove it.

Steve Ferraca, who is from Scarsdale, New York, was here Sunday night to ask for copies of my 35 mm Kodachromes taken at the Sun Dance. Mr. Mickelson walked in and said Mr. Ferraca is from some wealthy family with some political pull. The Washington Office wired in June asking if Education could hire him on the farm. They wired back, "No." The Washington Office wired back, "Find a place."

Joseph Lehner, the *waiscu* (white man) who lives with Edgar Red Cloud, is in the hospital. They just returned from the Sheridan, Wyoming, Indian Days where Reno took in $100 in prizes. Edgar didn't volunteer to give back the dollar I "loaned" him on request to get Reno there or the dollars from others in town. Joseph had been drinking wine with the old chief and had gotten sick. He even thought the time he ate peyote at Ira's might have had something to do with his illness. He told me about the colored fans and staffs and gourds he had visions of seeing when under the influence of peyote.

August 19, 1954

Last evening Steve Parks from Rosebud called to say he had a patient brought to him from Wagner. So he was sending him to us since he couldn't handle the man. He was fifty years old, with multiple fractures all over, including the head and face. He was draining spinal fluid from his nose. Lacerations on his face were not repaired before he got here, and it is too late to suture them now. The injuries happened to him on Tuesday night. There are fractures of a clavicle, ribs, and femur and a compound fracture of a tibia and fibula. I gave the news of the fractures to Emmaline Sauser for the newssheet since she called and asked about the man. I see she reduced the injuries to common terms. This case kept us up till midnight last night. I had been up most of Monday and Tuesday nights since I was on call for Bob Bragg and myself. So I'm pooped tonight.

I saw a note in yesterday's newssheet that many of the chronic complainers, including my friends James and Edgar Red Cloud, Charlie Yellow Boy, and Jackson One Feather, were in Mr. Reifel's office giving him hell on Wednesday. They were blaming school authorities for the poor behavior of students. They wanted the kids to stay out of school for two or three weeks to work in the harvest fields. And there were other complaints. When I took Edgar home, he said what all those guys were complaining about was that so many high school girls got pregnant last year while in school. And he says they believe that it is the school's fault. Mr. Reifel, to my notion, is right: the trouble lies in the home.

Mr. Reifel wrote that poor behavior of students was due to parents and grandparents. Then he wrote that the conference would continue in his office at 2:00 p.m. on Friday, tomorrow. I sure plan to get in on that discussion since he asked concerned branch chiefs to come. I thought that for a change they aren't squawking about Health. I want to get in on their foolishness. Then Emmaline asked me today to come.

I ran into Edgar. He asked me to take him home, so I did. On the way I asked him how they cured their chokeberries. He said they ground the cherries and seeds all together. Then they make cakes of them and put them out to dry. They turn them every few days. The dried cakes will keep several years. They can mix the cakes with corn and dried meat; they call it *wasna*. I can't understand why they grind up the seeds, but he says they add so much flavor. They are drying some now. Edgar gave me two cakes that look like well-cooked hamburgers. And they smell like a cookie of some sort.

I am afraid that all the chokeberry jelly and jam we made is going to have to be boiled again with more Certo. It is supposed to be one of the most difficult jellies to get to jell. Ours is sans seeds however!

I had heard from several sources that Mr. Reifel really gave a good talk at the dedication of Number Five Day School at Oglala the other day. Then tonight Mrs. Mickelson told me what he had said. First Mr. Sande, now in the Area Education Office, gave an opening talk. He told how he had personally had a hand in seeing the project develop. He talked about how the funds were requested and appropriated. He then turned the forum over to Mr. Reifel, who got up and said thank you for the key to the school, but he wasn't sure he ought to give it to the people of Oglala. He wasn't sure how they would treat it. He said that everywhere he went he saw initials carved in school desks and seats and in church pews even. He said he wasn't sure the people deserved the school. He said they acted like POLLYWOGS. Parents just didn't seem to get their kids in school. Lillian Mickelson said he really poured it on the Indians at Oglala.

Mr. Reifel seems to be trying to get to parents to rouse their concern. He is trying various ways now to make them accountable or to shame them. He is traveling a slow road, though I believe he has made a start.

What a drive tonight! We went over to the Mickelsons' to go down

257

to our garden there and pick beans to can. There had been a fire this afternoon at Herd Camp at the south pasture next to the Nebraska state line. The fire actually started over there and burned north coming into South Dakota and onto Herd Camp pasture.

Mick and Dick Oehmcke wanted to drive out and see the damage. Lillian was going and asked us to go. We did. The baby thoroughly enjoyed riding over all the bumps. We turned south on the road that goes by Charlie Yellow Boy's. Soon the road got narrower, then became only two tracks heading across the country until eventually there was no road. Nearly sixty acres of hills were burned off. On the Nebraska side there was still fire burning on a line about one-fourth mile long. No one was around, and the fire probably had started up again.

So off we went over the steep hills, down sharp hills, across rugged valleys and ravines into the Nebraska side, hit a dirt road into White Clay, stopping to warn Nebraska farmers. But no one was home. In White Clay all the Nebraska farmers were in drinking beer plus the fire chief from Pine Ridge, Mr. Case. No one seemed aroused or in a hurry when we drove in and Mr. Mickelson told them.

We sped to Pine Ridge, where in ten minutes there was action. The siren blew and blew. We went home because of the baby. I called Eddie Coker, acting superintendent. I called Holy Rosary Mission, since the fire appeared to be on Catholic farm land in Nebraska. Soon fire trucks, followed by about a dozen cars, drove off toward White Clay. Today the fire was reported to have been caused by lightning.

August 21, 1954

The meeting in Mr. Reifel's office yesterday afternoon must have been plenty good. He turned around to me once and said, "This is good. Wish you could get it." It was all done in the Sioux language and lasted for two and one-half hours. The points covered were there needs to be fewer pregnancies of school girls and more discipline. He told those present that discipline was up to the families. The school advisors were to be advisors and not disciplinarians. He pointed out that Indians want to keep their kids out of school to work in the harvest fields. They want to take money from estates before probated. They want to sell their land when they want to. They have no understanding of different types of allotments, cultivation, grazing, and so on and why things cannot happen when they want them to happen. The old chief sat there with his head bowed leaning on his long walking stick. Moses Two Bulls fell asleep once. John Lone Dog was the leadoff man.

August 23, 1954

We were all excited when Dr. Steve Parks from Rosebud received a copy of a letter from the Washington Office, a copy of one sent to Mr. Roberts, the Area director. We thought at first Steve, who is yelling for help over there, had sent in the original wire. Miss Simms called today to say that she had asked for more help, but they took one look at five doctors assigned to Pine Ridge and said two could go from here to Rosebud. With Dr. Bragg leaving, Dr. Gassman leaving the service, and Dr. Quint leaving on a two-month tour of North Dakota reservations, that will leave only two here, Dr. Walters and myself, and we can't both go to Rosebud. But the other day Mr. Kessis called to say a Dr. LaVizzio, a colored fellow who has just finished his residency in surgery, could be assigned here effective September 20. "Would we take him?" Mr. Kessis asked, and we both said "Yes." So he can be here alone. But then today Miss Simms called and said she wanted Dr. Walters to go to Cheyenne now when Dr. A. John Zumwalt takes his vacation.

I went through some of the files today. These Indians received allotment numbers with the Allotment Act, I guess before about 1900. There isn't much in their files, but I gathered some information.

Since the columnist Hal Boyle was here and syndicated his national column on Pine Ridge, Mr. Reifel has received several letters.[2] This is one, received on August 9, 1954, reproduced as it was received.

Mr. Reifel

Dear Sir I saw in my paper Where the indian are having a bad time. as you War saying. I am EX Soldier of War 1. and going on 54 but I dont

Look over 35. I Would like to get a indian Girl for a Wife. One that can have a Baby. I own my own home and 1, ACare Land. I lived here, by myself for 20 years, I did not get Married Because the Woman around here eather go to a Beer Garden then stay home and I dont Want a Beer soak. I like Beer But I don't get Drunk. I War Borned in Texas of German, and Swiss Parents. If some Indian Girl Wants to Write and send me her Picture I Will answer. She can be 25 to 35 but I dont Want None that cant have a baby. I get a Pension from the Gov for being Wounded. And I work in the auto shops some time. I think this is the Best Way to help Indian by Marring them off. let me know yours.

Rudolph C. Herbert.

August 25, 1954

I ran down to see Mrs. Forshey Monday night (August 23). She just got back from vacation. She was eagerly catching up on all news of the past three weeks. Boy, is she down on Edgar Red Cloud. Last year when her brother was here, he and her sister-in-law carted Edgar all over the Black Hills buying his dinners, and so forth. Then one day before they left, Edgar asked if they'd like to see Reno dance. They said yes. So Edgar took them to Loafer Camp and brought the old chief's costume and dressed them up and took pictures. Then Edgar took her brother aside and said, "We kept Reno out of school to dance for you today. We'll have to have some money for this." Mrs. Forshey said her brother didn't tell her until this year that he had done that. And how it came up is that this time Edgar brought a petition asking for donations for the Red Cloud monument. Congressman Berry has introduced a bill in Congress to build a monument. Under those circumstances, of course, the government pays for the monument. So the old chief and Edgar are running a racket. Mrs. Forshey calls them racketeers now.

By golly, that morning on my way to work who should come down the highway from Rushville but Wilson Brady with his camping gear on the top of his car. He stopped and wanted two dollars. I gave it to him since he didn't get the two dollars before. But that is the last donation I'm giving anybody.

When I told Mrs. Forshay about the petition that Edgar brought to me to get money for Reno she had a fit. Because Reno and Edgar also got more money in Sheridan than he told me, and not one cent did he offer to pay back.

Who should come in this morning but a well-known man with a welfare slip. He wants me to fill it out on his daughter, who was in the accident a few weeks ago. She is sixteen years old, has suffered an injury, and is surely incapacitated for work. But that girl is not a breadwinner! They think they can get paid just for being sick. They want money at every turn of the hat. They don't know what relief is.

We've had so many fractures lately. I was glad to see Mrs. Forshey's comments in the Pine Ridge bulletin not long ago. She said those who get fractures will not get relief if they were not working before they got their fracture since they are in no way incapacitated in their household. And I'd like to add that since they get all their medical needs cared for they have no idea just how fortunate they are.

We had four fracture cases from the rodeo Sunday and one head concussion and a fracture transferred from Rosebud. Yesterday I did a total thyroidectomy on a patient from Rosebud. Besides so much surgery in the house there is also GYN surgery. Now our gynecologist, Dr. Walters, is being called to the Cheyenne reservation. I tell you, this is the most discouraging situation I've ever been in. There just seems to be half a staff here at a time. Dr. Bragg and Dr. Gassman are both leaving the service. Mr. Kessis called about the new surgeon coming in September and that will help somewhat. Yesterday I took two Public Health nurses as well as Dr. Quint and Dr. Bragg, the dentist, and Mr. Manson A. Garreau, the sanitarian aid, to the school workshop on the request of Mr. Pyles to tell about our programs.

I was so upset with Miss Olinger. She gave her talk and then looked at me and said, "Dr. Ruby, shouldn't the toilets at Kyle be separated? The public uses the school toilets. One person out there is running around with VD." She dumbfounded me for a while. I finally said a school is a public building. You can't restrict a public toilet to certain ages. There are many people running around in our society who have VD but are not infectious. There is no need for restricting toilets. Anyone untreated should be reported, and we will turn them over to Law and Order since we are not disciplinarians. She is always doing some foolish trick like that. Afterward I talked with her, and she finally said that the reason she threw that in was because Mr. Morris Newkirk at Kyle wants the public, except for the students, not to use school toilets because his janitors just don't want to do all the cleaning up.

I got a program of the school workshop when I was there yesterday. I didn't have the time to read it over because I was too busy. I didn't even go through yesterday's mail until today. But here all branch chiefs were to be on a program this morning for a workshop as to how they coordinate with other branches. Mr. Reifle's secretary Emmaline called. But just before that this morning I had talked to Mrs. Forshey who was mad at having to go over. I told her I couldn't make it. So Emmaline called. I told her I was too busy. She said to send a representative. I said Miss Golden has been here one and a half weeks and is too new. I said call me back if he is insistent, but she didn't. That is the first meeting I've refused to go to. The honest fact is I'm so fatigued and have so much to do that I'm tired and sore all over. I can hardly move this morning. I'm afraid that what is going to happen is that I'm going to keel over one of these days.

Talk about not reading my mail. Both Public Health nurses came to see me mad as hops because Miss Golden wants to change the method for them to order supplies. She wants their supplies ordered separately. Both were crying. I really think they should be able to get supplies here for their clinics and not have to wait and such. But the situation has always been bad. The nurses here just don't have time to pick their supplies all the time. And they wanted intravenous solutions. Miss McGill put a note in my box to okay that. Well, I had forgotten, but on my standing orders to the nurses were that they can start ivs on patients in shock, without an order first.

I gave Mr. Pyles a jolt yesterday. In a meeting he told all teachers that he hoped we'd be able to help the kids and get glasses for them. He didn't want to be disappointed that some poor child couldn't get glasses. I said, "Mr. Pyles, I'm going to have to disappoint you more, but our budget has been cut, and we will be buying fewer glasses this year." Dr. Quint got up and, bless him for saying it, remarked: "The kids who have had to buy their glasses wear them. Those who have them given to them do not." And I know that is true. I was amazed so many teachers held up hands when asked if some of those children were buying their own glasses.

August 28, 1954

Edna Phyllis, the little clown, is growing every day. She has finally stopped that 2:00 a.m. feeding business now that she eats a small dish of fruit, vegetables, and cereal three times a day.

She looks all over and watches. Whenever we have company she embarrasses me by staring a hole thru them. She is a real doll. I'll be glad when you all can see her. It would be nice if you and Skin would truck back here after your rushing summer business is over.

I enjoyed your letter yesterday. Say, sometime ago we saw an article in the *New York Times*, which we read, that stated the Halls were going to this place in Pennsylvania.[3] I thought we had clipped it for you. But I guess not.

More problems. As you will probably read next time or when the installment gets to you, Dr. Walters is detailed in Cheyenne, and Dr. Bragg, who was at our house for a steak dinner last night, is leaving the service permanently. They have one fellow coming, but not till the weekend that Dr. Gassman leaves, and he is a surgeon. They called to ask if we wanted him. I jumped at the chance.

With so few doctors and so much work to do I'm worried. Then there is the clinic for the school kids. That was the subject of an hour's conference yesterday. We'll try having it at the school Tuesdays and Thursdays. Now I have to fix a list of drugs to take over there. Such work and carting around.

I went to quite a Yuwipi meeting last night that you'll eventually read about. Before they started the meeting they let me take pictures. Then I had to take my camera out or the spirits would tear it to bits, so I was told. But I'm afraid I didn't get good pictures. I couldn't see through the lens with only one coal oil lamp burning. I'm afraid I didn't do my focusing well enough.

Jeanne put up a basket or lug of peaches yesterday. We have most of our canning done. Left to do is pears, tomatoes, corn, and grape jelly. I'm afraid that we won't be able to put up tomatoes since all were ruined at Mission, where we get vegetables for practically nothing. And they are fresh. I like to can though.

August 28, 1954

I told Agnes Elk Boy a week ago that Mrs. Coker would like to attend a Yuwipi meeting. She brought Joe Elk Boy, her father-in-law, in for a shot yesterday morning and told Mrs. Coker she could come. We went out last night. Mrs. Coker picked me up at 7:45, and out we went to Chief Jim Red Cloud's home.

It was dark when we got to the frame and stucco structure in which Jim Red Cloud and a host of his relatives live. In the yard not too far from the house there was a bright fire over which Agnes was cooking a meal to be served after the night's meeting. Farther to the east was another fire in front of the sweathouse. The Red Cloud sweathouse had been altered earlier in the day and made larger so it could accommodate more men. Twenty men went in for a sweat bath. The medicine man, Plenty Wolf, conducted the ceremony. Women do not take sweat baths. This meeting was for Dick Elk Boy, Agnes's husband. Dick was going to sacrifice himself to the Great Spirit. Two of their children had died. Agnes had had one miscarriage. Their last child was born healthy and survived. Dick had made a promise to the Great Spirit that if they had a living child he would go up on a mountain hilltop for twenty-four hours without food and drink and would smoke the pipe to the Great Spirit. But first he had to take a sweat bath. It was necessary to renew his body and purify it of his wife's menstrual flow.

As soon as the sweat was over the men came out, dried themselves, and dressed. It had been unusually hot in the sweathouse. It was even a warm night outside of the sweathouse. After the men dressed Plenty Wolf offered a prayer to the Great Spirit. Women and children had joined the crowd. They stood with heads bowed. Then those present formed a line and went by and shook hands with Dick Elk Boy. His mother wept softly.

The night before many of these same people and Plenty Wolf had conducted an all-night meeting. Marie Hand had requested the all-night meeting to thank the Great Spirit. The previous winter her children had been sickly, but they survived the winter and recovered.

Two cars took Dick Elk Boy, the immediate family, and the medicine man and his helpers to the hills. Through a narrow gate, over a rough road, over ruts, over holes, through a bottomland of grass four feet high, across a clearing, over more rough road, through another bottomland of tall clover, then up a steep hill, across a clearing, and up another hill. The cars stopped. The party got out and walked up a steep hill, across to another steep incline, and then up another steep hillside to the highest hill on the range south of the Red Cloud lands. The party followed along the hilltop for a ways and onto a small projection. There a crowbar was used to dig four holes, each about five feet apart to make a square. A rosary consisting of a string of pea-sized pinches of tobacco, each wrapped in calico of various patterns several inches apart, was strung around the four holes in which branches of wild cherry limbs had been placed, each about three feet high. A yellow flag was put on the branch to the east, black on the west, white on the south, and red on the north. Along the line from south to west another hole was dug and here a taller cherry branch, about four feet high, was put in the ground. Four strips of cloth were tied to the branch, each a different color, white, yellow, black, and red. Around the base of the branch four small flags, each with a similar color of cloth, were stuck into the ground.

One of the helpers spread some sage on the ground. Dick went inside the enclosure, marked off by the long stringed rosary. Plenty Wolf gave him last-minute instructions. He then lighted a piece of braided sweet grass with a match and purified the inside of the enclosure. Plenty Wolf took Dick's shoes and handed them to Agnes. The women present had never been on this hilltop before. Plenty Wolf offered a prayer, standing in the same direction as Dick. Dick stood in front of the main cherry branch, facing it. The people were to his back. When Plenty Wolf began to pray, the men got down on their knees. The women squatted. Two songs were sung. The people got up. A few mumbled. They started off quietly back down the hill to the cars.

Back at the house the furniture had been moved out. Blankets were tacked up over the windows. Mattresses and pillows were piled around the room.

Plenty Wolf brought his suitcase in and sat it in the center of the room. One of the helpers brought in a bucket of hot rocks. He kept pouring small amounts of water over the rocks so that steam rose into the room. The people filed by passing through the steam as if taking a sweat bath. Jim sat near the door, greeting a few who came in.

Plenty Wolf placed four bottles of sand in the room to mark the corners of a rectangle five feet across the top and bottom and eight and one-half feet along each side. The top of the rectangle faced north. Here he made the altar. In the center he placed a larger glass jar of sand. In the four corner jars he placed the pieces of cloth, each in the rear was white, toward the east was yellow, to the west was black.

In the center jar at the altar was a tall flag three feet high with large streamers of black, yellow, white, and red cloth, and at the base of the stick were small flags each with a similar color, about a foot wide. On the big stick he tied two bunches of golden eagle feathers with laces of braided porcupine quills. The helpers tonight were Narcisse Wounded, son of Willie Wounded, and Weasel Bear, from Oglalla. Felix Greene, a Yuwipi helper, sat near the northwest corner of the room.

Plenty Wolf spread a one-foot square of cardboard at the front of the center bottle of sand. He poured sand out on the board, smoothed it with an eagle feather, which he laid down beside the board. He then strung a rosary of beaded tobacco around the corner bottles of sand. Narcisse Wounded took up several rosaries from those wishing to be treated. He handed them to Plenty Wolf and lined the center surface of dirt with them. He placed the peace pipe on the west side of the altar. He placed a package of Bull Durham on the east side. He laid a tobacco pouch and four gourds out. He put one at each corner of the front altar and two at the center. At the rear corner on the east Weasel Bear placed a white basin of water perhaps holding a gallon and a half.

Narcisse went around the room handing each person a small pinch of something, most likely sage. With this they rubbed their hands, arms, and faces. Then he handed out small sprigs of sage to each person. These they put in their hair, usually behind the ear.

Narcisse took a rope of braided sweet grass eight inches long, put it inside the single coal oil lamp to light it, and waved it above and around each person in the room and then about the inside of the enclosure. Plenty Wolf got out a blanket and a small rope. The ceremony was ready to begin.

Plenty Wolf sat in front of the altar after removing his shirt, belt, shoes, and a pocketknife from his pocket, which he handed to a member. He took a pinch of tobacco from the pouch and held in over the small curl of smoke from the burning braided sweet grass. Then he lifted his hand with the pinch of tobacco between thumb and forefinger, and his lips mumbled a prayer. He then put the tobacco in the pipe. He repeated this eleven more times. Then he took a small plug of sage and tapped it in over the tobacco. The peace pipe was handed to a woman at the northwest corner. She kept the pipe until the smoking began.

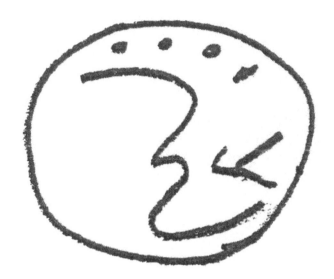

4. Message to Great Spirit at Yuwipi service, as observed and described by Robert H. Ruby on August 28, 1954. Drawing by Robert H Ruby.

Plenty Wolf drew a message for the Great Spirit in the sand. It was this.

Narcisse Wounded and Weasel Bear took their places at the center of the north wall at the head of the altar. They took up their drums and began to drum. Plenty Wolf handed the coal oil lamp to Jim Red Cloud along the east wall next to the entrance door to the outside. Jim put the light out. A song was sung. Then Plenty Wolf offered a prayer. The words came rapidly. He hesitated slightly once. The words came out like a well-known poem he might be reciting. Jim put the lights on. Plenty Wolf took a gourd, took out the cork on the underside, opened it to the room, and corked it up again. He took another gourd, took out the cork, and picked from it a small straight pin and a razor blade. Agnes Elk Boy got up from the west side of the building and walked along the outside of the front of the altar, along the east side inside the enclosure at the back and next to Plenty Wolf. He reached over to get the peace pipe. He handed it to Agnes, who held it, pointing it outward. Plenty Wolf stuck a pin into the skin of her left arm, elevating the skin. With the razor blade he took off a tiny fragment of skin, which he placed inside the gourd Narcisse Wounded was holding. He repeated this twelve times. Marie Hand, who had held the all-night meeting, came forward and went through the same process. Then Hazel Shield went through the same routine. Each time after taking the twelve pieces of skin Plenty Wolf whipped the arm with sage. There was considerable blood on Agnes's arm. The severed skin was a sacrifice. Each woman offered many pieces for Dick, for Jim Red Cloud, and for the medicine man himself.

After they had returned to their places, Plenty Wolf handed the peace pipe back to the woman next to Agnes and Hazel, who sat along the west wall near the north end. Marie was at the west wall near the south end.

Wounded and Weasel Bear came forward. They threw the blanket over Plenty Wolf. Wounded had first tied Wolf's hands behind him with a short length of small rope. Then they took a much longer piece of narrow rope, tied it about his neck, looped it about his shoulders, then the waist, and then below the hips and below the knees. They laid him face down on a mat of spread sage branches. He made a few muffled sounds.

Then Jim doused the coal oil lamp after Narcisse Wounded and Weasel Bear had taken their places at the drums.

During the ceremony at intervals small sparks flashed, almost always near the northeast side of the altar. The gourd traveled around, and broad flashes of light flashed around the room, not in rapid succession.

Between songs the spirits kept up a continual noise. As the gourd kept making noise the spirits imparted knowledge to Plenty Wolf, who in turn told the messages from the Great Spirit to those present. The gourd noise was so much louder when the Great Spirit wished to emphasize a point or show his enthusiasm for something.

One of the men being treated was Peter Stands Up. He had come out of the hospital the day before. He had gone in the agency hospital on Tuesday evening and was out two days later. Peter wouldn't or couldn't talk when he went in the hospital. But he was talking the next morning in the hospital. Now he had come to have Plenty Wolf doctor him. He wasn't up to snuff yet.

Plenty Wolf said two spirits had left the meeting. One went to the Sioux Sanitarium and one went way back east. There is a Weasel Bear woman in the Sioux Sanitarium with tuberculosis and a Weasel Bear man back east working. The spirits went to get reports on these people. They each brought back favorable reports of those they went to check on.

Two songs were sung for Dick up on the hill. Then Plenty Wolf told the crowd that the spirits would leave the house after the meeting and go up on the hill with Dick. The bad spirits were leaving the bodies of those being treated. Presently they went upward, leaving the room. As they left the music or songs and drumming was softer. A quick cool wind of the rushing spirits passed through the room. It was a pleasant respite. The room was hot.

All the while the medicine man had talked in a muffled voice. But then when the spirits untied him just before the last song, his voice no longer sounded muffled.

James lit the lamp. Plenty Wolf was sitting on the floor, his hair rumpled where the blanket had been pulled from over his head. The rosary around the room was gone. The small individual rosaries of those being treated were gone. Gourds were lying around. There were empty jars. The flags were down. There was no semblance of order about the enclosure and its objects. On the dirt was another message, this time from the Great Spirit to Plenty Wolf.

The woman with the peace pipe lit it and puffed, saying "Me-tau-que-essen."

Each responded "How."

Then she handed it to the person next to her, who puffed and said "Me-tau-que-essen," and all responded with "How."

And so on as the pipe went around the room.

Plenty Wolf took a basin of water. He said a few words over it and placed a sprig of sage in it. Then Narcisse passed it with a dipper from person to person. Each person said "Me-tau-que-essen," others responded "How," and then the person drank.

A meal followed, not dog. Tonight the same party will go after Dick Elk Boy. A meeting will be held at the conclusion of which dog meat will be served.

Some of the highlights of last evening were when Vincent Red Cloud was supposed to have taken Dick up to the hilltop. He ran off. So I looked at Nell Coker. We were standing around the sweat bath yet, and I asked her if we should volunteer to take Dick up. She said, "Yeah." Then I offered that we would do that. Plenty Wolf said okay. So Nell brought the car over, her Oldsmobile. We took Dick, who was sacrificing himself, and Plenty Wolf, the medicine man, Dick's mother, another woman, Hazel Shields, who was our guide for the night; plus there was Nell and myself. It was dark. The view was pretty from the top of the hill. We stumbled, slipped, and stepped on the sharp Yucca plants; maybe some of it was cactus. I couldn't see worth a darn. Since we left Dick on the mountaintop, we had more room coming back. The car scraped its oil pan on bumps.

Plenty Wolf has tattoos all over his arms, forearms, chest, and back. I think he was nervous at first. He is supposed to not have been in the "profession" very long. And it hasn't been long that he has been having himself tied up in the blanket and then getting out. I think he was nervous at the presence of the *waiscu*. But he didn't harangue us like Poor Thunder had on the merits of the profession and how he came to obtain it and just how dignified a profession it was. He didn't say such to us. We called him over, and Nell and I each gave him a dollar because he let us take pictures of the altar.

Hazel Shields sat next to me. She guided Nell and me around all night. As our guide, she got to go up on the hilltop. It was the first time she and Agnes had been up there. She is the loudest singer I remembered from the previous meeting I attended. She got hoarse last night.

She talked to me throughout the meeting. She wanted to know what

Peter Stands Up had when he was in the hospital. I told her a head cold. I guess I should not have said that because I kept asking her what the spirits said Uncle Pete had, and she said, "He (the spirit) hasn't said yet." Finally it dropped. Then after the meeting I asked her again. She said he only told Peter. So the spirits must have found something else wrong with him. She wanted to know if he had "run away" from the hospital, as she put it. I told Hazel no. He was discharged. She said the spirits said he was wet when he got home and that he had walked home. I had just supposed Brady came after him, so she said he must have walked straight across and crossed White Clay Creek and gotten wet.

As I walked in the building, I stopped to say a few words of greeting to Jim Red Cloud. I was asked to take a sweat bath by telling me I'd better do it. Taking a sweat bath before meeting is simply walking by the steaming rocks in the sweat house. But the whole house was like a sweat bath house, with no ventilation on a hot night and thirty or more souls cooped up in that space. I could feel the water simply run down my face and neck, I was so hot. Plenty Wolf did a good job of panting himself behind the blanket in which he was tied up for the two hours the meeting lasted. The sparks that flew during the meeting were always near Felix Greene. I would never have known, but he is a Yuwipi helper.

Several ahead of me had not drank the water, but merely took the bowl from which everyone drank, said their "Me-tauqui-essen" and handed it back to Narcisse Wounded, the son of Willie Wounded without drinking. I did the same thing. Hazel came after me. She took several long drinks and then turned to me and said, "You should drink some of that water."

"Why," I asked. "Isn't it the same as any water?"

"No," she said, "That is holy water. It will make you healthy."

Right away Agnes corrected her, "More healthy."

"Yeah," said Hazel, "I mean MORE healthy."

Mary Ann Red Cloud, Edgar's daughter, was there. This was the second Yuwipi she had been to. She sat next to Mrs. Coker and was as scared as could be. She kept hanging onto Nell's arm and asking, "Aren't you afraid?" At the end Plenty Wolf threw his blanket in her direction, and the gourd hit her in the head; she screamed.

What was particularly interesting to me is the way in which these people trust and accept me more and more to see their things. Letting government employees into those meetings and sharing the peyote is so new since it has never been done before. And really, taking skin off people isn't considered according to Hoyle. I had a feeling of sincerity on their part. Or a place for Yuwipi.

It is 8:00 p.m. Poor Yetta Gassman just called. Felix Walking is in their house and drunk. Harvey is gone. Felix wanted to talk to me so she called me on the phone. He wanted me to bring the peace pipe I have that needs fixing. But he is drunker than a skunk. What he wants is money. So I headed him off. Then he wanted to know where "his friend, Dr. Walters, is." I had called Dr. Stephen Parks earlier at Rosebud, and he said Dr. Walters was there, so I told him he was in Rosebud. What will poor Felix do for more money tonight to get his liquor?

I had a full hour's session with Mr. Mickelson yesterday. He doesn't want to bring kids from school to the clinic at 3:30 each day as was done last year. I don't really want to go over to the school. He wants us to go over there twice a week for the clinic. It may be better in some respects. But what I tried to get across to Mick is that we can never be sure that we can get there each time. Tentatively the clinic will be on Tuesday and Thursday at 1:00 p.m. That would be a mess to have someone over there. Surgery will run into that hour, as it did just this past Tuesday and Thursday. And poor Miss Golden is on her high horse. It means she will have to get more drugs from the storeroom to keep over there. That school clinic is really one grand mess. And so much unnecessary stuff. We'll see how it works out.

Fourteen. September 1954

I'll be darned if Sister Aquinas didn't call from the hospital in Hot Springs and say that a seventeen-year-old woman had to be transferred down here. Her father and mother are constantly drunk. Sister said the father was there two days ago. He was drunk. This girl was a patient in Omaha several years ago. The paper got a hold of her story and published about the poor little girl who didn't have any visitors. Mrs. Forshey and Frances Cottier of Welfare told me checks came in from all over the United States. The girl actually got thousands of dollars in gifts. Her folks got ahold of every bit of it and spent it on liquor and lived high for a time. Isn't that the most pitiful story? Pathetic, these people, disgusting. The girl was in Hot Springs under the Crippled Children's Program, but Dr. Bailey there has left. So now they want to send this invalid here. But Mrs. Forshey said they are no longer residents. She said the problem should be shoved right in the father's face. That is right, but the girl would suffer.

September 1, 1954

School started Monday. Kind of nice to see school kids around town again. Poor Mr. Mickelson is run ragged. I went over to see him and his wife Monday night. He didn't get home until 10:30 p.m. The rest of us were eating. So last night I started studying for my surgery boards, and they came over, ate, and left at 11 p.m.[1] But he floored me. He said he had an extra man put on his pay list whose services he doesn't receive: Boob Janis. I told him that was impossible. That I'd been paying Boob's salary and car expenses for a long time.

A family situation here. The mother and father lived together for years and raised a family. Eventually they got married and raised more kids. He drinks habitually and won't work. The entire family lives off of the old-age check of one of the family members' folks. One daughter has got infectious hepatitis. I took her out of school. Her mother said she had nothing to feed her since I told her to eat an elaborate diet. Her husband, the father, is very unconcerned. He wouldn't go to work to care for his little girl. Mrs. Forshey would not give the family money to buy food for the girl because others in the family would eat it up.

So Mrs. Forshey gave the child to Linda Unsigned with enough money to buy food. We went over to see her tonight. The kid is doing fine. Linda built her own home in back of her husband's. She won't live with her husband because he drinks and gets drunk. Linda's family is about the only Indian family in Pine Ridge with an electric refrigerator. Linda dressed up this morning and went over and gave Mr. Reifel a piece of her mind. He has ordered his police to shoot all barking dogs. The cops came in her yard last night. Then the dogs started to bark, and the police shot at her dog but missed. She told Mr. Reifel that they had better not do that again. She said her dog was going to bark if anyone comes in her yard. She told him if he wanted to do something he should get rid of all the bootleggers around her. She had to have her dog for protection at night. We keep Captain in at night. They have shot quite a few dogs around our place. Mr. Reifel doesn't like dogs that bark constantly all night. I don't either, but it is only reasonable that dogs, any of them, will bark if someone comes into a person's yard.

I just went over to Mrs. Forshey's place. We sneaked over to Linda Unsigned's tonight. A knock came at her door. She knew it was Edgar, so she didn't go to the door. Then when he went around to the back, we left the house. She is sure upset with Edgar and his father, and I don't blame her. Edgar bawled her out for telling her brother not to donate to the Red Cloud monument that is going to be built. Boy is that a graft. Congressman Berry is trying to get legislation through Congress to build a monument, for which, of course, Congress would pay, but Red Cloud is going around collecting money for it. Mrs. Forshey told him point blank, "If I gave you some money you'd buy liquor." Edgar said, "The old chief does that."

All of Reverend Orchot's vegetables were stolen from his garden. He is a Presbyterian minister. Then today I learned that $80 had been stolen from the Catholic Church.

Dr. Bragg is gone. Only Dr. Gassman and I are left. Dr. Quint does strictly eye work and is no help on the messy things, like school physicals, athletic physicals, emergency room and Relocation physicals, and such stuff that occurs throughout the day. Dr. Walters has been sent to Cheyenne to help out while Dr. Zummwalt is on vacation.

I got out of here at 7:00 tonight to go home and eat and then go to Mrs. Forshey's for the trip to Katie's. I'm sick of all the physicals coming up. It looks like the end of elective surgery. Then what use is there for me here?

I'll be darned if Sister Acquinas didn't call from the hospital in Hot Springs and say that a seventeen-year-old woman had to be transferred down here. Her father and mother are constantly drunk. Sister said the father was there two days ago. He was drunk. This girl was a patient in Omaha several years ago. The paper got a hold of her story and published about the poor little girl who didn't have any visitors. Mrs. Forshey and Frances Cottier of Welfare told me checks came in from all over the United States. The girl actually got thousands of dollars in gifts. Her folks got ahold of every bit of it and spent it on liquor and lived high for a time. Isn't that the most pitiful story? Pathetic, these people, disgusting. The girl was in Hot Springs under the Crippled Children's Program, but Dr. Bailey there has left. So now they want to send this invalid here. But Mrs. Forshey said they are no longer residents. She said the problem should be shoved right in the father's face. That is right, but the girl would suffer.

I had a meeting in Mr. Reifel's office today. A Mr. William H. Kelly, professor of anthropology at the University of Arizona, was his guest. I think Mr. Reifel put on a show for him. He brought all department heads to tell about the reorganization of the BIA, SMCO [Soil and Mois-

276

ture Conservation Operations], and consolidating the Grazing and Farm agents into one branch, now the Land Operations branch. He used the words *bastards, hell, damn,* and the like in front of the ladies present. The council had representatives present as well. They are certainly against Relocation. They seem to fight it. They had a fund on loan to the Relocation Department and took it back this year.

We talked about education and getting school kids to classes on time. Education gets $700,000 here. There are 1,500 school kids on the reservation. About 1,200 are now in school. I believe that includes the Mission, which started school today. Then there are some kids in public schools and others in denominational schools.

The same stuff was talked about: TIME, and its value in the Indian culture. The warhorse, Mr. Grueb, talked of getting all people off the reservation and closing up lock, stock, and barrel. Mrs. Forshey urged that Relocation be pushed, but was less aggressive about it than Mr. Grueb. Mr. Pyles pulled the other way. He said that kids where families live off the reservation should be brought back to school if they want to come here. This is not allowed now, but he used to send Mrs. Whirlwind Horse after kids off this reservation.

And me suturing kids. Trying to answer dizzy requests such as a telegram asking payment for the hospital bill of Melvin and Serena Spider and Moses and Maine Bull Bear in Sterling, Colorado. Looks like they were in a wreck or a drunken brawl. To hell with that noise. When I got my budget for this fiscal year, they said no funds were to be used for off-reservation medical care.

One of our mothers needs a cesarean section now. I got Dr. Crum from Rushville to come over and do it. But I'm sure paying that bill. If that damn Area Office can take Dr. Walters, they can just pay to have someone come and do that surgery.

September 2, 1954

All Pine Ridge is up in arms. For the first time since Mr. Reifel arrived at Pine Ridge and set Ethel Merrival in her place, she is up in arms again.

As my neighbor Butch Stoldt (half Oglala and half German) says, "She has always sorta been my political enemy, but now we see eye to eye." Ethel has called a mass meeting over the dog situation.

When I came to Pine Ridge, I had never heard of any complaints registered against dogs prior to that. There were some dogs that barked all night long, but no one seemed to complain. Since Mr. Reifel arrived, he has been harping continually about barking dogs. For about one week now he has given his men orders to shoot all barking dogs.

One of the first dogs shot belonged to the chief of police. His wife registered a complaint against the shooting of her dog. Maybe it's by coincidence, but anyway I've been told for that reason the chief was relieved of his position, and another man was made the chief of police. The old chief was demoted to just a policeman. Butch said the chief was so drunk in Rapid City the other night that Butch had to help him home.

It seems the situation is very much out of control. The police are shooting into yards at dogs. Dogs, dead, are left lying around where they fall. Injured dogs are being left to themselves. It is said that Sydney Young ran over a dog and didn't kill it. So he clubbed it and then shot it.

I heard today that our neighbors' dog was shot. He never barks. So I went over tonight. Sure enough, old Chang was shot twice, but is going to live. Butch has gone out and gotten a lawyer. Apparently he will make something of it.

After all, in cities dogs are picked up and kept several days for someone to call for them, before they are euthanized. They are not shot.

Keva Goings, cook at the hospital, said some of the cops are going to be beaten up when they leave the force. She said she'll swear that she saw cops with flashlights going through Joe Horn Cloud's place looking for his dogs the other night.

Edgar is always the joker. He says the Indians are going to bring their dogs up to the hospital to have their voice boxes removed.

I sure laughed at Katie Chief. The police shot at her dog in her yard.

Katie's family use their dog as a warning against prowlers who steal clothes from her clothes lines and against drunks from her neighborhood bootleggers. She went down to talk to Mr. Reifel the other morning. She told him she had only complained to a superintendent once in all the time she'd been here, and she must be in her sixties. And that was to Mr. Powers. This is the second time. She was indignant that they shot at her dog that never leaves her yard and only barks if someone comes around. She said he told her to keep her dog in her house. Then she added, "He'll be telling us the dogs are bringing in germs." I laughed until I was sick. Mr. Reifel is trying to spread the consciousness of germs.

Another gal complaining the other morning wanted to be in the clinic. She had no appointment. "Where is your number?" asked Mr. Reifel. "I don't need one, Ben Reifel," said old Mrs. Hudspeth, now from Hot Springs. "I knew you as a kid when your dad used to drag you around and you ate dog meat."

He really has made great complaints against dogs. He told Katie Chief he didn't like them. Katie told him, "I don't think you are a Sioux. All Sioux love dogs." Mrs. Forshey thinks he has so identified himself with white men that his past gives him a persecution complex, and he has a compulsion to get rid of dogs.

Ethel is calling a meeting of everyone she sees on the street. So the old warhorse is on the warpath again. It is rumored that some people are going to go around and collect all the dead dogs and throw them on Mr. Reifel's lawn.

Butch really told Mr. Reifel off. Butch said Reifel responded, "Just a minute, Butch, don't get so heated." But all of Butch's kids were bawling the other night, and Butch said he isn't going to stand for that. His dog will make it, however. Mrs. Two Dogs had two of her dogs shot right in her yard and killed. She'll be another one raising a real fuss.

Mrs. Forshey wants to get in on the meeting. As do I. But she almost asked Ethel when and where the meeting was going to be held. Butch told me tonight it will be on Monday.

I went to school this afternoon for the first clinic over there. We were up till midnight last night operating. We had to get Dr. Crum over from Rushville to assist. Rosebud wanted to send a strangulated hernia case. I told him we couldn't take it. He wanted to send a patient with a fracture today. I told him it was impossible. We have two problem obstetric cases in the house. It just seems too much work, not enough nurses, and too little help. Well, the crux of the thing is that Aberdeen told me not to have a clinic now at school. But I'm going to go ahead anyway. It will be a benefit for Mr. Mickelson, and I do want to help him. It might also help us. Last year we had ten to fifteen kids there every afternoon.

Mr. Mickelson has warned his staff that the cases sent must be emergencies. And as happens, we get nothing but dermatitis cases. So Mr. Mickelson is calling a meeting tomorrow of advisors and matrons, and I'm going over to talk to them.

September 4, 1954

I checked with Weldon Rolfe, acting in Mr. LaCourse's position since he left. Boob Janis was taken from my payroll, but I'm going to get someone in his place and pay his salary. Mr. Bertch will be putting on someone I see.

Guess WHAT!!!!! Our dog, Captain, the collie, is going to Washington DC to represent the dogs of Pine Ridge. Yesterday quite a notice was put up in the post office. There is speculation as to who did it. Some think Ethel Merrival, but she is not that clever. Some think Mr. James LaPointe of Rehab did it. That is Mrs. Forshey's guess because it sounds like his memoranda. Some think Jake Herman. It sounds like him, but it couldn't be. I had him in the clinic yesterday, and he sounded too cool to the whole dog business when I talked to him about it, and that was before I even considered that he might be the one.

Here is the bulletin posted in the Pine Ridge post office and other places around town:

K-9 NEWS

ATTENTION ALL DOGS

The time has come to do something about our lives and our little master's hearts. There is an undeclared war against us and the night raiders are unmercifully mowing us down in cold blood nightly. It is another Pearl Harbor, another Wounded Knee massacre, another Custer's Last Stand. It is tactics used behind the iron curtains of Europe and Asia only.

This is all one man's doing (sounds like Red China). The night raiders or D-Men are shooting us down under pressure from the mighty. It is either us or their jobs. Our supreme sacrifice only will preserve their jobs. Some of our dear masters have made that supreme sacrifice in World War II and Korea so that the mighty and the rest of the human beings in these United States, a free country, can live freely and do as they please within the laws and not get shot down on the command of one man as they do behind the iron curtain countries overseas.

What is this town coming to next? We heard that ever since Pine Ridge first set down, no one has ever seen or heard of a Pearl Harbor attack on us dogs as it is now. What have we done that was so terrible? Are we bootlegging, cattlerustling, or are we practicing illicit cohabitation for the purpose of obtaining more ADC funds from the state? These are what the mighty and his D-Men should check and try to stop. They are more important to the human welfare than shooting down dogs. The sidewalk from the club building on the corner, past the agency office and to the tribal office are so full of weeds protruding from the north fence that people have to squeeze single file to get to the office. On Tuesday afternoon, a young lady had an epileptic attack in front of the agency office and had to go to the sidewalk. Two hours later she had another attack in one of the grocery stores and hit the floor again. These are what the mighty and his D-Men should be looking after instead of shooting down dogs.

This is breaking the hearts of many little boys and girls to whom some of us belong and you cannot blame them as they were taught at school, be kind to animals. So what are we anyway? Something must be done quickly or it will be the horses next and then perhaps kids next, as we heard, the human birth rate is already annoying the big boy. We only hope our little masters do not grow up to be dog killing cops for their bread and butter, or worse yet, a dog despising big shot. We need help. Isn't there a state humane society? A national humane society?

Maybe we should organize. Elect an executive board of five members and two representatives from each fire zone. Select a delegate to go to Washington and get the low down on this uprising and get help from the national humane society. We want to all remember that we must send a big intelligent dog. My choice will be the big collie from fire zone 4. I think he can get time off from his internship to help us and maybe Pine Ridge once more will rest peacefully as of bygone days and not like an old wild west town of the 80's with shooting keeping people awake all night. As for us, we are leading a very normal life. Dog's life, that is.

Hoping no human is accidentally shot down from the stray bullets of a D-Man.

Scotty.

Member—A Society for the Preservation of the
Dog World from the Deadly Guns of D-Men.

September 9, 1954

I entered Mrs. Forshey's office this last Tuesday, maybe it was Monday. I heard her in the most animated conversation. Presently she said, "I'm not being sarcastic!" A few "uh-huhs" followed, and then with the voice on the other end going at full speed, she hung up loudly. It was a man who is an advisor at the school. He has for some time now been managing the students' personal funds. He is the one who came out of college money ahead. He is the one who used to bring Mrs. Mickelson some fresh vegetables because she had given him something. He would bring her two fresh tomatoes, or one cucumber. He is the one who asked Dr. Walters to operate on his wife and to put down "a small operation" so he wouldn't be charged too much.

Well, Mrs. Forshey has known that he takes kids to certain stores for clothes and then has an arrangement to get a tie or pair of socks, and so forth. Or he used to take the ADC checks some kids got, get groceries for their family, and then walk out of the store with groceries for himself. Mrs. Forshey said one grocer in White Clay told her Rider would take a basket, go around and pick out a basket of very expensive items, show them to the grocer, and then walk out. She has suspected he takes pennies here and there from kids' accounts. He is so eager to get a hold of money. He went into the bank the other day and got some money for two kids not even in OCHS. They are out at another school, out at Slim Buttes.

Mrs. Horn Cloud told him when he came for the money that he should call Mrs. Forshey. "Oh, no, it's all right," he responded. Later she heard about it. I don't know whether Mrs. Forshey called him or he called her. But the conversation must have been heated. Then that very afternoon he had to bring the money back. She, Mrs. Forshey, happened into the bank. He waved the money in her face and shouted, "See, I brought it back." Then he shouted and raved. He accused himself by telling her, "I suppose you think I was trying to steal it." He told her, "You have all the money around here. Your program is no good. It's lousy."

Mrs. Forshey says he is so paranoid and has such a persecution complex that he is a mental case. He shouted so loudly she was sure Mr. Reifel would hear and come over.

Mr. Reifel seems to have been shoving so much stuff onto other branch chiefs. He said when he came he was going to have a good time. Now that Eldon LaCourse is gone, he has to do more work. It is getting to him. He has more memos to write, and because Emmaline is behind, it frustrates him, so he is writing some of them in longhand.

He wrote a memo to Mrs. Forshey on that family who are living at Slim Buttes and that were kicked out of Chadron, who are from Fort Yates and tied in with a family from Rosebud. He asked Mrs. Forshey in the sake of humanity to do something for two families because Mr. Coker had told of their horrible mess living in tents at Slim Buttes. Well, a lot of Indians live in tents. But they are residents here. Chadron should have taken care of them as residents. Well, anyway, Mr. Reifel added on her memo, "(my kinfolk)." So he has a sense of humor. They should be related to him in a way. He is a Rosebudder.

Mrs. Forshey has been watching Mr. Coker. She thinks he is trying for a superintendency. I know there was a political deal afoot. When they broke up smco, Forestry, Grazing and Farm Agents departments and put them all into one just recently, a month ago perhaps, Mr. Reifel asked to have Mr. Coker stay here and Mr. Mast be moved. Mr. Mast is probably a better worker. I was for it myself because we need Mrs. Coker at the hospital as a nurse. We are far too short of nurses as it is.

This morning a woman jumped out of the window at the hospital and fell two stories without breaking anything. Tonight she is nutty and more active than ever. She is a woman in her forties with a postpartum psychosis. She married a man from Rosebud; he died of tuberculosis a few months ago. She said she had no children but actually had six. She was a resident of Gordon three and a half years ago, I guess, when Mrs. Forshey came here. She was getting welfare and had an able-bodied husband then. When Mrs. Forshey investigated the husband, he said he did not know she was becoming mentally disturbed. She got checks and spent the money herself. Anyway, she delivered last Saturday and a day later developed the postpartum psychosis. She has had nurses on guard every minute because she has wanted to get her baby and leave the hospital. This morning she took the plunge when not watched. I tried to get a hold of the chief of police last night to put her in jail just so she'd be locked up. But he didn't come around until today. He had a better suggestion. He'd send a prisoner up to watch her. So now we have a prisoner up to sit there and keep an eye on her.

I went to see Mr. Reifel the other night. I had seven cases of vene-real disease over the weekend and one today. I told him there were so many that I didn't have time to locate the contacts, and so forth. So I told him I wanted a policeman to bring certain people in to me. He brought back one today who went off the other day without treatment. A policeman is going to bring in two girls in the morning. Half of the infections are coming from our boys who go to Rapid City. I saw in the Rapid City papers the other morning that 90 percent of the loose women, white and Indian, being picked up on the streets in Rapid City have been found to have VD.

The Gildersleeves of Wounded Knee are a fright. They are always trying to get the ADC and OAA (Old Age Assistance) checks to the detriment of people. One case from Manderson was an old man who never ran up bills. Mrs. Gildersleeve tried to get him to run credit there at the Gildersleeves' store in Wounded Knee and then she went to Welfare and tried to have his address changed to have his checks sent to her. Mrs. Forshey said she wouldn't allow or let a man start to run credit where he'd not done that in the past. If he wanted to get his checks and then go and spend cash, all right. But the habit of letting a person run credit is not good. The Indians do it all the time. The stores know who they are but take the gamble. For instance, one man was having a land sale check coming for $100. So, it was a few years ago, Svara's let him run up an $800 bill. And so did another store in Whiteclay. That person told each place it was the only place he was trading. So each place collected about half of the check.

Everyone seems to be fed up with the Indians' lack of responsibility. Mrs. Mickelson was telling me today about a family that is so large that three little girls have to sleep in the car each night. When the family goes out for a night with the car they have to wait to get into bed. Then Mrs. Hemingway told Mrs. Mickelson that Relocation offered a man a job in Los Angeles. They told him he'd have to take it and support his many kids. "What," he screamed. "I'm not going to support them." So he dumped them in Holy Rosary and the boarding school.

Mrs. Forshey is sure off on the number of people coming to her with their rodeo injuries and expecting to get relief. They never worked or were not working before their injuries, so they haven't been incapacitated. Besides, they get all their medical expenses free.

Mr. Reifel is on the defensive now. It is the first time since he's been here. He is trying hard to keep face on his dog deal. He has had so much criticism. How naive can a man get? Or how much does he think he can fool someone? I was amused. In the news sheet for Wednesday, the day after the dog meeting, he announced it was a special meeting called by Mrs. Merrival. Then he announced it was called for Health, Education, and other aspects of the coming visit of Commissioner of Indian Affairs Emmons. Then he said unfortunately Mrs. Merrival had to leave, and about the only thing that received discussion was the dog problem. He really knows the truth, I hope. The meeting was called for nothing but that purpose.

Mr. Mickelson is going round and round with a woman who is a teacher at school, an Indian, and very Indian in her habits, undependable. She used the excuse she had to take an uncle of hers to the bus. Then after that she went to the dog meeting. There were repercussions from other teachers who would love to have gone. She and her husband both have jobs. Her husband was once canned from civil service because he drinks his money up each weekend. She has one daughter. Yet the woman always wants to borrow money from school accounts like the Student Fund. Mr. Mickelson has his troubles with her.

Another woman seemed a little different from other Indians around here, even though she hasn't a brain in her head. She was the bum deal Mr. LaCourse pawned off on me, the poor excuse for a secretary last November and December. Her mother is head of commissary and did give the young woman a year of work after high school. Well, anyway, the young woman is pregnant and not married. Her mother isn't upset. It is a common thing here.

I did school physicals yesterday at Kyle in the a.m. and at Porcupine in the p.m. Mrs. Olinger helped me, and she pulled a stunt on me in the teachers' workshop meeting. Everywhere we went yesterday she kept needling the teachers and then, when they were out of the rooms, telling me how horrible they were. I certainly don't like to work with her.

All schools take preschool kids, or beginners. They are really kindergarten material. One tiny child came up to Porcupine. I learned that his family haven't anything to eat in the home. So they send their kids to school hungry. The father is a perfectly able-bodied man who tried hard to get relief. He couldn't because he doesn't qualify, and now he won't go out and work.

Mr. Reifel and others said time and time again that parents call and say, "You do something with my kid." Mr. Reifel tells them they are the parents and must take responsibility for their children. Yesterday Mr. Schindelbower showed me a note he received from a mother because he threatened to send the law out if she didn't get her child in school. The mother said she tried hard and couldn't do a thing with her daughter. "You do it," she wrote to Mr. Schindelbower. What people.

I spent a while this week with Mr. Pyles making a schedule for the mobile X-ray unit to be here in October. He is weak and needs a dormitory supervisor. I need nurses. But he had to turn them down because he has no housing. Yet he is afraid to turn out Sidney (Buddy) Miles, who does not work for the government but lives in an Education house on campus. Mr. Miles is on the tribal council.

September 11, 1954

Our work has slowed down in the last few days. Baby Edna does something new each day. Her coordination is so much better. Night before last she reached out and took hold of her nipple. First time I've actually seen her reach and take something she had her eyes on. Usually babies' little hands wobble all over. We had her walking with us outside yesterday. I picked one of our marigolds and put it in her fingers. The next time we looked she had it in her mouth.

Jeanne chopped off our big morning glory. They make a background of blue by the kitchen window and up over that old oil drum in back.

There are others there, and after a vine is all dead they may cover up the dead vines, and it will look better, but I do enjoy the blooms in the morning.

Lil and Mick (Mickelson) were over for dinner Wednesday. Jeanne gave a dinner for the Masts, who are leaving. Tonight Lil is giving a dinner for the Masts, and we are going over there. Tomorrow Edna Phyllis is going to be baptized, and afterward Reverend Orchot and the Mickelsons, who are going to be the godparents, are coming over for dinner.

September 16, 1954

Mr. Reifel just suffered another defeat. The first was on the dog issue. The second involved a plan of his, exclusive of the Social Services Department, to give welfare or relief money to families going potato picking.

So now Mr. Reifel is hammering to get kids in school. He has been talking it up for some time. Mrs. Forshey said she did not know about promises made the last few days to communities. Mr. Reifel blamed her for not assisting him introduce his plan. But he made promises to families to give relief money to them or people who would care for children of families going to the harvest fields.

A similar plan carried out last spring showed that more families than usual went out to work when they received money for going or received money for keeping their kids in school. Now Mr. Reifel wants to subsidize a similar program. Mrs. Forshey wrote him a memorandum listing many reasons why such a plan should not be done. It was caustic, but to the point. He asked her why she couldn't pick up the phone and call him. She told him because she couldn't reach him half the time and because it was difficult to talk to him. It is. He does most of the talking. But, of course, he called her three times yesterday. She hid out at her home where she prepared the memorandum. I think, though, that these people sometimes get Mr. Reifel down, and it was his way of keeping the kids in school.

But several facts have to be weighed. There would have been families galore tramping through the welfare office. Because money was being given out, more families would have been leaving. That is all right, but the reason is wrong. And I also wonder, "How long are you going to subsidize these people to get an education?" They should want an education for their kids, and the kids must want it. They can go elsewhere where there is work all the time if they wish. No one is keeping them here. They can put their kids in public schools, too.

Well, Mr. Reifel told Mrs. Forshey he would call Aberdeen at 8:00 a.m. and for her to be in his office. What does he do? He calls Aberdeen at 7:00 a.m. here (8:00 a.m. in Aberdeen), but they wouldn't go along with his plan either, but for other reasons. Contracts would have to be made for foster homes. Only two or three weeks away, too many cases, and no time. So Mr. Reifel backed down on relief funds, but he called in Mr. Pyles, who had been in on the other plan and told Mr. Pyles he would have to arrange with the day schools to supply three meals a day for those kids. And folks keeping the kids could come to the schools and eat also. Now if that isn't something for Mr. Pyles. It is still subsidizing education.

To make it as simple and brief as possible, this is my version of the deal. The pattern around here is for families to go to the harvest fields to pick potatoes each fall. They haul the entire family, taking the kids from school, often for an average of two to three weeks. They go to the fields and the kids are made to do as much as, and many times more than, the parents, who have a vacation, often resting the entire time as the kids work. What money is made is spent as soon as it is made. A great deal of it goes for liquor.

Near Scottsbluff, Nebraska, last fall thirty men were thrown in the jail one night on drunken charges. Each man was fined $20. That netted that city $600 in one night, and the farmers nearby also got their fields harvested. The city would not allow the families to stay in the town after the work was done, and I should say after the money was spent because it is spent as soon as the work is over. The city won't take responsibility for ill-health or other problems.

A parent is responsible for his own kid. He should want to see that kid in school and make sure the kids are there. But there won't be so many going harvesting. The day school teachers will hate it since they usually have a picnic for several weeks when half the kids on average are gone. This affects day schools greatly, but not boarding schools. Mrs. Forshey spent three hours at our home last night telling about her tangle with Mr. Reifel.

Wouldn't you know it? People have to come here and live to understand that Indians are not storybook characters. Joseph Lehrner, the white boy from Pennsylvania who has been staying with the Red Clouds, sure learned about it. I've commented on him before. He is the one who, when he came here in June with all of his five months of earnings, would say to Edgar, "I want to hear some more Indian talk." He is eighteen years old. Yesterday he sent a wire home to his father, "Send me 50 dollars to get back on. I will pay you back." He had wanted to buy some beadwork. He doesn't have a cent. He is even hungry. He now has only the clothes on his back and no extra clothes. Agnes and Dick Elk Boy borrowed $30 from him that he is trying to get back. He never will. He has bought food all summer for the Edgar Red Clouds. Besides that, Reno and Edgar have made several hundred dollars working in the movie, dancing, selling beadwork, and enlisting donations for the monument to Red Cloud that is going to be paid for by the federal government anyway if it is sculptured. So now Joe hasn't got a penny. He did wise up. It took him a long time to learn about his "storybook" Indians.

I get very disgusted at times with folks who have so many irresponsible habits, with those who not only don't want to work, but won't work. The Oglala Sioux are the worst I have ever encountered. I'm sick and tired of them trying to get relief and taking my overworked time so I can't expend it where it is needed. Another woman was on relief from Welfare. She had a land sale of just under $10,000. Every bit was gone in under six months. So Welfare won't take her on again for the period of time in which a normal person would spend that much money wisely. So she tried to get a disability pension for medical reasons, but that didn't work. She had elective surgery, thinking she'd get a disability check monthly. To top that, she said she was getting clinic treatments for her operation. That was the three times she had to come back. How do you like that? It happens every day. It disgusts me.

I did physicals at OCHS. I covered the first eight grades, excepting the seventh, which I couldn't find. I took only those who weren't examined last time, which means last year. I thought today, if I had a choice again, were I to make a decision again on a profession, I'd like to be a teacher of young children. I'd like to work with them. They are cute kids. The outer garments were fair to very nice. The underclothing in some cases was flour sacks. This is unnecessary in this day and age for anyone with a parent who is able to get out and do a day's work.

September 18, 1954

We have quite the conversationalist in our home. I sit and talk to Edna Phyllis, and she talks back, screws up her little mouth, and mutters all sorts of sounds, and then just smiles and smiles. We take a daily walk around the yard at noon. Then in the evening we sing.

Captain has gotten something. He just scratches and scratches. We flea-powdered him and even salved him, but he still scratches, so we need to get him to the Vet.

A nice fall day, and I have lots of little chores to do and don't know where to start. We can't get tomatoes to can. There just aren't many around. I got ahold of some green ones that we are canning as soon as they get pinkish and as soon as they get soft. They aren't nice and red but will be okay for use in cooking, I guess.

Dr. Walters gets back this weekend from Cheyenne, but then in a week Dr. Gassman leaves, so there still will be two of us unless the new guy comes in, but I don't expect him until I see him.

We took Edna Phyllis to church last Sunday and had her baptized. The Mickelsons are the godparents. She was an angel all through the meeting. The minister and the Mickelsons came for dinner after church. I was going to leave with her after the baptism, but she was good so I just stayed there with her. The hurricane in New England is called Edna, you know. That's our baby.

September 18, 1954

The following are not isolated instances. They are everyday happenings. A man is in the jail here awaiting transfer to a federal prison after being sentenced in the federal court for assault with a deadly weapon. He came up to the hospital last night complaining of pain in his chest. I asked him if he might not have some anxiety because of the present position he is in, though to be sure, I didn't use those words. No, he didn't care, he said. It didn't worry him. Yes, he had a wife and three children, but that didn't make any difference either. I've had two or three applications submitted in the past year for positions at the hospital by people who have police records or arrests. Such things don't bother the Indians.

Another man is six months out of the army and is going to be married soon. But he has no job or means to support a wife. He wasn't concerned. My next patient was a woman from Wounded Knee. She is eight months pregnant and nineteen years old and not married. My third patient fits the same slot.

After the clinic I looked over my correspondence. Two women had left St. Joseph's Hospital in Omaha on their own before their treatments were completed, so Dr. Eagen's office returned their train tickets. I went to the expense of sending them down with a car and driver. I got train tickets for their return and sent them down. I authorized their hospitalization. Well, if and when they come to this hospital again I'm not going to see them. A doctor in private practice wouldn't put up with such nonsense, and I am a firm believer that the way to help these people is to develop some standards, to deal with them as with other people, and stop the coddling and nursing and wooing of them. So let them handle their problems on their own.

The weather still manages to be unpredictable, with flash floods and hail. Today is a typical fall day. It is sunny, but there is briskness in the fall wind. The trees down at White Clay Creek have taken on a tint of yellow, and the wood vine has taken on a tint of red here and there. This is football weather. The boys this year at OCHS are certainly small.

Dr. Gassman has one more week before his tour of duty is through. He has been writing various places for a job. One clinic wrote back, "We hire only Protestants. If you fit this make application." Dr. Gassman is Jewish.[2]

September 22, 1954

Two of the three Lame Deer Indians who participated in the Sun Dance and who remained behind will probably be here forever. Now one fellow is going to get married. He is going to marry the woman was in the terrible wreck that killed a woman and injured others. He is twenty-three. She is twenty-eight.

Uncle Orrin was at the horse races in Alliance and met Posey Eccofey down there. He has race horses.

One of my old friends had a land sale. He has two new cars, a 1954 and a 1953 in front of his shack. Can you imagine? Now his $6,000 will be gone in no time. He has a son from a previous marriage who is on ADC in Montana. But does he support that kid with all his money? No. The taxpayers do.

Well, school is well underway. The sores are getting scrubbed up and healing. Our supply of Toposide is well reduced, and so are the head lice.

Vincent Red Cloud is going to get married to a sixteen-year-old girl. Edgar doesn't know it. Edgar has tried to keep him from getting married for so long. Now he won't have his chauffer or car. Poor Edgar.

And Joe Lehrner, the young white man who stayed with them through
the summer and who blew all his money from five months of work for
food for all of them, was finally kicked out. He left what few belongings he still has at Mrs. Forshey's office and went to the potato fields to
work to get money to go home. I guess his father refused his request
for a loan. Vincent stole his bow and arrow and pawned it for money.
Joe bought scads of beads for Mrs. Red Cloud, who promised to make
him beaded things. She told him she never sews during the hot summer months. Joe felt sorry for her and bought her a cooking stove. Her
old one was in shambles. But, of course, though Edgar and Reno made
lots of money, it was all consumed in liquor. That young man had to
learn in a terrible way that Indians are not the fascinating people por-
trayed in storybooks.

Glenn L. Emmons, the commissioner of Indian affairs, was in town
yesterday. He spoke to the teachers' institute. I couldn't get there for
the banquet, but I went down for his talk.

Mr. Reifel introduced me. Our conversation went like this:

"How do you spell your name?"

"R-U-B-Y."

"I knew some Rubys from Alabama."

"My father's folks are all from upper New York State."

"The Alabamans were rebels." Ha ha.

"Yes."

He talked later about two things in Indian affairs that he was interested in improving: health and education. But he didn't ask me one
question about the hospital or its operation here.

We had a frost two nights ago. Froze all our flowers and froze everything excepting the tomatoes. I had covered them. The fall days are nice.
The agency whistle blows everyday at 8:00, 12:00, 1:00, and 5:00.

Life goes on, but what an existence. A woman was just in with nothing serious. She said she had a bad cold. She put up such a horrible
story that Dr. Walters fell for it and recommended her son stay home

fifteen days extra on his army leave. He can't hold out against their songs and dance.

September 26, 1954

On Thursday the 23rd I did school physicals at Red Shirt Table, where I had lunch with the Shaws, the teachers there. We ate the same lunch as the school kids did. At each place I've been to, conducting school physicals, we have been fed macaroni and cheese. The lunch at Red Shirt Table was no exception. One child was Todd Fast Wolf, who played the young Crazy Horse in the movie this summer. Mr. Shaw tells me the movie people used his office and phone to call Hollywood. I don't understand how they could. I can't even call from the phone at Red Shirt Table to Pine Ridge and understand what is being said.

I then went to Day School Number 6. Mr. Friesly is the teacher there. There were approximately fifteen kids at Red Shirt Table, twenty-five kids at Day School Number 6, and twenty at Day School Number 4, Mr. Roy Martin's school.

These people sure know where you are or what car it is. At Day School Number 4 a man came to the school and said his grandfather was ill. He wanted to know if I would come and see him. After I got over there, then he wanted me to look at the baby. It had cried all the night before. The grandfather had gastritis, the baby nothing. This is what I observed. The house was a one-room affair. There were two beds and a cot. The cook stove was in the center of the room and in homes like this one is used for heat as well as for cooking. Flies swarmed around in droves. Paint was peeling from the furniture. Only a few chips of paint were on a few chairs. The baby was dirty. Secretions were running from the nose to the lips. The grandmother had sore eyes. The great-grandfather of the baby was sitting on the caked and hardened soil by the side of the flimsy frame and stucco house. The great-grandmother was sitting on one bed, not bothered by the multitude of flies and puffing on a long-stemmed Indian pipe. The floor was dirty. The boards were worn into ridges and littered with junk. There were a few metal cans and boxes on the floor. A scraggly pup or two sauntered by. Everything seemed greasy and soiled. The walls were shabby, and the wallpaper was torn and fly specked. There were enamel pans that were battered and rosetted by the cracking and flaking enamel. The curtains were stiff and black from filth. There was a small table, wooden, plain, nonpainted, and showing hard use.

I have had numerous cases where people, Indians, take off their casts before they should. A rodeo rider was one of the worst I've had. At the Pine Ridge Rodeo this twenty-three-year-old male broke his right radius. The ends were overriding. Three of us struggled, and finally we got a good closed reduction, and put a cast on it. He had his wife cut that cast off before a week was past because he wanted to ride in rodeos. The rodeo folks wouldn't let him compete with a cast on. So he took it off for that reason. He has made good money. Several hospital employees have seen him since then ride and take prizes.

Of course, the bones slipped. This man's arm is nicely curved, and he still can't supinate or pronate it. His wife told Dr. Walters last Friday that after two more rodeos he was coming in to see what could be done. When he comes in, if he does, he is going out that door as fast as he came in. I won't have a thing to do with him. He can take some of the money he made in the rodeos and have his arm fixed elsewhere. I'm writing letters to Welfare and the Social Services (relief) office that he is able to work full capacity, if he can ride in rodeos, and is not to get rehabilitation or relief for such nonsense as that.[3]

Chief Red Cloud came to the house on Friday to borrow money. We had him eat with us. He likes wieners and sauerkraut.

This is the most beautiful time of the year. And to spend a weekend in the Black Hills amid their fall splendor is an opportunity. We spent Saturday night with Uncle Orrin in his cottage. Saturday afternoon we visited Bob (Gold Bug) Nelson and Florence Nelson. We dined at the Sylvan Lake Hotel. Sunday we drove the highways and visited the zoo and Game Lodge where both presidents, Coolidge and Eisenhower, have had summer white houses. It was an interesting visit.

September 28, 1954

I remember the other day at the dinner for Commissioner of Indian Affairs Glenn Emmons that Mr. Reifel introduced the dignitaries present: Representative Berry of the U.S. House of Representatives and the secretary for Senator Mundt, among others. Then he introduced Chief James Red Cloud. James had on his Indian suit and feathers. He looked glorious, but the dignitaries had no idea that he comes from a hovel and is a beggar. Speaking about Red Cloud, Mrs. Forshey got together with Mr. Mickelson and told him Agnes and Dick owe Joseph Lehrner $30. They called Dick in at pay time and took it from his check after cashing it. Mrs. Forshey said Agnes and Dick tried every trick in the book to sneak out of it. Even when waiting right there, Agnes tried to sneak away twice. She has power of attorney to sign Dick's check. She signed her name and then laughed and said, "Oh, I've signed it wrong." She thought she had them stumped, but then Mick erased it and had her sign Dick's name.

Some white people, perhaps most white people, think Indians are storybook people. They don't know of all the things that Indians get away with. How some people might visit homes and remark about a bare cupboard. They don't know what "grub trunks" are and that all these people keep their food locked up in trunks so visitors won't eat it, Indian visitors, that is. They don't know that these people are the biggest thieves, cattle rustlers.

I really got into two deals today. Yesterday Mr. Reifel called Emma Nelson when I wasn't available. She told him that Mrs. Barnes, the social worker at Alliance, Nebraska, was bringing a baby to the hospital for us to keep awhile. The baby is the child of a white man and an Indian mother who lives in Nebraska. She has been married to three white men. She won't care for this child. So Mrs. Barnes, the social worker, pulled a fast one. The county court of Box Butte County at Alliance took the child from the mother. Mrs. Barnes got a family at Manderson to care for the child, but they apparently made no arrangements to pay for the care. After all, the child is not a resident, and the father is not an Indian. But they dumped the kid in the hospital. So I'll bill the county court in Alliance. Anyway, I doubt that Alliance will pay, because they expect Pine Ridge to do so. If they don't, Mrs. Forshey will go with me to take the baby back to Alliance.

A still bigger deal I got into was when a letter came to Mr. Reifel asking that we arrange to transfer a female patient from the Hastings State Hospital in Nebraska to the Yankton State Hospital in South Dakota. The letter was from Dr. Herbert A. Huggins, the new Area medical officer. Mr. Reifel sent the letter to Mrs. Forshey. She told him I ought to know about it since it involves Health funds. He laughed and laughed. Well, back of all this is the fact that this patient has been out of South Dakota for years. But she never stayed one place in Nebraska, so Nebraska won't consider her a resident even though she has been in the state for years and in the Nebraska mental institution for four or five years, as well as in the state reformatory or some penal institution. She is promiscuous and a drunkard, a burglar and a public menace. Now she has epilepsy and mental deterioration. Mrs. Ruth K. Heineman, the Area social worker, goes down there and gives Nebraska lots of promises to spend Health funds to bring her to South Dakota.

There is more to it than that. I am certain Mrs. Heineman gave some phony line to Area Director Roberts because all I know about him leads me to believe he is a man of principle and not political shenanigans. Mr. Reifel penned a note to Mrs. Forshey that Area Director Roberts wanted us to send Lenore to Yankton so there won't be any adverse publicity. And he told Mrs. Forshey this is an election year and so there is politics at play. I don't believe Director Roberts knows that in July 1951 the state's attorney for Fall River County, to which Shannon County is attached, ruled the patient was not a resident of South Dakota and that in May 1951 Graham Holmes, the Area legal advisor, ruled the patient was not a resident. I don't think he would go along with the deal. Well, what did I do? Mrs. Forshey first of all called me in on it. So I called Dr. Yohe, the superintendent at Yankton State Hospital, to arrange for transfer of the patient. I gave him her background and also the information contained in various documents in the Social Services Department. He said since a county court had to commit her or send her there, it had to be the county in which she was a resident. He wouldn't take her since she was not a resident of South Dakota and that as far as he was concerned the matter was through. I wrote that up in a memorandum for Director Roberts. I think it will cause some disturbance.

Fifteen. October 1954

Last Thursday the parents of a girl came to me and said they had gotten a letter from the Department of Crippled Children in Pierre to take the girl to Dr. Ahrlin, a bone and joint specialist in Rapid City, on Friday for an appointment at 2:30 p.m. They didn't have gas money and wanted to know if I could do something about it. I reminded them that their daughter has a short leg and *equina talipes varus*, probably the result of an old polio leg. Now she has a chance to have medical attention and get something done to help her to walk better. I explained that I had made all the arrangements for them to get this free medical care, but they had to take their daughter to Rapid City. I reminded them they go into Nebraska and distant places for dances. Now the least they could do was to get their child to the doctor in Rapid City. The parents have no sense of responsibility. No sense, period. When I was a youngster, my father would have walked and carried me to Rapid City under such circumstances. But I can't understand people who won't make the effort.

October 2, 1954

I'm working this weekend. I have already admitted six patients for Saturday, mind you, besides seeing others as outpatients. What a beautiful day. It is so autumnish.

Already we are beginning to think about our trek back home. The movers were here to move Dr. Gassman and gave us an estimate on poundage. But darn it, we have jars, including pints and quarts, of fruits and vegetables and their trucks are not heated. Besides, our stuff will have to be in storage for a short while so it could all freeze and burst.

That means, I guess, that we will have to haul it with us and stay at night in a hotel with a heated garage.[1]

We will leave approximately the middle of December. If we go to McCall first we will be camped at your place for Christmas. If we go on out to Jeanne's mother's home, then we will come back for a visit later. Would you all be willing to drive back about the time we pack and drive out home with us with all your expenses paid?

Poor Jeanne. She has little Edna Phyllis, age three and three-quarter months, Vicky Mast, age eleven months, and Lorie Mast, age six years, at home today. The Masts went off for the day. The Masts are the ones who kept Edna last weekend for us while we went off the reservation.

October 10, 1954

I performed an appendectomy on a nine-year-old kid from Rosebud because his appendix ruptured. Charlie Yellow Boy dropped in to get some medicine. He is an elderly gentleman. He never asks for money or other things, just medicine so he won't have to go to clinic and wait, I guess. I accommodate him. The mother of Kenneth Ghost Dog was here at the house. Her boy is one we are sending to Omaha in the morning for care. I get so fed up with these Indians. Sometimes you can't do enough for them. I'm beginning to show fatigue.

Last Thursday the parents of a girl came to me and said they had gotten a letter from the Department of Crippled Children in Pierre to take the girl to Dr. Ahrlin, a bone and joint specialist in Rapid City, on Friday for an appointment at 2:30 p.m. They didn't have gas money and wanted to know if I could do something about it. I told them that their daughter has a short leg and *equina talipes varus*, probably the result of an old polio leg. Now she has a chance to have medical attention and get something done to help her to walk better. I explained that I had made all the arrangements for them to get this free medical care, but they had to take their daughter to Rapid City. I reminded them they go into Nebraska and distant places for dances. Now the least they could do was to get their child up to the doctor in Rapid City. The parents have no sense of responsibility. No sense, period. When I was a youngster my father would have walked and carried me to Rapid City under such circumstances. But I can't understand people who won't make the effort.

Then Mr. Mickelson called me at 9:00 p.m. and said the girl's folks had been to the school wanting to know if somebody there wouldn't take her up to the appointment. It was a no go, so they left her in the dormitory. I happened to realize something I hadn't thought of in the afternoon. I had a car going up to take two patients to the Sioux Sanitarium the next day, Friday. I told Mick I'd take the child up then. I'm fed up with Indians.

They have no integrity and don't know what friendship is. Mrs. Forshey has for years fed, given money to, and otherwise befriended Edgar Red Cloud. He gave her a drum. Now I know what an "Indian giver" is. Edgar was in and out of her home for the drum. When she finally wore out and got sick of his meanderings and begging for donations, she gave the drum to Joe Lehrner. Edgar brought Joe into Mrs. Forshey's office when he kicked Joe out of his home after Joe supported the family all summer. Then they went down into the potato fields. Edgar should have been a writer of melodramas. He wrote a letter to Mrs. Forshey, and I saw it. He mentioned the word *drum* twenty-eight times in four pages, two sheets of a letter. He has the drum now because Mrs. Forshey finally got it from Joe again since Edgar raised such a fuss about it and shoved it out to him. But he must be trying to justify it. In a letter he says when they let Joe and the drum out, Reno and he, Edgar, looked at each other with tears in their eyes. Reno said, "Dad, should I quit dancing?" Brother, did that go on and on in the letter. I laughed and laughed when I read it.

A tribal elder got some medicine from Dr. Walters the other day. He wouldn't take it until I saw it and said it was okay. He wanted a shot, the second time now. He's been getting placebos. He was out near our house here on Thursday gathering wood from the burned building. I was going to snap a picture, but by the time I saw him and got ready, he was gone.

October 13, 1954

I am trying desperately to study for my board examinations, which I am to take in Denver on October 27. I'm not ready and shall not be ready by then. As soon as I get back from there I go to Aberdeen for an Area Medical-Dental meeting. Then I get back from there and go to Atlantic City for the annual American College of Surgeons convention to receive my fellowship in the ACS. I had to drive up to Slim Buttes so Mr. Jamruska could take a photograph of me for the ACS to use.

The roads around the hospital are torn up. Duane McDowell, Senator Mundt's secretary, said they were torn up in 1940 when they tried to get funds for the project now being done. I remember that when McDowell visited the hospital two weeks ago I asked him if he were going back to Washington DC to sit in on the Senate hearings over the McCarthy censure. He said no, but his boss was. His boss is Senator Karl Mundt, chairman of the Army-McCarthy hearings. I asked him if the Senate would adopt the censure recommendations of the Watkins Committee. He said probably, not because anything like that would set a precedent, and the senators wouldn't want to be caught in such a move.

Several schools are closed while Indians take their kids and go to Nebraska to go potato picking. Then they come home after serving their jail sentences for being drunk, and they come back without any money. The kids of school age aren't enrolled in the schools down there either.

Butch Stoldt told about one Indian who boasted, "I don't have to go potato picking. They are going to pay me to stay here to keep my kids in school." That was before Mr. Reifel was overruled by Aberdeen and told he couldn't take welfare funds to pay families to keep them here and keep their kids in school. Subsidization of education has gone far enough. If they don't want an education, let 'em go.

I have new duties. Now that Dr. Gassman, is gone we have no internist. So I'm running down VD contacts. Fortunately the hospital load is very light right now.

I tried to get Mrs. Dolores H. Klinker, the anesthetist from the VA hospital in Hot Springs to come down and give an anesthesia for a gastrectomy to be done next week, but she doesn't feel she can come. Dr. Walters will give it instead. The Aberdeen office people will be here that day. With everybody busy it should be an eye opener for them.

As my tour of duty draws to a close and with only two months left, it seems that there are a million things to do. I have little lists all over as I plan and think of things that will have to be done before leaving.

October 16, 1954

Yesterday, Friday, was a nice day for the OCHS homecoming game. There was a large crowd. The team played the Hay Springs team. The Indians were dressed nicely. The yell leaders and baton twirlers were in style. A queen was crowned, Charlene Brewer. A parade preceded the football activities, and a dance was held in the gym last night. I was asked to be one of the three judges of the floats at the parade. The others were Mrs. Theise of Whiteclay, Nebraska, and Mr. Hagel of Pine Ridge. I called them all as chosen. We agreed unanimously, the three of us, for juniors as number one. Two of us chose freshman for second place, one vote for number five, Oglala. And two of us chose seniors for number three, one for the birthday cake made by the elementary children.

To anyone witnessing the football game it looked like an ordinary school team, with lots of spirit and nice clean kids. But take the football boys, and it's a different story. For instance, one boy has been in jail for beating his mother. There are a couple of boys who are the fathers of illegitimate children. There is a youngster whose relatives were just thrown in the clink in Rapid City again, repeaters for habitual drunkenness. That isn't his fault, of course, but he has run off from school several times and taken another player with him. Some of these kids have been in the tribal jail. There is the youth who was thrown in jail last winter for trying to get into the girls' building at the school while drunk. He was recently dishonorably discharged from the Marine Corps. I could go on. There are probably some situations such as this among any group of children anywhere, but not to the extent that it is here.

The percentage must be much higher here. I can't imagine it being that high all over the country.

The day before the game it was cold. Seems it was our coldest day. On Thursday they held a horse sale at the school. There were horses there sired by Morgan Gold and Red Correl. Morgan Gold is in the hall of fame of horses. But the horses went so cheaply! Miss McGill bought several. Mr. Mickelson bought a couple. I wanted to buy some too and would have except that it wasn't practical. Where would I keep them or how would I keep them or how would I get them home when we go?

More communications were received today from the Sioux Sanitarium. A female patient is out of the sanitarium and at home living with her children. She has far advanced active tuberculosis. Oh, what a grand day. And I'm on call. This would be a day to go out somewhere. The old chief, Peg Leg, hailed me in town on my way to the football game. He wanted some more tincture of belladonna. I told him I was on my way to the school. He said he'd ride with me. I had to leave the game at 3:00 p.m. to get to the clinic. There he was by my car. He wanted me to take him home. I dropped him off near the corrals, the closest I got to his home. I guess he was surprised. But I told him if I had the time that evening I'd run some medicine out to his place. I did. I went out about 5:30 p.m. He was gone again. He went to Martin to a Republican meeting, Agnes said.

If Aberdeen thinks we don't do anything, we'll give them a show when they get here this week. They are to spend Wednesday here. We won't have a chance to talk because we are going to do a gastrectomy here that day. The purpose of the trip is for Miss Wayne to orient Dr. Herbert A. Hudgins to the Area. Dr. Hudgins is our new Area Office medical director.

I have an invitation from Mother Grace for Jeanne and me to have dinner with the nuns at the Holy Rosary Mission on Sunday evening, tomorrow night, and then go to the show with them there to see the film *Quo Vadis*.

Are we having a time. Just over a week ago Edna Phyllis found she could make some sort of a sound that had a whinny flavor. That was run into the ground. Now about three days ago she found something that smacked of a bullfrog sound crossed with the growl of "Cappie" [Captain]. Now she sounds like a base viol whenever she wants to get our attention. And I'm telling you that gal lives to stand. I hang onto her hands and she pushes herself up. I have to hold her to keep her from toppling. I steady her; I don't hold her up. She does all the work and stands herself. And she is only four months.

We shot the works. It is going to cost us well over a thousand dollars to have a book published that we wrote on the Indians. But we decided to do it. It is being published by a cooperative publishing house. I don't actually have confidence that we will recover all our money, but we thought it would be to our credit to just have a book published. Maybe you can all get some wholesale to sell it to tourists there next summer. Ha. Anyway, I hope when the time comes you will order at least one copy for $2.50 from the publishers. They are Vantage Press, Inc. If anyone is interested, give them the address. The name of the book will be *The Oglala Sioux Indians.*[2]

Jeanne didn't say a word, but she was disappointed at not being able to go on to her home at Christmas, as can be expected. So we may go on to her home in Chelan for Christmas. We haven't decided yet.[3] But we do wish you would come back, both Skin and you, and leave with us. We could have a good time.

October 17, 1954

I'm pretty disgusted. Most every place I've been there is good and bad. But it seems that this week there has been nothing but the BAD.

A well-known man has had his daughter out of the hospital for five days. She has been in twice and near death each time. The last time she was ready to go home days before he arrived and got her. It didn't bother him that we had to wait days for him to come and get his baby when we needed beds so badly. He was in again yesterday with the baby sick again. I'd been here all morning and noon, and I told Mrs. Coker to tell the man that it would be about an hour before I got over there. He left in a huff. He couldn't wait one hour. Boy, he must be a high-powered person to be so much in a hurry. He was begging Mr. Reifel for some money and a handout not long ago. He and his wife have each been to our house on several occasions, and we've given them food. No more. The fellow has now worked a couple of days in Nebraska and made a little money. The result: he was drunker than a skunk yesterday. Yet his kids are still starving.

Mrs. Olinger called me once to say a reservation family had gone away and deserted their kids. They live at Kyle. Well, they came in here a few days after that. They had been in Montana, and the hospital had to admit the father with alcoholic gastritis. Well, their son has been here for over a month now. He came in for surgery. The family was in to see him once and said they'd be right back to take him home. They did come back all right, this weekend, and said that they would get the kid only when they got good and ready. Such people!

There is the rodeo cowboy who took off his cast after one week and ruined a perfectly good reduction of a hard-to-reduce fracture of the radius and wrote to us about it. Or that woman with a lipoma on her back who thought she'd get welfare from Hawkins in Martin. No soap, so now she is going to try Mrs. Forshey in the relief office here.

I have discovered people here who typify the term *Indian giver*. I know where it comes from. I have seen the criminal instincts pop out of people I thought were reliable. In fact, there is not one Indian on this reservation who I think has integrity and self-respect and complete control of himself. My last example went up in smoke last night. The best worker we have at the hospital went off his rocker last night. He got mixed up with another guy who has just been in town for a few days from the state penitentiary with three other men that made up their group. They were drunker than skunks, throwing beer cans all over the streets in town. The cops chased them to the state line down by White-clay. The cops were Sid Young, Gordon Jones, and Dennis LeCompt.

Dennis got in on it in some way and also Joe Swift Bird. Well, those guys beat our cops up but good. Sidney has a well-socked face and a possible broken jaw. He has contusions all over his body. Joe got his shirt torn open and got marched down the street by one of the hoodlums who got ahold of the only gun the cops had, the one Sid had. Gordon got busted in the forehead a couple of times with the butt end of the gun. Dennis, of course, wouldn't get a scratch on him. There goes my best worker, anyway. And I liked him.

Then a woman came in. Her husband beat her up, lacerated her head and leg. He has done it before. Her stepson is the one who killed a girl and wrecked several cars in July when he was so drunk. Well, I kept her here, and later her husband came to the hospital with a gun to try and kill her. Fortunately the door was locked, and he couldn't get in. And that isn't all. She is going back to live with him. Such nincompoops.

And that wasn't all of my weekend. Who should they first call me about today but a couple of characters dragged over from Nebraska. I also get sick of Nebraska. They don't hesitate to drag over the drunken bums that need hospitalization, but they sure keep those in jail who pay the fines and fill the city treasuries. Well, anyway, they brought in a man who has only recently been out of the jail. Well, he and others chased the China-Burma-India campaign hero of World War II. Several of them beat the stuffing out of him. They were all drunk. So was our war hero, for that matter. Then after several of them beat him up they scrammed, but they turned their car over. One of them really got banged up in the turnover. So they brought him here. The veteran was also brought in. He is unconscious and has a broken jaw and is a real mess. I'm sick and tired of this place.

Jeanne and I kept the invitation to join Mother Grace, Sister Bernard, and Father Lawrence Edwards of Holy Rosary Mission for dinner. Then we went to the show there, *Quo Vadis*. We had to leave early, but Father Edwards told me that one of the OCHS boys was drunk and came out there and beat up one of their kids. He was a guy who was in the hospital not long ago. Then Mr. Mickelson told me the same boy had beaten up his mother several times. So they called Mick and then the cops, who came after him.

And just as soon as I got back, a woman who comes in periodically with "nervous spells" arrived. Tonight she rode back from Hot Springs with Pierre LeGrande Jr., and he was so drunk, she said, that it made her nervous to ride with him.

I must add that the police here have no guts. Another family who leaves their babies at the hospital have been hanging around the jail and town all day, but the police wouldn't make them come and get their baby, who has been laying around up here for ages. I called the jailor and said that a woman wanted to file a complaint against her husband and would he come to the hospital and take her complaint. The jailor said he would but never showed up.

Father Edwards told me tonight that he never goes around without a gun. He goes early Sunday morning off across that road—landing east just this side of Whiteclay at the state line. He always carries a gun. One time he met a carload of drunks ready to ambush him. They had a row of whiskey bottles strung along the road with the tops broken off. He also told me one night he went to Smithwick in the middle of winter to pick up a lady teacher and bring her back to Holy Rosary.[4] He wasn't far out of Smithwick when he saw three Indians who flagged him down. Then he saw their car stuck in a snow bank. A pickup came along at the same time, and Father Edwards said the men asked the driver for a ride. The driver of the pickup said he wouldn't give the Indians a ride. So Father Edwards stuck them in the back of his rig. Presently one of the men started to bother the lady teacher. Then he put Father Edwards in a neck lock and turned off the ignition. Father Edwards said the man was drunk and told him to turn and drive the opposite way. He talked big, but Father Edwards started up and came on into Pine Ridge. A little ways north of the mission the three asked to get out. The character who once threatened Father Edwards was too drunk to get out and run. He called after the others to come and get him, but they kept going. So Father Edwards took this character on into the jail. Shortly after getting back to Holy Rosary Mission, a special investigator came up to him and inquired about the men, saying those three had stopped a lady, hit her over the head, threw her out, and took her car, and stranded it in the snow bank.

Mr. Carr said not long ago someone tried to stop him up near Red Shirt Table. They were moving when he first saw them so he knew they had no car trouble. I've learned my lesson. I'll never stop for drunken Indians or for any of them now. It is simply too dangerous. This has been perhaps an unusual weekend, but it seems there has been a lot of hooliganism, crime, and plain cussedness and irresponsibility.

I thought we had at least a halfway decent worker in one man at the hospital, but I learned from the nurses that even he has to be herded, and it's the same thing with the sanitarian aid. They never do a solid thing on their own.

October 21, 1954

The Aberdeen brass came rolling in Tuesday night. Dr. Hudgins, Mr. Lindstrom, the head of sanitary engineering, and Miss Wayne. I had made a reservation at the hotel ahead of time, but they came in and went over to the newest motel. They had requested I get them a reservation, too. If that wasn't the limit, after I promised the hotel faithfully they'd be here.

Wednesday morning we did a gastrectomy. So the visitors saw the full force in swing. And thereby hangs a most disastrous happening. When the patient went back to his room, his Levine Tube had come out, and so he had an emesis of bloody fluid, not unusual with the Levine Tube out. Probably the most excitable nurse we have, Miss Vera Stomley, came running out of the room and screamed down the hall to another nurse, Miss Verna Cadotte, "Call the priest immediately." And she did. When I got up there later, I was in the room and Father Edwards from Holy Rosary Mission came running into the room. I thought he was there on a routine visit. The condition of the patient was very good. He hesitated because I was irrigating the new Levine Tube that was just put down. I just said, "Come on in," still thinking he was just visiting. He said he could wait until I finished. Then he told me he was told to come immediately. I could have sunk through the floor. My spirits and my soul did. Under a six-hour strain of operating, that was a blast. I exclaimed, "Father, this man is not critical." Father Edwards then left.

I was so mad I couldn't see straight. Miss Stomley had not asked the condition of the patient from other doctors. Their opinion was the same as mine, that he was fine. So I called Miss Stomley in and told her she was way out of order. She tried to justify it by saying, "We Catholics do that." I said, "You do not call the Father for every patient operated on." Then she said, "You told Father not to give that man Last Rites." I told her I had not. She maintained I had. That, I think, is a serious offense for someone who is supposed to be an adult. Well, I knew I hadn't, so I went out to talk to Father Edwards later that night.

When he knew I was there he came running down the hall with a look of terror on his face. I said the patient was all right. He sighed. Then I asked him point blank if I told him not to administer Last Rites to that patient. He said I had not. If I had, he responded, he would have told me to go jump in a lake for telling him how to run his business. I asked, "Did I tell you 'he does not need Last Rites?'" which would have been a far different connotation. That being dictating his business. He said I had not. He said, "You told me the patient was not critical." But Miss Stomley has persisted in her lies. Father Edwards told me further last evening when he was there that he noticed when he went in the room that the patient immediately got a look of concern on his face. So actually, after the terrific bodily strain of six hours of surgery, that uncalled-for circumstance created by the nurse put even more strain on him. She'll get a memorandum you can be sure.

Dr. Hudgins told me my letter about a political deal to get a patient back into South Dakota squelched an unethical attempt to move her around. Dr. Hudgins admitted it was a political deal, and he told me, "I was just passing the buck on down." He wanted to know if we could take tonsils out of six kids at the Pierre Indian School. Heavens, we can't even do all the tonsils we have here to do.

October 23, 1954

I have been studying like mad for my board exams. I'm going to Denver on Tuesday to write them. I'm not ready, but I am as ready as I'll ever be.

A patient from the Turtle Mountain Reservation on whom we performed a gastrectomy last Wednesday is doing wonderfully.

Well, if I didn't get the news from Mrs. Forshey. Mrs. Chief, the Indian social worker at Rosebud, gives welfare to all councilmen over there for political reasons. One councilman even went into Mr. Pitner and asked him why he was getting welfare money. Mrs. Chief is to be fired, finally. All the correspondence is dated November 3, which is after the election to keep politics out of it. Otherwise that meddling Congressman E. Y. Berry would have Mrs. Chief rehired to look good for the voters.

I was certainly interested in a column in the October 16 *Journal of the American Medical Association*. It refers to large groups of persons of little or no Indian blood who persist as PROFESSIONAL INDIANS (a wonderful term) in "freeloading" at government expense under the guise of being incompetent Indians. Of course, a great deal of this is done, or on such reservations as this it is the practice since there is not the personnel in the hospital to find out degree of blood, residence, and so forth.

Edgar Red Cloud is back from potato picking. He says that they had a Yuwipi meeting last night at the home of Hazel Shields. But he says two drunks were there and kept things in an uproar.

Sixteen. November 1954

Mr. Reifel called Dr. Quint to ask him if three days was enough for him to take off to spend in New York redoing a part of his boards. He said yes. Then Mr. Reifel asked him if it was okay to put it in the newssheet. That is the first time I know of that he has asked anyone if he could put something in the newssheet. Dr. Quint said he didn't think that Mr. Reifel should use the same wording as before: that Dr. Quint was away, and his wife and child were staying home alone. Mr. Reifel said, "Yes, I wonder if anyone will ever take their vengeance out on my wife when they know I'm gone and she is home alone."

November 1, 1954

I leave tomorrow evening or Wednesday morning for Aberdeen for the Area Medical-Dental conference. When I get back, I have three days, and then I will be off again for Atlantic City for the American College of Surgeons convention.

The old Indian custom for waving is to raise two arms in the air, not just one, as is the white man's custom.

Indian children play with all sorts of animals. Long ago they used to run down skunks. After the skunks were skinned, the skunk fat was cooked, boiled, skimmed from the top when the water cooled, and that was put aside for colds. A teaspoon of skunk oil was enough to cure anything, I guess, from what the old timers say about the taste.

I see by a note from the Area Office that the central office has arranged for the transfer of a female patient from San Haven to the Sioux Sanitarium. San Haven is way up in North Dakota. The woman has written both me and Mr. Reifel to get us to transfer her. Of course, the reason we didn't is that every time this woman gets to the Sioux Sanitarium, she runs out of there. She is loaded with tuberculosis. Really there are times when the central office ought to mind its own business.

There have been so many people who left the Sioux Sanitarium against medical advice, many failing to keep appointments, people not picking up their family from the hospital, and whatnot that my memos have been hot and heavy. The best that ever happened was one I sent to Moses Schindelbower about one patient. Mr. Schindelbower took it personally, or else he was on the defensive, or perhaps he is paranoid, maybe even has a persecution complex. He is the teacher at Porcupine. Anyway, he wrote a note saying he couldn't figure out why I was reprimanding him. I asked Mr. Reifel about it since he had seen a copy of the correspondence. He said, "We sure have a lot of thin-skinned people around here." I asked Mr. Pyles how he took it, and he viewed the letter as just for information. That is what it was intended for.

Mercy! Another case dumped on us. A mental case and a bum from Julesburg, Colorado. The sheriff from that place brought the man up here. He has been away from the reservation for ten years. People think that just because people are Indians that we should come and get them and care for them when they've been away from here for ten years. The guy is really a bum. He drinks constantly, and that, I think, is the basis of his mental deterioration. He left his wife and kids ten years ago and wouldn't support them.

Aggie Iron Cloud made an observation that I share. All the young nurses we have are cheerful. They come in and eat and work and leave and have a good time. But all the older, longtime unmarried, old-maid nurses are always "bitching" about something from the food to everything on the floors. And it sure is a fact.

Miss Golden, who came here in August from Rosebud, went back again Saturday. She was to have been able to stay here, but Miss Pawluk, whom I don't know yet, is to return. She had military leave to go to the army for seventeen months. I sure hated to see Miss Golden leave. (This is not Miss Holden. Miss Golden replaced Miss Holden when she left in July.) I don't care who comes. Just so that someone comes. But not Miss McGill. I can't stand her much longer.

November 9, 1954

We voted today in Pine Ridge. We had not registered but were allowed to vote on signing some sort of a statement that we had not registered and were not voting elsewhere. One week ago tonight we left for Aberdeen. We stayed at Rosebud, leaving Pine Ridge about 6:30 and arriving at Rosebud at about 10:30 after blowing a muffler and nearly gassing us, baby, and dog. Jeanne and I made it okay except when I got lightheaded. We got the car fixed at Martin, South Dakota.

Our conference began on Thursday. Pine Ridge presented the scientific portion of the program. I talked a bit on ruptured spleens. Harley Quint spoke on eye conditions, and Joe Jackson, the obstetrician and gynecologist, on prolonged labor.

Friday I spent an entire half day in personnel concerning the fracas here with the tribal police that occurred on October 17th. The big question was whether to get rid of an employee who was involved right away, which could have been done with no question at all since his year-long probation was not up until Monday, November 8th. During their probationary employment any person can be separated without any fanfare or repercussions.

I talked to Jakes because Nelson was out sick. I told him to let the guy work until federal action proved the man guilty. Then if there is a sentence, that would take care of him.

Monday before 8:00 a.m. Mr. Reifel called me. He said he had to call Aberdeen about the fight. I told him how I felt, but I added since it had to be decided today whether or not to get rid of the offender that I wouldn't make it difficult for him and stand in his road since I knew his policies. Well, I see the man is still with us. So any effort as of today to separate him would be a long-drawn-out and costly affair. Costly in the sense of words, of course.

All the roads that are to be improved around the agency have been finished. How nice to have a good oiled road around the hospital.

Ethel Merrival is now asking that the tribal council ask for commodities for cattle owners and cattle loan clients since the welfare commodities cannot be handed out to them. She'll spend hours of effort to get a few pounds of cheese and a few cakes of butter. If she spent all that energy in a salaried job, she'd be able to buy so much more than she gets by pleading. She wants commodities to give to cattle clients since her husband has sixty-five head, I believe. She is trying to kick old chief James Red Cloud out of distributing the commodities in his community. She wants to put Burns Prairie in that district as distributor. She doesn't like the chief and vice versa.

Mr. Reifel visited the hospital on Sunday, the first time in six months that he had been up there to visit the patients. There was a delicious letter circulated to him to stay home and quit running all over speaking. It said that he should devote himself to helping the Indians. There was no name on it, but it may be that Mr. Reifel knows who sent it.

Jeanne and I went for a walk last night over the hill back of our place. We took the road that goes down to White Clay Creek. There was frost all over the ground. There was plenty of light and a big moon. The frost sparkled over the ground in the moonlight.

I leave Thursday for Atlantic City, New Jersey, to get my fellowship in the American College of Surgeons.

November 28, 1954

I have been back from Atlantic City a week ago tomorrow. We have a new administrative officer, a Mr. Dexter, who came from up in Wisconsin or Minnesota. I didn't meet him until Wednesday when we had a meeting in Mr. Reifel's office. He introduced himself after the meeting and said, "I've heard so much about you, even before arriving here, that I expected to find an old man with white hair."

Mr. Reifel called Dr. Quint to ask him if three days was enough for him to take off to spend in New York redoing a part of his boards. He said yes. Then Mr. Reifel asked him if it was okay to put it in the news-sheet. That is the first time I know of that he has asked anyone if he could put something in the newssheet. Dr. Quint said he didn't think that Mr. Reifel should use the same wording as before: that Dr. Quint was away, and his wife and child were staying home alone. Mr. Reifel said, "Yes, I wonder if anyone will ever take their vengeance out on my wife when they know I'm gone and she is home alone."

There was a potluck dinner last night for Joe Jackson. Very few people were there.

Mary Ann Red Cloud wants clothes from Mrs. Forshey. Mrs. Forshey told her long ago she could have clothes if she worked this summer. Mary Ann didn't work, but she sent a note down that she wanted some clothes and that she would surely try to help herself next summer. This is the same old story. Then she added that she wished she could just have the bones to eat from the turkey that Mrs. Forshey would have for Thanksgiving. That is a dirty crack, but I wonder if she realized how nasty it was. Of course, there are several things about it. Mrs. Forshey is working for her salary. Mary Ann's family could do the same. And Mary Ann's father drinks up what little bit he gets.

Charlie Yellow Boy and Edgar Red Cloud nabbed me yesterday and did say that they wanted to come over to the house for a powwow before we leave.

Our new chief nurse is not to my liking. She is making too many changes that would be changed back if I were staying here, but since I'm not, I shan't go into it with her. I'll let Dr. Walters do that, and he can surely do it. She is not a warm person, no personality, just a blank. She is efficient though. Things are clean and up, but, of course, the census is lowest right now and has been for some time, affording her time to distribute her workers so they can keep things clean.

And it's a good thing because there are only Dr. Quint and myself here. Dr. Walters went on leave as soon as I got back. And Dr. Quint leaves for a number of days the last of this week, so I'll be by myself. Here we are supposed to have a complete staff with replacements. Where in the world are they?

There is so much going on here I can't keep up on all of it. The Masts were to leave and go to Rosebud to head the new Land Branch. That was decided months ago. Now I find just lately the Masts could stay here, and the Cokers would have to leave and go to Rosebud. Anyway, the Masts are toying with the idea of going to South America.

At the school, one teacher's wife left at the same time that another man did. She returned a few days ago, and the second man went to the state sanitarium. I had been treating the second guy for ulcers. Now I know what the difficulty was. And the teacher had been his best pal. Well, well.

November 30, 1954

The latest is that one man, a Sisseton Sioux employed at the boarding school for a short time, had it out with Manning Rider and then quit. Now he is hanging around here trying to get Rider fired. He has really dug up all dirt on Rider, and he is interviewing all those who have had trouble with Rider and who don't like him.

It's real messy. I still can't find out why things have been changed. I don't know why Mr. Coker is to leave now and Mr. Mast to stay as head of the new department incorporating smco and Forestry and Grazing. Mr. Mast is probably going to South America anyway. Mr. Coker is apparently on the outs with Mr. Reifel over something, I don't know what. But the change in Mast over Coker to stay is not local. I wish I knew the answer to that. Mr. Reifel used to ask Mr. Coker to serve as acting superintendent most of the time when he was gone, but he now asks Mr. Mast.

Boy, I have always said that Mr. Pyles was a namby-pamby and a fence sitter. That is the only reason he could be here as long as he has been. His people finally got rid of a man because he is such a horrible worker, and the man put up such a howl about having arthritis. Now Mr. Pyles is in the process of hiring the guy back as a bus driver. The man says he doesn't have any more trouble with his joints. Boy, if that isn't something. And another thing, there is a terrible shortage of houses. Education is as hard up as anybody for the need of houses. Sydney Mills, a representative to the tribal council and a nongovernmental worker, has an Education house on the campus. Mr. Pyles is afraid to hurt his feelings or step on his toes. He won't kick him out of there. It has finally gotten to Mr. Reifel, so the other morning in a conference Mr. Reifel asked him how they were for houses and if Mr. Mills should be moved out soon. Mr. Pyles said, "No hurry." Pyles is such a weakling.

He doesn't hesitate to impose on others. He wants to know if my nurse will move from the clinic's house to a trailer house at Wanblee. Mr. Pyles must be nuts. He wants trailers to be used as dormitories for nurses, and he'll use buildings for kids. Now today he wanted the nurse to cart school kids in to the eye clinic. I said I'd ask her only because I thought she may be coming in today. But I didn't get a hold of her anyway.

I received a letter from Eva Nichols, the Indian troublemaker in Omaha, Nebraska. She wants me to pay the bills of two people who went to hospitals in Omaha and received outpatient treatment. She wants their room rents paid. One is not on the rolls here, and we didn't send her down. The other one is on our rolls, she says. I sent down a woman. I told Mrs. Nichols that I sent her down with the idea she would pay her own rent, and I wouldn't for the life of me pay the rent with federal funds. In polite terms, I told her to mind her own business and quit writing me because all I can do for these people is arrange for their trips to Omaha.

Mrs. Forshey asked me if this setup was a matriarchy around here. When a family wants welfare, the man is head of the family, but he sends his wife in to do the dickering with Mrs. Forshey while he sits in the car. I see this happen on other reservations, too. Mrs. Forshey won't talk with them. The husbands are bashful, say the wives. That, of course, is true. Mrs. Forshey is writing a speech she is going to deliver in Denver. I gave her a word to use. She said she didn't like to say out and out that these people are lazy. I told her a nice word to use instead is UNAMBITIOUS.

Seventeen. December 1954

So now we bid "goodbye" to Pine Ridge and start our journey to Washington State to set up a private practice. The movers have taken our belongings, and what was left over is packed in our new Chevrolet station wagon.

December 4, 1954

Government service is sure the nuttiest business. In the first place politics plays a crazy role. Nobody, but nobody, will say anything about anybody else, even if it is on the direst of terms. I should say they do not make statements or put things in writing. Yet when all is said and done, plenty of talking is done by those who take sides. I'm thinking about this man whom I've never seen in my life, but who is reportedly the guy who is trying to get Manning Rider fired.

And talk about government service. You can't get any work done here without a permit from Congress. Yet the Area Office calls in the state sanitary engineer and aids and hospital accreditation committee or safety groups to go over the hospital. Their recommendations for safety—physically and medically and sanitary wise—cover pages and include suggestions by the score. A copy goes to the commissioner of Indian affairs and to the Area Office as well. What has been done about it? Absolutely nothing. What has been done from this end? Absolutely nothing. However, we have made changes on sheets of paper with the justifications. Nobody pays any attention. Maintenance is particularly good at ignoring the orders coming out of the Area Office.

Agnes Red Cloud Elk Boy finally had her baby. They have gone to the medicine man so much during her pregnancy. They have appealed to Yuwipi so much, and her husband Dick Elk Boy has gone through numerous sacrificial rituals. He has been out all night praying on the hilltops, and so forth. They have lost so many children. Agnes has lost all of hers before term. This new birth is their first term baby, and he is doing okay, I guess. I just saw Edgar. He says it is a very big boy.

It is probably a good thing that I'm not going to be here long. Miss Pawluk, RN, is back and has things in a real mess. The first day that I was able to talk with her I discussed her changes and said that if she had others to make that would be fine, but I wished to know about them first. Well, everything from all floors up and down is changed over so that I can't find anything, and neither can others, but I am just not going to do anything about it. I'll be out of here soon. If I were staying on, I would do something about it. Dr. Walters is on leave. Dr. Quint is in New York taking a board exam. I'm the only one here. I had to perform an appendectomy on a person with a ruptured appendix last night. I practically had to do it by myself. Miss Pawluk was going to pull the nurse from the floor to scrub and assist, mind you, and leave only the assistant nurse there to run the floor and send only a circulating nurse over. I called her and soon fixed that. I got another nurse to come over who scrubbed so that I could have both an assistant and a scrub nurse.

A day hardly goes by in which I'm not called to the phone. The first thing I hear after answering is, "How is my boy?" or "How is she?" I presume Indians believe in mental telepathy or some sort of thing. I invariably have to ask "Who is calling?"

December 12, 1954

Peter Bald Eagle Bear couldn't stand the new pressures, so he resigned from his job as tribal judge. There were the old pressures from families and relatives, which he could have handled in the old way, and he did, by letting arrested family persons off. But then lately there have been other pressures from the other side, urging stiffer punishments. Anyway, one of the men who substituted was Henry Big Boy, who all but told Mrs. Coker to go to hell when we tried to get him to come and care for his daughter. The mother came a couple of times to see the baby and when we told her the child could go she would hurry away, each time saying she was going to get the kid some clothes first. And old Henry said he'd get his little girl when he got good and ready. Gee, what an outfit.

Mrs. Olinger left a present at the hospital for Jeanne and me. The mothers and sisters of Holy Rosary Mission gave us a going-away gift. Thursday night the agency held a going-away party. They gave us $25 collected from the agency. There were a large number at the dinner. I had to leave right after the potluck dinner with Dr. Quint and Miss Sim, the anesthetist from the Aberdeen Area Office, to do an emergency gall-bladder operation. But the night before, Wednesday, the day we drove to Chadron and picked up our new car, the Indians came over. Jake Herman did the translating tonight for Edgar Red Cloud. It is usually Edgar who does the translating for Chief Red Cloud. As Mrs. Forshey told me Saturday (last night), Edgar wants the chief to die so he will be the prestigious Chief Red Cloud. And people will translate for him. Since his father was not there, he acted in the chief's place with all the ceremony of having someone translate his words.

Indians are born entertainers and are adept at telling stories. One real trait was evident. Edgar kept poking fun with stories about his brother-in-law. But in the old Indian custom a boy must never tease his sister. One is apt to come over and pull his ears very hard. Edgar can, of course, speak better English than many white people, or at least as good. But he has to play the eminent part of protocol of being the chief. He told me his father couldn't come because he had loaned his feathers and buckskin out. He would be out of his costume. So the next day the chief came to get a donation for some Christmas party or something. I gave him a dollar. He asked me, "You had a party here last night with the Indians?" "Yes," I said.

At the going-away party Jake Herman presented us with beaded moccasins for Edna. Frank Afraid of Horses gave Jeanne a beaded wristband,

and Edgar gave Jeanne some beaded earrings from Mary Ann. This is the first time in the history of Pine Ridge in which any group of Indians has come to send off a white government employee, so I am told. But we were the first to socialize in our home with the Indians here. They made very flowery speeches. Joe Sitting Hawk (not Oglala Joe with the tape on his nose and the peyote user) came to join the party, but he said Captain barked and scared him, so he just dropped in Thursday night to wish us goodbye. Those here also were Leroy White Whirlwind and Reno and Vincent Red Cloud, Dick and Ira Elk Boy, and Ira's wife, the Blue Bird woman. Charlie Yellow Boy was to come, but he got sick, and the family took him to a Yuwipi meeting to get cured. Ha! Joe Mast came over with his projector and ran off some movies that I took around here of the Sun Dance and Hearst ceremonies. Of course, on Friday Mr. Mickelson called Edgar and Mr. White Whirlwind to school to lecture to them since Reno and Leroy had taken girls from the dormitory and got ahold of wine and gotten drunk.

So now we bid "goodbye" to Pine Ridge and start our journey to Washington State to set up a private practice. The movers have taken our belongings, and what was left over is packed in our new Chevrolet station wagon. We're taking clothing, suitcases with things needed while traveling, and a new baby basket for Edna that fits behind the front seats, where we can get to her easily. And a place for Captain, too. We will arrive in McCall probably before you get our last letter from Pine Ridge. We will stay a couple of days before proceeding on to Chelan in time for Christmas with Jeanne's mother.

Editors' Postscript

As is usual for a memoir, this is a report of observations more than a critical analysis. Memoirs are written from the perspective of an interested party, leaving the analysis for others. Dr. Robert Ruby's memoir contains a wealth of information for use by scholars. As a participant in the operation of the Pine Ridge Indian Reservation, Ruby observed the lives of his patients as well as his agency staff and townspeople, forming opinions about all of them that he shared with his sister.

The Pine Ridge Indian Reservation and the operation of the hospital have evolved over the past half century. When Ruby arrived in 1953, discrimination was much more overt in American society, and one of the African American physicians at the hospital was unwelcome at some restaurants and hotels in Rapid City. The Indian Health Service employed African American physicians and nurses and a Jewish physician at the Pine Ridge hospital during Ruby's tenure. A social structure was quite evident at the hospital—white physicians and administrators were the institutional standard. This began to change while Ruby was there, as the holder of the superintendent's position transferred from a white man, Mr. O. Sande, to an enrolled American Indian, Benjamin Reifel. The change continues to the present. The Oglala Sioux Tribal Health Administration is largely composed of enrolled tribal members.

The community of Pine Ridge itself has changed in some ways over fifty years, though the underlying problem of poverty remains. Today there is an air strip south and east of Pine Ridge. Paved roads lead in and out of the town, and traffic lights have been installed on U.S. Route

18. A Pizza Hut franchise is operating, and a large gas station and convenience store, Big Bat's, appears to be thriving.

The Holy Rosary Mission, located a few miles north of Pine Ridge, has become the Red Cloud Indian School. The school has developed a good working relationship with some colleges and universities, and students who succeed in their studies are now bringing their skills and education back to the reservation.

An aggressive program to combat alcoholism and smoking, to encourage better child care, and to foster better health is being promoted by the Oglala Sioux Tribal Health Administration. A fleet of ambulances is in operation, providing much better service to the reservation's families than the converted station wagons of the 1950s. Perhaps it is only symbolic, but it is worth noting that the old hospital, managed by Ruby, was located overlooking the town, but with the front of the buildings facing away from the town of Pine Ridge. The new hospital's front entrance faces the town of Pine Ridge, implying a welcoming attitude.

Readers should know the limitations of a memoir of this kind. The viewpoint of a young surgeon from a white, middle-class background who had entered a respected profession was probably quite different from the viewpoint one might obtain from an Oglala Sioux living at Pine Ridge in the 1950s. Historians know all too well that sources are often fragmentary and may focus on only one aspect of a complicated situation. Although Dr. Robert Ruby's memoir provides a good look at life on the Pine Ridge Indian Reservation and at some of the issues confronting the Bureau of Indian Affairs and the management of Indian health care, it is obviously a work from the perspective of a white physician. Historians will have to wait for a study of these issues and times from a Sioux perspective to gain a fuller understanding of the intricacies that are introduced in Dr. Ruby's memoir. We can hope that other writers will add to the scope of our understanding of Indian health care from multiple perspectives, including that of the Oglala Sioux.

Appendix

Books by Robert H. Ruby

The Oglala Sioux: Warriors in Transition. New York: Vantage Press, 1954.

Books by Robert H. Ruby and John A. Brown

The Cayuse Indians: Imperial Tribesmen of Old Oregon. Norman: University of Oklahoma Press, 1972.

The Chinook Indians: Traders of the Lower Columbia River. Norman: University of Oklahoma Press, 1976.

Dreamer-Prophets of the Columbia Plateau: Smohalla and Skolaskin. Norman: University of Oklahoma Press, 1989.

Esther Ross, Stillaguamish Champion. Norman: University of Oklahoma Press, 2001.

Ferryboats on the Columbia River, Including the Bridges and Dams. Seattle: Superior Publishing, 1976.

A Guide to the Indian Tribes of the Pacific Northwest. Norman: University of Oklahoma Press, 1986.

Half-Sun on the Columbia: A Biography of Chief Moses. Norman: University of Oklahoma Press, 1965.

The Highland Runners: A Tale of the Okanogan. Wenatchee: North Central Washington Museum, 1992.

Indian Slavery in the Pacific Northwest. Spokane: Arthur H. Clark 1993.

Indians of the Pacific Northwest: A History. Norman: University of Oklahoma Press, 1981.

John Slocum and the Indian Shaker Church. Norman: University of Oklahoma Press, 1996.

Myron Eells and the Puget Sound Indians. Seattle: Superior Publishing, 1976.

The Spokane Indians: Children of the Sun. Norman: University of Oklahoma Press, 1970.

Notes

Introduction

1. Personal information for this book was compiled during the years 2003 to 2009 and is based on personal interviews, telephone calls, and correspondence between the editors and Robert H. Ruby. Audiotape and typed transcripts of interviews are available to researchers at the Eastern Washington University Archives, Cheney, Washington, as are copies of all correspondence. The original letters that make up this memoir are contained in the Dr. Robert H. Ruby MD Collection (acc. L-2002-29, MS 170), Pine Ridge Series, Box 2, Folders 96–97, Northwest Museum of Arts and Culture, Eastern Washington State Historical Society, Spokane, Washington.

2. Ruby, interview.

3. Ruby, interview.

4. Ruby, interview. Recent studies of the Pine Ridge reservation include Pickering, *Lakota Culture, World Economy*; Wagoner, *"Just Like Indians"*; Robertson, *Power of the Land*; Frazier, *On the Rez*; Kurkiala, *"Building the Nation."*

5. On the Indian New Deal, see Biolsi, *Organizing the Lakota*; Rusco, *Fateful Time*; and Kelly, *Assault on Assimilation*; on termination and relocation, see Fixico, *Termination and Relocation*.

6. See endnote 1 above. Background on Ruby's life, particularly his career as a writer, is documented in Collins and Mutschler, "Great Spirits." See also Collins and Mutschler, "'Thank God They Did What They Did.'" Marion (Ruby) Johnson recalls that her father never failed to invite Yakama visitors into his home, that they took meals at the dinner table with the Ruby family, and that the elder Ruby instilled in his children the deepest respect for the common humanity of all people; Johnson, interview.

7. Johnson, interview.

8. Johnson, interview.

9. Johnson, interview.

10. Johnson, interview.

11. Wilkinson, *Blood Struggle*, 8–9.

12. Wilkinson, *Blood Struggle*, 9.

13. Wilkinson, *Blood Struggle*, 8–11. On Sun Dance at Pine Ridge, see Mails, *Sundancing at Rosebud and Pine Ridge*.

14. Wilkinson, *Blood Struggle*, 12.

15. Indispensable sources for background on health services provided to Indians by the American government are U.S. Department of Health, Education and Welfare, *Health Services*, and *Indian Health Program*. See also Davies, *Healing Ways*; Rhoades, *American Indian Health*; Keller, *Empty Beds*; Steeler, *Improving American Indian Health Care*; Massing, "Development of United States Government Policy." Finally, Francis Paul Prucha furnishes an invaluable overview of the development of Indian healthcare, particularly from the standpoint of federal policy initiatives in *Great Father*, 2: 841–63, which was based partly on the findings of Putney, "Fighting the Scourge."

16. U.S. HEW, *Health Services*, 86.

17. U.S. HEW, *Health Services*, 87.

18. T. J. Morgan to Secretary of the Interior, September 5, 1890, U.S. Commissioner of Indian Affairs, *Annual Report*, 1890, vol. 19 (hereafter ARCIA). A biographical sketch of Morgan's career as Indian commissioner can be found in Prucha, "Thomas Jefferson Morgan."

19. Trennert, *White Man's Medicine*, 64–73; quotation on 64.

20. Morgan to Secretary of the Interior, ARCIA, vol. 20.

21. Morgan to Secretary of the Interior, ARCIA, 1890, vol. 20.

22. Morgan to Secretary of the Interior, ARCIA, 1890, vol. 20.

23. Morgan to Secretary of the Interior, ARCIA, 1890, vol. 21.

24. Morgan to Secretary of the Interior, ARCIA, 1890, vol. 22.

25. Morgan to Secretary of the Interior, ARCIA, 1890, vol. 20.

26. Morgan to Secretary of the Interior, August 27, 1892, ARCIA, 63.

27. Morgan to Secretary of the Interior, ARCIA, 1892, 63.

28. Raup, *Indian Health Program*; and Trennert, *White Man's Medicine*, 201–17.

29. Kuschell-Haworth, "History of Federal Indian Healthcare."

30. Kuschell-Haworth, "History of Federal Indian Healthcare." See also Kunitz, "History and Politics."

31. Chas. G. Penney to D. M. Browning, October 9, 1893, ARCIA, 289.

32. J. Ashley Thompson to V. T. McGillycuddy, August 20, 1884, ARCIA, 211. For a modern treatment of Oglala Lakota methods of healing, see Lewis, *Medicine Men*.

33. Thompson to McGillycuddy, August 20, 1884, *ARCIA*, 211.

34. Thompson to McGillycuddy, August 20, 1884, *ARCIA*, 211.

35. Thompson to McGillycuddy, August 20, 1884, *ARCIA*, 211.

36. Eastman, *From the Deep Woods*, 76.

37. Eastman, *From the Deep Woods*, 76–77.

38. Eastman, *From the Deep Woods*, 78–79.

39. Eastman, *From the Deep Woods*, 79–81.

40. Eastman, *From the Deep Woods*, 87, 119–20.

41. Eastman, *From the Deep Woods*, 87–88.

42. J. S. Pede to D. M. Browning, June 30, 1893, *ARCIA*, 292.

43. Pede to Browning, June 30, 1893, *ARCIA*, 292.

44. Z. T. Daniel to D. M. Browning, July 8, 1893, *ARCIA*, 291.

45. Z. T. Daniel to D. M. Browning, September 3, 1894, *ARCIA*, 290.

46. James McLaughlin to Cornelius Bliss, August 4, 1897, Roll #37, M1070, RG 75, National Archives, Reports of Inspection of the Field Jurisdictions of the Office of Indian Affairs, 1873–1900.

47. Province McCormick to Hoke Smith, November 29, 1894, Roll #36, M1070, RG 75, National Archives, Reports of Inspection of the Field Jurisdictions of the Office of Indian Affairs, 1873–1900.

48. Z. T. Daniel to D. M. Browning, September 3, 1894, *ARCIA*, 290–91.

49. Daniel to Browning, September 3, 1894, *ARCIA*, 291.

50. Daniel to Browning, September 3, 1894, *ARCIA*, 290.

51. Daniel to Browning, September 3, 1894, *ARCIA*, 290–91.

52. Daniel to Browning, September 3, 1894, *ARCIA*, 290.

53. Southerton, "James R. Walker's Campaign," 117.

54. W. B. Dew to W. H. Clapp, August 14, 1896, *ARCIA*, 295.

55. W. H. Clapp to W. A. Jones, August 21, 1899, *ARCIA*, 335, 337.

56. 1910 Pine Ridge Agency Report, Roll #106, M1011, RG 75, National Archives, Superintendents' Annual Narrative and Statistical Reports from Field Jurisdictions of the Bureau of Indian Affairs, 1907–1938 (hereafter SANSR).

57. Southerton, "James R. Walker's Campaign," 107–26.

58. Southerton, "James R. Walker's Campaign," 112.

59. Southerton, "James R. Walker's Campaign," 112–13.

60. Chalcraft, *Assimilation's Agent*, 224.

61. Southerton, "James R. Walker's Campaign," 122.

62. Southerton, "James R. Walker's Campaign," 122.

63. Southerton, "James R. Walker's Campaign," 122–25. Contributing to Walker's difficulties in formulating and submitting an outline for a sanato-

rium was the fact that, despite his best efforts, he had failed to unburden himself of his daily duties. In 1908 he wrote, "My time is fully occupied as a physician, and I could only work at this plan piece meal at night time, hence the delay"; James R. Walker to Architectural Department, Interior Department, December 17, 1908, File 863-1908-Pine Ridge-721, Box 537, RG 75, National Archives, Washington DC, Central Classified Files, Bureau of Indian Affairs, 1907–1939 [hereafter CCF].

64. 1912 Pine Ridge Agency Report, SANSR.

65. 1916 Pine Ridge Agency Report, SANSR.

66. 1914 Pine Ridge Agency Report, SANSR. The specific location in Pine Ridge for a general hospital or sanatorium was selected in 1907; see Memorandum from Chief of Land Division to Education and Health Division, June 22, 1915, File 82134-1915-Pine Ridge-721, Box 537, CCF.

67. 1916 Pine Ridge Agency Report, SANSR.

68. 1914 Pine Ridge Agency Report, SANSR.

69. Report of Pine Ridge Reservation and Schools by Joseph A. Murphy, Medical Supervisor, February 29, 1916, File 25151-1916-Pine Ridge-700, Box 534, CCF.

70. Quoted in 1910, 1912, and 1914 Pine Ridge Agency reports, SANSR.

71. 1919 Pine Ridge Agency Report, SANSR.

72. 1919 Pine Ridge Agency Report, SANSR. Emblematic of the depth of the crisis was the situation that unfolded in Gordon, Nebraska, twenty miles south of Pine Ridge. Acting on reports of many Indian deaths having occurred there, the agency superintendent dispatched boss farmer Judson Shook of Manderson district to investigate. At the Gordon cemetery, he discovered seven unburied wooden caskets containing Indian bodies. Shook went back to the reservation, notified relatives, and returned with them to retrieve the remains of the deceased. Influenza continued to take its toll in Gordon—it was known as "the city of the dead"—and several subsequent trips were made. The final estimate of Indian deaths in the town ranged between sixty and seventy; Centennial Book Committee, *History of Gordon, Nebraska*, 38–39.

73. 1922, 1923, and 1927 Pine Ridge Agency reports, SANSR.

74. 1919 Pine Ridge Agency Report, SANSR.

75. 1922 Pine Ridge Agency Report, SANSR.

76. 1923 Pine Ridge Agency Report, SANSR.

77. 1925 Pine Ridge Agency Report, SANSR.

78. 1924 Pine Ridge Agency Report, SANSR. See also endnote 69 above. An extensive survey of reservation conditions in 1916 showed that of school-age

children, 9 percent suffered from trachoma, 6 percent from corneal scars (1 percent were blind in one eye), 35 percent from decayed teeth, and 44 percent from diseased tonsils. Nineteen percent showed evidence of tubercular infection of the lung; see endnote 69 above.

79. Merriam, *Problem of Indian Administration*.

80. James H. McGregor to Charles J. Rhoads, January 25, 1931, File 5634-1931-Pine Ridge-721, Box 538, CCF.

81. Woodworth-Ney, "Diaries of a Day-School Teacher."

82. Woodworth-Ney, "Diaries of a Day-School Teacher," 199, 200.

83. Woodworth-Ney, "Diaries of a Day-School Teacher," 199.

84. Woodworth-Ney, "Diaries of a Day-School Teacher," 199–200.

85. Woodworth-Ney, "Diaries of a Day-School Teacher," 200.

86. Woodworth-Ney, "Diaries of a Day-School Teacher," 200.

87. Woodworth-Ney, "Diaries of a Day-School Teacher," 200.

88. Woodworth-Ney, "Diaries of a Day-School Teacher," 201.

89. U.S. Congress, *Report with Respect to the House Resolution*, 1328.

90. See endnote 1 above.

91. See endnote 1 above.

92. Background on the 1955 transfer can be found in Kunitz, *Disease Change*, 146–52; Riggs, "Irony of American Indian Health Care," 1–22; Bergman, Grossman, and Erdrich, Todd, and Forquera, "Political History," 577; U.S. Department of Health, Education and Welfare, *Health Services*, 94–97.

93. See 92 above.

94. See 92 above, 572–73, 578.

95. Robert H. Ruby (hereafter RHR), letter to editors, March 18, 2006.

96. Ruby, *Oglala Sioux*.

1. August 1953

1. Pocatello ID had a population of 26,131 in 1950. U.S. Census Bureau, *Census of Population and Housing*, 1960.

2. Captain, the Rubys' young collie, joined the family earlier in 1953. Robert Ruby purchased Captain as a puppy from a registered kennel outside St. Louis approximately six weeks before completing his residency. He shipped the puppy to Jeanne as a gift approximately six weeks before returning to Washington to marry her. Following the wedding, the three began the drive to Pine Ridge. RHR to editors, April 29, 2006.

3. Red Lodge MT had a population of 2,730 in 1950. U.S. Census Bureau, *Census of Population and Housing*, 1960.

4. Hettinger ND had a population of 1,762 in 1950. U.S. Census Bureau, *Census of Population and Housing*, 1960.

5. Aberdeen SD had a population of 21,051 in 1950. U.S. Census Bureau, *Census of Population and Housing*, 1960.

6. The population of Pine Ridge SD was under 1,000 at the time the Rubys lived there. U.S. Census Bureau, *Census of Population and Housing*, 1960.

7. Siegfried Reinhardt (1925–1984) was a world-renowned artist who lived in St. Louis for most of his life. The Vatican Museum permanent collection holds some of Reinhardt's work. He produced a sketch of Ruby while Ruby was in St. Louis. By then Reinhardt was already a recognized artist, having been reported on in *Life* magazine in 1950 and 1952. *Life*, March 20, 1950, pp. 84, 93; *Life*, March 24, 1952, pp. 88–90; *New York Times*, October 26, 1984.

8. Ruby grew up outside Mabton WA.

9. Ruby reports the system for communication with the police and summoning emergency assistance evolved over time. In the period when Valentine McGillycuddy was agent, there were no telephones between the agency buildings or offices. A bell tower was built on the roof of the agency building, and a rope ran down from the bell, through the roof and ceiling. The bell was audible for a mile. Bell signals called specific people: one ring was the signal for the agent to return to his office if he was out of the building; two rings summoned the captain of police; and three called the chief of police. McGillycuddy, *McGillycuddy, Agent*, 147. By the time Ruby came to Pine Ridge, some offices had telephones, but the red light on the hospital served a function similar to the bell in use a half century earlier. RHR to editors, January 11, 2006.

10. "Chowder" is a family nickname for Ruby's sister, Marion. She and her husband LeRoy live in McCall ID. In 1950 McCall had a population of 1,173. U.S. Census Bureau, *Census of Population and Housing*, 1960.

11. Chadron NE had a population of 4,687 in 1950. U.S. Census Bureau, *Census of Population and Housing*, 1960.

12. "Skinny" is the family nickname for LeRoy Johnson, Ruby's brother-in-law.

13. William O. Roberts was serving as the regional director at Aberdeen when Ruby arrived at the Pine Ridge hospital.

14. Ruby's sister Marion's mother-in-law, Stella (Mrs. B. T.) Johnson.

15. The large frogs were planted in the Denby reservoir by Bob Grooms in the early twentieth century. In the 1960s the pond was poisoned to kill off undesirable fish; the frogs were eliminated as well and have not been restocked. The original Denby Store was, at one time, operated by relatives of television

personality Bob Barker. The existing building was constructed in 1939 as a replacement for the old store, which burned. The store was later sold to a Mr. Davis, but it is now closed. This information was received by Robert Ruby in an interview with Pat Grooms (Bob Grooms's great-nephew) at Denby SD on June 25, 2006.

16. This is Holy Rosary Mission, now named the Red Cloud Indian School.

17. Karl E. Mundt (1900–1974) was an educator, real estate investor, and member of Congress. Born in Humboldt SD, Mundt, a Republican, was elected to the U.S. House of Representatives in 1938. He served until December 1948, when he was appointed U.S. senator for South Dakota. Mundt was re-elected to the Senate in 1954, 1960, and 1966 but chose not to run in 1972. He was in his first term in the Senate when he visited Pine Ridge in 1953. U.S. Congress, *Biographical Directory*, 1549–50.

18. Spearfish SD had a population of 2,755 in 1950. U.S. Census Bureau, *Census of Population and Housing*.

2. September 1953

1. RHR to editors, February 2, 2006.

2. Jeanne Ruby had a college degree in home economics.

3. Public Law 277, 83rd Cong., 1st sess., codified as Section 1161 of Title 18 of the United States Code. The result was not uniform legalization of alcohol sales on Indian reservations. Some tribes legalized the sale of alcoholic beverages; others did not.

4. American Indians have served with distinction in wars fought by the United States. Prucha, *Great Father*, 835–36, 1003–5. Also see Franco, *Crossing the Pond*. The military service of Indians as "code talkers" using their native language to communicate in a way that was unintelligible to the enemy during World War II has received considerable treatment, both scholarly and popular. The Navajos served in the Pacific Theater, and their story is covered in Paul, *Navajo Code Talkers*. Comanche work in Europe is the subject of Meadows, *Comanche Code Talkers*. *The Wind Talkers*, a 2002 motion picture starring Nicholas Cage, fared poorly in both critical reviews and at the box office. Ruby gave a series of public lectures in Washington State on the Navajo Code Talkers, who served during World War II. RHR to editors, April 29, 2006.

5. Because the incident occurred on an Indian reservation, which was under federal criminal jurisdiction, the matter was referred to the federal prosecutor, rather than county authorities. Prucha, *Great Father*, 679–81.

6. Rapid City sd had a population of 25,310 in 1950. U.S. Census Bureau, *Census of Population and Housing*, 1960.

7. At the time Ruby joined the Indian Health Service, the Bureau of Indian Affairs had been developing a policy for gradual elimination of the federal-tribal relationship. This was formalized in 1954 as the Termination Policy, which was intended to bring American Indians into full-fledged citizenship and end the relationships between tribal entities and the federal government. Spicer, *Short History of the Indians*, 125–26, 139–40.

3. October 1953

1. Withdrawal was the precursor to the Termination policy, intended to end the relationship between tribes and the federal government. Prucha, *Great Father*, 1032–34.

2. The Native American Church combines elements of aboriginal and Christian religious practices. Strongly resisted by whites in general and especially by the federal government, the church developed after 1890. The ritual use of peyote, a hallucinogen, was of particular concern to the bia. Spicer, *Short History of the Indians*, 119–22. For a brief history of the Native American Church, see Hirschfelder and Molin, *Encyclopedia of Native American Religions*, 197–98. A more detailed study of the religious use of peyote is Stewart, *Peyote Religion*.

3. Robert Bragg was a pediatrician. rhr to editors, April 5, 2005.

4. Ruby recalls that Sheppard was a dentist. rhr to editors, April 5, 2005.

4. November 1953

1. The relocation program was instituted in 1948 by Commissioner of Indian Affairs Glenn L. Emmons, with the goal of encouraging Indians to move from rural reservations to urban areas. It was believed that this would enable people to find better employment opportunities in the expanding industrial economy following World War II. The project began in the Southwest and was expanded to include offices in Chicago, Denver, and other cities. Relocation was controversial, but the program officially continued into the late 1970s. The bulk of relocation took place between 1953 and 1960. Prucha, *Great Father*, 1079–84.

5. December 1953

1. States generally apportioned school funds on a per-pupil basis. A census of school-age children was taken periodically to determine for how many ᵁs each district was to receive state funds. This is the census Ruby mentions, and not the U.S. census.

2. Gerald L. K. Smith (1898–1976) was a conservative evangelist, three-time presidential hopeful, and dissident. His religious intolerance and political views are amply covered in Ribuffo, *Old Christian Right*; and Jeansonne, *Gerald L. K. Smith*.

3. Oveta Culp Hobby (1905–1995) was President Eisenhower's secretary of health, education and welfare when it became a cabinet agency. She was the first secretary of HEW and the second woman cabinet head after Frances Perkins. Born in Texas, she graduated from the University of Texas Law School in 1925 and became parliamentarian for the Texas legislature. In 1931 she married former governor William Hobby and began a career in journalism. As Colonel Hobby, she commanded the Women's Auxiliary Army Corps (WAAC) from 1942 until 1945. She was appointed by Eisenhower in 1953 and resigned in 1955 due to her husband's ill health. See Sutphen, "Conservative Warrior."

4. James Douglas McKay (1893–1959) was Eisenhower's first secretary of interior. He was born in Portland OR and served in the Oregon state senate and as governor of Oregon before being appointed as secretary of interior by Eisenhower in 1953. He resigned in 1956 for an unsuccessful bid for the U.S. Senate seat from Oregon. See entries for James Douglas McKay in *National Cyclopedia of American Biography*, 50; 477–78; *Who Was Who in America*, vol. 3.

5. Ellis Yarnell (E. Y.) Berry (1902–1999) was the Republican congressman representing the western district of South Dakota from 1951 until 1971. Berry was born in Iowa but grew up near Philip SD and graduated from the University of South Dakota Law School in 1927. U.S. Congress, *Biographical Directory*, 615.

6. RHR to editors, December 22, 2005.

6. January 1954

1. Benjamin Reifel was born September 19, 1906, near Parmelee SD. His father was a German American; his mother, Lakota Sioux. His Lakota name was Lone Feather. Although his father saw farming as more practical, Ben's mother encouraged him to obtain more education. He attended South Dakota State College, where he was commissioned a second lieutenant in the U.S. Army Reserve in 1931 and earned a BA in chemistry and agriculture in 1932. In 1933 he married Alice Janet Johnson and joined the staff of the Bureau of Indian Affairs. Reifel was called to active duty in 1942, served in the European Theater of Operations, and left active status in 1946 as a lieutenant colonel. He returned to the Bureau of Indian Affairs. In 1949 Reifel took a leave of absence to attend Harvard University. He earned an MA in public administration

in 1950 and a PhD in the same field in 1952. After serving as superintendent of the Fort Berthold Reservation, Reifel became superintendent of the Pine Ridge Indian Reservation in January 1954. He was the first Indian to occupy that post. In 1955 he became Area director for the BIA in Aberdeen SD. He resigned from the BIA in 1960 to run for Congress on the Republican ticket. He served five terms in the House of Representatives, retiring in 1970. Reifel was selected by President Gerald R. Ford to be his commissioner of Indian affairs, a post he held briefly at the end of the Ford administration. President Ford selected Reifel for the post because of Reifel's personal integrity and because Ford wanted to "clean up the mess" at the BIA. Commissioner Reifel died on January 2, 1990. His papers are held by the library at South Dakota State University. U.S. Congress, *Biographical Directory*, 1705; Gerald R. Ford to Charles V. Mutschler, telephone interview, September 16, 2004.

2. "The Bimson Report" appears to have been written in 1953 or early 1954 and may draw its colloquial name from Walter Reed Bimson, an Arizona banker who was active in civic affairs. Bimson's interest in economic development on Indian reservations is implied in notes in several archival collections but is not specifically referenced in a brief biography of Bimson. Walter Bimson played an active role in the Small Business Administration during the Truman administration. Schweikart, *Banking and Finance*, 25–30; Schweikart, *History of Arizona Banking*, 123–24.

7. February 1954

1. The Native American Church combines elements of traditional American Indian origin with elements of Christianity. This included the sacramental use of peyote. Controlled by Indian spiritual leaders, the Native American Church gained acceptance among American Indians between 1880 and 1930. During this same period white Christians actively opposed the Native American Church. The official incorporation of the Native American Church was in 1915. Spicer, *Short History of the Indians*, 119–22.

2. Ruby describes the drum used in the peyote ritual as being a cast iron pot about eight inches in diameter, covered with a piece of tanned hide. The hide is tied to a series of knobs around the outside, near the top. Before the covering is secured, a small amount of water is poured into the pot. The tone is altered by tilting the drum to allow a certain amount of water to reach the tanned hide. RHR to editors, December 22, 2005.

3. Lewis, *Medicine Men*, 84, contains the hypothesis that the sparks are made with a cigarette lighter.

4. Ruby reports that the scout is responsible for preventing unwanted interruption to the ceremony by preventing persons from disrupting it at inappropriate times. RHR to editors, December 22, 2005.

5. Ruby reports that the framework for the sweat house was made from a series of willows or other pliable saplings stuck in the ground in a circular plan. The saplings are bent across and over the circle and tied down on the other end, making a frame like an inverted bowl. This frame was then covered with blankets, canvas, animal skins, or brush. RHR to editors, December 22, 2005.

6. Lewis, *Medicine Men*, p. 84.

8. March 1954

1. In 1954 passenger service between McCall and Cheyenne was offered by the Union Pacific Railroad.

2. According to Ruby, the soil in this area is a clay that acquires a slippery, gumbo-like consistency when wet. This clay is probably part of the White River clays, which occur on the Pine Ridge Indian Reservation. Gries, *Roadside Geology of South Dakota*, 124.

3. Orrin Holmes was Ruby's uncle, his mother's brother. Holmes lived in the Black Hills, where he owned property for many years.

4. Sculptor Korczak Ziolkowski (1908–1982) was originally associated with Gutzun Borglum carving the Mt. Rushmore sculpture. *Who Was Who in America*, 1985, 8: 440. Ruby reports that his uncle, Orrin Holmes, knew Ziolkowski fairly well. He said that the artist enjoyed frequent gatherings with his friends. According to Holmes, the artist was an early proponent of new mothers leaving the hospital in one or two days instead of the then standard practice of a week-long bed rest for new mothers.

9. April 1954

1. Ruby grew up near Mabton WA. His parents' farm was some 150 miles northwest of the Umatilla Indian Reservation.

2. The Termination policy was being implemented at this time, with the intent of bringing tribal members into full citizenship. The theory was that this would allow the federal government to terminate the federal-tribal relationship. A good overview is contained in Prucha, *Great Father*, 1013–84.

3. Valentine McGillycuddy (1849–1939) served as the agent at the Pine Ridge reservation in the late 1870s to mid-1880s. See McGillycuddy's biography is by his wife, Julia B. McGillycuddy, *McGillycuddy, Agent*. The South Dakota Historical Society has a small quantity of McGillycuddy family papers that relate

to McGillycuddy's tenure at Pine Ridge. The McGillycuddy biography provides another white observer's look at life on the Pine Ridge Indian Reservation, approximately seventy years before Ruby's memoir.

4. Ruby notes: "This says a lot. Sande saw Jim Red Cloud and romanticized him as the offspring of a celebrated mid-19th century Indian leader. But the title and lineage did not impress Reifel, who was also an Indian. This says one reason why Jim Red Cloud was my friend. I also was impressed with him as a relative of *the* Chief Red Cloud, and I gave him lots of attention. I felt as if I was touching history." RHR to editors, July 21, 2005.

5. Ruby reports that Mrs. Elk Boy informed him that the pipe had belonged to the original Red Cloud. Ruby offered her the option to pawn it but informed her that she had to pick up the pipe before he and his family left the reservation. He reminded her on several occasions to come and pick up the pipe, but she never returned for the red calinite pipe. RHR to editors, February 8, 2006.

6. Officially called the 5307 Composite Unit (Provisional), the all-volunteer unit included Sioux and Japanese Americans, under the command of Brigadier General Frank D. Merrill. The name "Merrill's Marauders" was never used officially. The unit was deployed in the China-Burma-India theater of operations and captured the Myitkyina airfield in northern Burma on May 17, 1944. Officially the code name for this volunteer force was GALAHAD. See Dear, *Oxford Companion to World War II*, 424.

10. May 1954

1. Ruby recalls that the school still had a few government-owned horses. RHR to editors, August 6, 2005.

2. The program seems indicative of federal efforts to move toward implementation of the Termination policy to ultimately end the federal-tribal relationship.

11. June 1954

1. Casino gambling has changed the nature of the communities of the Black Hills since the 1950s when Ruby was there.

2. John Lund, born 1913. Lund quit acting in 1962. Ragan, *Who's Who in Hollywood*, 1012.

3. Robert Warwick (1878–1964) began his career in silent films and was one of the relatively few silent actors to make a successful transition to motion pictures with sound. His film career, which began in 1915, continued until 1959. Truitt. *Who Was Who on Screen*, 749.

4. Victor Mature, born 1915, began starring in films in 1939. He was in a number of westerns, including this one, *Chief Crazy Horse*. Ragan, *Who's Who in Hollywood*, 1084.

5. Suzan Ball (1933–1955) had a very brief acting career. Although she was attempting to return to acting following the loss of her leg, she died of cancer in 1955 at age twenty-two. Ragan, *Who's Who in Hollywood*, 80.

6. Public Law 568 (HR 303) 68 Stat. 674. The bill was enacted into law on August 5, 1954. *United States Statutes at Large*.

12. July 1954

1. Ruby reports that coolers were commonly used for cooking in the summer. These structures consisted of four poles in a rectangular shape that supported a wire top on which were piled pine branches. It was a cooler place than inside a house or tipi to cook or perform other work. The term commonly used in the 1950s when Ruby was in South Dakota was "Squaw Cooler."

2. The American College of Surgeons was organized in 1913 to provide professional support for this branch of the medical profession. Walton, Beeson, and Scott, *Oxford Companion to Medicine*, 745. The ACS publishes a bulletin that includes articles about the activities of its members. Ruby was featured in the November 2005 issue. Sandrick, "Surgeon Chronicles Native American History," 14–19.

3. Karl E. Mundt was a U.S. senator from South Dakota from 1949 through 1972. Between April and June 1954 Senator Mundt chaired the Senate Permanent Subcommittee on Investigations during the Army-McCarthy Hearings. These televised hearings were conducted from April 22 through June 17 at the instigation of U.S. Senator Joseph McCarthy (Wisconsin). McCarthy, who was to have chaired the hearings, wished to act as interrogator and thus passed the chairmanship to Senator Mundt. Senator McCarthy claimed that the army and federal government in general had been corrupted by communist agents, but his tactics angered many citizens who saw the hearings on television, and his credibility faded. U.S. Congress, *Biographical Directory*, 1549–50.

4. Crookston NE was a very small town west of Valentine, on the Chicago and Northwestern railroad line. *Rand McNally Atlas*.

5. Deloria, *Speaking of Indians*. The book is about the Dakota and Teton tribes and was re-issued in 1979 by the University of South Dakota Press.

6. Weston does not appear in U.S. Congress, *Biographical Directory*, suggesting that he was a state senator and not a member of Congress.

7. The Janis family originally spelled the name with a double s, *Janiss*. The

family descended from Chief Red Cloud's sister, who married a white man named Nick Janiss. Valentine T. McGillycuddy recorded the name spelled with the double s and notes that later the family simplified the spelling. McGillycuddy, *McGillycuddy, Agent*, 109.

8. Steven B. Karch, M.D., *Drug Abuse Handbook*, Boca Raton, Florida: CRC Press, 1998, pp. 17–18.

9. Boyle, "Black Hills Residents"; Boyle, "Sioux Sun Dance Dying Tradition"; Boyle, "Young Braves Prefer."

10. Warren Morrell, "Thru the Hills," *Rapid City Journal*, July 29 and 30, 1954.

13. August 1954

1. Ruby reports that Janis was not "Bob" but was always known as "Boob" by the people at Pine Ridge. He does not know if this was a nickname or Janis's given name. RHR to editors, September 4, 2005.

2. Boyle, "Sioux Sun Dance Dying Tradition"; Boyle, "Young Braves Prefer to Do Jitterbug."

3. William and Lucy Hall were friends of Ruby's sister Marion and were teachers. RHR to editors, April 29, 2006.

14. September 1954

1. Ruby is referring to medical board examinations.

2. Overt bigotry was not uncommon in the mid-1950s. Many communities had real estate covenants that forbade the sale of homes to African Americans, Asians, Catholics, and Jewish people. Gassman's experience was probably not unusual. Furthermore, Ruby recalls that Bragg and he were refused service at one of Rapid City's better restaurants, and the two of them had to find a less attractive eatery that would serve African Americans. Blacks, even physicians, were not universally welcome in Rapid City in 1954. A half century earlier, women physicians would have experienced similar hostility. Susan Anderson MD was unable to situate her practice in an urban center like Denver and had to settle for a remote ranching town in west-central Colorado. Her experience is recounted in Cornell, *Doc Susie*.

3. Ruby's frustration with the problem of alcohol abuse seems to show through at this point. The matter was severe, as Indians sought ways to raise money for liquor. In a telephone interview, Joe Svara, who was a store owner in the area in 1953 and 1954, reported that Indians seeking money for liquor were frequently accused of vandalizing federal attempts to build homes for

them by stealing plumbing fixtures from the unfinished houses, which were then sold to raise funds for alcohol. Svara, telephone interview.

15. October 1954

1. Ruby appears to have been getting exhausted and was showing his disgust with the complications arising in his efforts to move.

2. Ruby's book on the Oglala Sioux was the start of his prolific scholarship on American Indian history. Some articles were authored independently, but many of the books were co-authored with John A. Brown, professor of history at Wenatchee Valley College. Mr. Gildersleeve, who ran the store at Wounded Knee, sold Ruby's book *The Oglala Sioux*, for many years, periodically writing Ruby to order additional copies. RHR to editors, January 1, 2006.

3. The Rubys did return to Chelan after leaving Pine Ridge. RHR to editors, January 1, 2006.

4. Smithwick SD is a small town in Fall River County located north of Oelrichs, west of the Pine Ridge Indian Reservation.

16. November 1954

No notes.

17. December 1954

No notes.

Bibliography

Primary Sources

National Archives and Records Administration. Washington DC. United States Bureau of Indian Affairs. Record Group 75.

Central Classified Files, BIA, 1907–1939.

Microfilm Set M-1011.

Microfilm Set M-1070.

Ruby, Robert H. Papers. Northwest Museum of Arts and Culture, Spokane WA. Accession No. L-2002-29, MS 170.

Secondary Sources

Bergman, Abraham B., David C. Grossman, Angela M. Erdrich, John C. Todd, and Ralph Forquera. "A Political History of the Indian Health Service." *Milbank Quarterly* 77, no. 4 (1999): 571–604.

Biolsi, Thomas. *Organizing the Lakota: The Political Economy of the New Deal on the Pine Ridge and Rosebud Reservations*. Tucson: University of Arizona Press, 1992.

Boyle, Hal. "Black Hills Residents Fond of Good Yarns." *Rapid City Journal*, July 30, 1954.

———. "Sioux Sun Dance Dying Tradition." *Rapid City Journal*, August 1, 1954.

———. "Young Braves Prefer to Do Jitterbug." *Rapid City Journal*, August 4, 1954.

Centennial Book Committee. *The History of Gordon, Nebraska*. Dallas: Curtis Media, 1984.

Chalcraft, Edwin L. *Assimilation's Agent: My Life as a Superintendent in the Indian Boarding School System*. Ed. Cary C. Collins. Lincoln: University of Nebraska Press, 2004.

Collins, Cary C., and Charles V. Mutschler. "Great Spirits: Ruby and Brown, Pioneering Historians of the Indians of the Pacific Northwest." *Pacific Northwest Quarterly* 95, no. 3 (Summer 2004): 126–29.

———. "'Thank God They Did What They Did When They Did': Ruby and Brown and the Writing of American Indian History." *Journal of the West* 46, no. 2 (Spring 2007): 3–10.

Cornell, Virginia. *Doc Susie: The True Story of a Country Physician in the Colorado Rockies*. Carpinteria CA: Manifest, 1991.

Davies, Wade. *Healing Ways: Navajo Health Care in the Twentieth Century*. Albuquerque: University of New Mexico Press, 2001.

Dear, I. C. B., ed. *Oxford Companion to World War II*. New York: Oxford University Press, 1995.

Deloria, Ella C. *Speaking of Indians*. New York: Friendship Press, 1944.

Eastman, Charles A. *From the Deep Woods to Civilization: Chapters in the Autobiography of an Indian*. Boston: Little, Brown, 1916.

Fixico, Donald. *Termination and Relocation: Federal Indian Policy, 1945–1960*. Albuquerque: University of New Mexico Press, 1986.

Ford, Gerald R. Telephone interview with Charles V. Mutschler, September 16, 2004.

Franco, Jere Bishop. *Crossing the Pond: The Native American Effort in World War II*. Denton: University of North Texas Press, 1999.

Frazier, Ian. *On the Rez*. New York: Picador, 2001.

Gries, John Paul. *Roadside Geology of South Dakota*. Missoula MT: Mountain Press, 1996.

Hirschfelder, Arlene, and Paulette Molin, eds. *Encyclopedia of Native American Religions*. Rev. ed. New York: Facts on File, 2000.

Jeansonne, Glen. *Gerald L. K. Smith: Minister of Hate*. New Haven: Yale University Press, 1988.

Johnson, Marion (Ruby). Interview with editors. Pine Ridge SD, June 25, 2006.

Karch, Steven B., M.D. *Drug Abuse Handbook*. Boca Raton FL: CRC Press, 1998.

Keller, Jean A. *Empty Beds: Indian Student Health at Sherman Institute, 1902–1922*. East Lansing: Michigan State University Press, 2002.

Kelly, Lawrence C. *The Assault on Assimilation: John Collier and the Origins of Indian Policy Reform*. Albuquerque: University of New Mexico Press, 1983.

Kunitz, Stephen J. *Disease Change and the Role of Medicine: The Navajo Experience*. Berkeley: University of California Press, 1983.

———. "The History and Politics of US Health Care Policy for American Indians and Alaskan Natives." *American Journal of Public Health* 86, no. 10 (October 1996): 1464–73.

Kurkiala, Mikael. *"Building the Nation Back Up": The Politics of Identity on the Pine Ridge Indian Reservation.* Uppsala, Sweden: Academia Ubsaliensis, 1997.

Kuschell-Haworth, Holly T. "A History of Federal Indian Healthcare." Excerpted from "Jumping through Hoops: Traditional Healers and the Indian Health Care Improvement Act," *DePaul Journal of Health Care Law* 4 (Summer 1999): 843–60. Available online at http://academic.udayton.edu/Health/02organ/Indian03.htm.

Lewis, Thomas H. *The Medicine Men: Oglala Sioux Ceremony and Healing.* Lincoln: University of Nebraska Press, 1990.

Mails, Thomas E. *Sundancing at Rosebud and Pine Ridge.* Sioux Falls SD: Center for Western Studies, 1978.

Marquis Who's Who. *Who Was Who in America, 1951–1960.* Vol. 3. Chicago: A. N. Marquis, 1960.

Massing, Christine. "The Development of United States Government Policy toward Indian Health Care, 1850–1900." *Past Imperfect* 3 (1994): 95–128.

McGillycuddy, Julia B. *McGillycuddy, Agent: A Biography of Dr. Valentine T. McGillycuddy.* Palo Alto CA: Stanford University Press, 1941.

Meadows, William C. *The Comanche Code Talkers of World War II.* Austin: University of Texas Press, 2002.

Merriam, Lewis. *The Problem of Indian Administration: Summary of Findings and Recommendations.* Baltimore: Johns Hopkins University Press, 1928.

Morrell, Warren. "Thru the Hills." *Rapid City Journal,* July 29 and 30, 1954.

National Cyclopedia of American Biography. Vol. 50. New York: James T. White, 1968.

Paul, Doris A. *The Navajo Code Talkers.* Philadelphia: Dorrance, 1973.

Pickering, Kathleen Ann. *Lakota Culture, World Economy.* Lincoln: University of Nebraska Press, 2004.

Prucha, Francis Paul. *The Great Father: The United States Government and the American Indians.* 2 vols. Lincoln: University of Nebraska Press, 1989.

———. "Thomas Jefferson Morgan: 1889–1893." In *The Commissioners of Indian Affairs, 1824–1977,* ed. Robert M. Kvasnicka and Herman J. Viola, 193–203. Lincoln: University of Nebraska Press, 1979.

Putney, Diane T. "Fighting the Scourge: American Indian Morbidity and Federal Policy, 1897–1928." PhD diss., Marquette University, 1980.

Ragan, David. *Who's Who in Hollywood.* New York: Facts on File: 1992.

Rand McNally Atlas of the World. Chicago: Rand McNally, 1942.

Raup, Ruth M. *The Indian Health Program from 1800 to 1955.* Washington DC: U.S. Public Health Service, 1959.

Rhoades, Everett R. *American Indian Health: Innovations in Health Care, Promotion, and Policy.* Baltimore: Johns Hopkins University Press, 2000.

Ribuffo, Leo P. *The Old Christian Right: The Protestant Far Right from the Great Depression to the Cold War.* Philadelphia: Temple University Press, 1983.

Riggs, Christopher K. "The Irony of American Indian Health Care: The Pueblos, the Five Tribes, and Self-Determination, 1954–1968." *American Indian Culture and Research Journal* 23, no. 4 (1999): 1–22.

Robertson, Paul. *The Power of the Land: Identity, Ethnicity, and Class among the Oglala Lakota.* New York: Routledge, 2002.

Ruby, Robert H. "Indian Peyote Cult." *Frontier Times*, 36, no. 19: 30–39.

———. *The Oglala Sioux: Warriors in Transition.* New York: Vantage Press, 1955.

Rusco, Elmer R. *A Fateful Time: The Background and Legislative History of the Indian Reorganization Act.* Reno: University of Nevada Press, 2000.

Sandrick, Karen. "Surgeon Chronicles Native American History." *Bulletin of the American College of Surgeons* 90, no. 11 (November 2005): 14–19.

Schweikart, Larry. *Banking and Finance, 1913–1989.* New York: Facts on File, 1990.

———. *A History of Banking in Arizona.* Tucson: University of Arizona Press, 1982.

Southerton, Don. "James R. Walker's Campaign against Tuberculosis on the Pine Ridge Indian Reservation." *South Dakota History* 34, no. 2 (Summer 2004): 104–26.

Spicer, Edward H. *A Short History of the Indians of the United States.* New York: D. Van Nostrand, 1969.

Steeler, William C. *Improving American Indian Health Care: The Western Cherokee Experience.* Norman: University of Oklahoma Press, 2001.

Stewart, Omer C. *Peyote Religion: A History.* Norman: University of Oklahoma Press, 1987.

Sutphen, Deborah. "Conservative Warrior: Oveta Culp Hobby and the Administration of America's Health, Education and Welfare." PhD diss., Washington State University, 1997.

Svara, Joseph. Telephone interview with Cary C. Collins, January 2, 2006.

Trennert, Robert A. *White Man's Medicine: Government Doctors and the Navajo, 1863–1955.* Albuquerque: University of New Mexico Press, 1998.

Truitt, Evelyn Mack. *Who Was Who on Screen*. 3rd ed. New York: R. R. Bowker, 1983.

United States Statutes at Large. Washington DC.

U.S. Census Bureau. *Census of Population and Housing, 1960*. Washington DC: Government Printing Office, 1960.

U.S. Commissioner of Indian Affairs. *Annual Report of the Commissioner of Indian Affairs*. Washington DC: Government Printing Office.

U.S. Congress. *Biographical Directory of the United States Congress, 1774–1989*. Washington DC: Government Printing Office, 1988.

————. *Report with Respect to the House Resolution Authorizing the Committee on Interior and Insular Affairs to Conduct an Investigation of the Bureau of Indian Affairs*. House Report 2503, 82nd Cong., 2nd sess. Washington DC: Government Printing Office, 1953.

U.S. Department of Health, Education and Welfare. *Health Services for American Indians*. Public Health Service Publication No. 531. Washington DC: Government Printing Office, 1957.

————. *The Indian Health Program from 1800–1955*. Washington DC: Government Printing Office, 1959.

Wagoner, Paula L. *"They Treated Us Just Like Indians": The Worlds of Bennett County, South Dakota*. Lincoln: University of Nebraska Press, 2002.

Walton, John, Paul B. Beeson, and Ronald Bodley Scott. *The Oxford Companion to Medicine*. 2 vols. New York: Oxford University Press, 1986.

Wilkinson, Charles. *Blood Struggle: The Rise of Modern Indian Nations*. New York: W. W. Norton, 2005.

Woodworth-Ney, Laura. "The Diaries of a Day-School Teacher: Daily Realities on the Pine Ridge Indian Reservation, 1932–1942." *South Dakota History* 24, no. 3 (Fall–Winter, 1994): 194–211.

Index

Page references in italics indicate illustrations; photographic inserts are listed in italics by the text page preceding the insert followed by the photographic plate number.

Aberdeen SD, as BIA Area Office, xii, *lxxiii*, 2, 10, 53
Adams, A. M., 194, 247
Adams, Alex, 46
Adams, Joe, 46, 64
Adams, Mr., 89, 90
adoption ceremony, 230
Afraid of Bear, Mrs., 171
Afraid of Horses, 84
Afraid of Horses, Amos, 209
Afraid of Horses, Frank, 38, 209, 323
Afraid of Horses, Pugh Young Man, 209, 222, 251
Ahrlin, Dr., 300, 301
Aid to Dependent Children, 78, 82, 204, 283, 285
Aid to Families with Dependent Children, 129, 172
Alaska, 94, 107, 250
alcohol, xv, 12, 25, 134, 135, 168, 274, 275, 325
alcoholic gastritis, 307
Allen, Mr., 167
American College of Surgeons, 222, 303, 313, 316, 341n2
American Horse, 242
American Horse, Ben, 65, 84, 118, 214
American Red Cross, liii
amputations, 11, 29
Anderson, Marian, xvii

aortic valve murmurs, 24
apnea, 57
appendectomy, 69, 107, 211, 301, 321
Aquinas, Sister, 274, 276
Army-McCarthy hearings, 225, 303, 341n3
Artichoker, Johnny, 194
Ashley, Victoria, 128
asthma, 218
automobiles, xxvii, xlv

Baca dancers, 244
back pain, 198
badger, 50
Bad Wound, 65
Bailey, Dr., 274, 276
Bald Eagle Bear, Peter, 322
Ball, Suzan, 214
Barnes, Mrs., 297–98
beadwork, 61–62, 188, 290, 323
Beard, Dewey, 221–22
Bear Robe, Charles, 179–80, 237, 239
Bear Runner, Oscar, 74, 102, 103
Bear Shield, 84
Bergen, Bill, 141
Bernard, Sister, 308
Berry, E. Y., 73, 80, 90, 172, 260, 275, 297, 312
Bertsch, Otto G., 95, 131, 204, 215, 216
Big Boy, Henry, 322
Big Road, Mark, 216
Big Thunder, Joseph, 12
"Bimson Report," 97, 100, 124, 199, 338n2
Black Crow, Ada, 188
Black Elk, xiv, 125
Black Elk, Ben, 125, 126, 133, 158

Black Elk, Henry, 109

Black Feather, Mrs., 117

Blindman, Nettie, 22

Blood Struggle: The Rise of Modern Indian Nations (Wilkinson), xix

Blue Bird, 323

Blue Bird, Julia, 170

Blue Bird, Mrs., 170

Blue Horse, 80, 155, 156

bone fractures: car accidents, 26, 100, 109; finger, 133; horse riding accidents, 27; Indians removing casts, 296, 307; intramedullary nail, 71; jaw, 308; leg, 196, 256; open reduction with plate, 38; rodeo injuries, 12, 13, 118, 261

Booth, Edwin, 16

bootleggers, 25, 70, 154, 158, 171, 177, 275

Bordeaux, Sophie, 232

Bores a Hole, George, 196

Borglum, Gutzon, 21

Borglum, Lincoln, 21

boss farmers, xix–xx, 147, 167

Boyle, Hal, 241, 243, 259

Brady, Wilson: borrowing money, 260–61; as cedar chief, 184; as dancer, 178; in full costume, 244; hiding and locking up food, 177, 245; at peyote meetings, 171, 176, 180, 182, 189, 207, 216, 219, 233, 240, 272

Bragg, Jubie, as dentist, 128, 194

Bragg, Robert: emergency cases, 192–93; ending tour at Pine Ridge Hospital, 252, 263, 276; professional meetings attended, 251; temporary duty on other reservations, 231, 250; tour as Pine Ridge Reservation physician, 42, 45, 194

Brands, Allen J., 68–69, 251, 252

Brave, William, 241

Brennan, James, xli, xlv, xlvi, liv, 230

Brewer, Charlene, 304

Brewer, Mrs. Joe, 88

Brown, Georgie, 211

Brown, John A., lxii, lxiii, lxvi, lxix; *Esther Ross*, lxvi; *Half-Sun on the Columbia*, lxvi

Brown, Victor, 211

Brown Bull, Vera Mae, 224

Brown Eyes, Philip, 128, 171

Brust, Mr., 128

Bryde, John, 205

Buckingham, Earl, 241, 248

buckskin, 59, 62, 64, 212, 323

Buechel, Father Eugene, 132, 136–38, 153, 229, 230

buffalo: in Custer State Park, 150, 151, 220; historic slaughter of, 69; jerky, 229; skulls and heads, 138, 240; Sun Dance symbol of, 240, 246; as warrior meat, 64; from Yellowstone Park, 73

Buffalo Bill's Circus and Wild West Show, 118, 242

Bull Bear, Maine, 277

Bull Bear, Moses, 277

Bunch, Wayne, 206

Bureau of Indian Affairs (BIA): Education Division, xxii, xxviii, 39; hiring reservation doctors, xxiv; Maintenance Department, 95; Medical Division, xxii, xxviii, 39; memoirs of officials, xvi; national hospitals and sanatoria, lviii–lix; Native American Church not recognized by, 125; pay and patient load of physicians, xxv; Rehabilitation policies, 165; Resources group, 247; Ruby's experiences with, xiii; supervision of Indian health care, liv–lx; transfer of Indian health care to Public Health Service, lix–lx, 68; yearly costs for Pine Ridge, 201

Burns Prairie, 316

Cadotte, Verna, 310

Calamity Jane, 206

cancer, 155

Captain, 112–3; accompanying Rubys to and from Pine Ridge, xi, 1–2, 323; as "Cappie," 306; on day trips with the Rubys, 225; dragging in trash, 19; as gift to Jeanne, 333n2; gunshot injury of, 91–92; itchy skin of, 291; representing dogs of Pine Ridge, 280, 282; staying inside at night, 275

car accidents, xxvii, 308

cardiac failure, 133

Carey, Walter R., 166, 251

Carlile, William K., 165, 166

Carlisle Indian Schools, xxviii, xxxix, xlii

Carr, Lyman J., 26, 45, 49, 95–96, 124, 125, 244, 310

Case, Mr., 258

cataracts, 220

Catches, Joe, 184, 188–89, 190

cedar, 159, 185, 188, 189, 234, 235, 236

Celilla, Carmine A., 175, 231

cellulitis, 40

cerebral vascular accident, 47, 123

Chadron NE: eye specialist, 72; Indian populations in, 171, 175, 283, 284; supplies and services in, 10, 19

Chalcraft, Edwin L., xliii–xliv

Chang, 278

Chemawa Indian School, xxviii, xliii, xliv

cherry wood, 42–43, 265–66

chest pain, 90, 292

Cheyenne Indians, 234, 235

Cheyenne River Agency, 87

Chief, Ben, 214

Chief, Katie, 278–79

Chief Crazy Horse (1955), 212, 213–14

child abuse and neglect, lxx, 134, 136

childbirth, past tribal practices, 63

Chips, Joe Ashley, 48

chokeberries, 257

Clapp, W. H., xli

Clifford, Mrs., 75

closed reduction, 296

Cody, Buffalo Bill, 47, 49, 51, 60, 118

Coker, Ed, as head of Soil and Moisture Conservation, 117, 118, 154, 155, 167, 200, 241, 258, 284, 318

Coker, Nell: as acting director of nursing at Pine Ridge Hospital, 213, 220, 226, 233, 284, 307, 322; observing a peyote meeting, 233, 234, 237, 264, 271, 272–73

conjunctivitis, lviii

Conoyer, Mr., 207

constipation, 138

contusions, 308

Coolidge, Calvin, 20, 241, 297

Cooper, J. M., 90, 165

corn, 176, 230

Cornelius, Mrs. John, 62

coronary occlusion, 90

Cottier, Frances, 274, 276

Crazy Horse, 20, 46, 47, 208, 221

Crazy Horse (Sandoz), 197

Crippled Children's Program, 274, 276

Cross Fire peyote sect: altar of, 176; designated chiefs, 159; feud with Half Moon, 104, 160, 180, 193; healing ceremonies of, 253; members of, 126, 171, 193, 239; using the Bible, 104, 108, 160, 190

Crum, Dr., 109, 277, 280

Daniel, Z. T.: on Oglala beliefs and values, xxxvi; on overall health of Oglalas, xl; as reservation doctor, xxxv; safe water concerns, xl; tuberculosis as prime cause of death, xxxvii–xxxviii; views on off-reservation boarding schools, xxxix

Dean, Dr., 84, 86

DeBenedetto, R. L., 138

deer, 55

Deloria, Ella: *Speaking of Indians*, 229

demoralization, lxx

dental problems, lv, lviii, 123, 332–33n78

dermatitis, 280

Dew, W. B., xl–xli

Dexter, Mr., 316

diabetes, 85

discrimination, 203

dogs: barking, 275, 278–79, 281–82; as meat for ceremonies, 111, 115–16, 122, 176, 246, 271; painting and baptism of, 115–16; pulling travois, 62

Dreamer, George, lv, lvi

Dreamer, Marion Billbrough, liv–lvii

dropsy, 183

drums: as gifts, 302; in Half Moon ceremonies, 185, 186–87, *187*, 188; in Indian dances, 84, 240, 242; in peyote meetings, 108, 338n2; in Sun Dance, 240, 242; in Yuwipi ceremonies, 110, 121, 191–92, 234, 235, 269

Dupuytren's Contracture, 229
dysentery, xlii

Eagen, Dr., 293
Eagle Dance, 241
Eagle Heart, Matthew, 207, 253
eagle leg bones, 62
Eagle Nest district, 15
eagles, 160
ear splitting ceremony, 232
Eastman, Charles, xxvi; examining patients,
    xxxii, xxxiii; *From the Deep Woods to
    Civilization*, xxxi; as Indian Service doctor,
    xxxi, xxxii; language ability and empathy,
    xxxiii, xxxiv; making horseback rounds on
    the reservation, xxxiv; as Santee Sioux, xxxi
Eckert, Bruce H., 205, 210–11, 216
Eckert, Mrs., 210–11
Ecoffey, Frank (Posey), 293
education. *See* schools and education
Edwards, Lawrence, 93, 140, 308–11
Eisenhower, Dwight D., 20, 125, 157, 234, 297
electrocution, 216, 217
Elk Boy, 114, 115, 155, 156
Elk Boy, Agnes: attending peyote meeting,
    233; borrowing money, 290, 297; delivering
    healthy baby boy, 321; participating in
    Yuwipi ceremonies, 115, 116, 264, 268;
    pawning a pipe, 169, 340n5
Elk Boy, Dick: ankle sprain, 219; borrowing
    money, 290, 297; farewell to the Rubys, 323;
    sacrifices for healthy children, 264–65, 266,
    270, 321
Elk Boy, Ira, 219, 234, 239, 252, 323
Elk Boy, Joe, 264
Elk Boy, Louise, 233
Elk Boy, Richard, 121
Ellsworth Air Force Base, 242
Emmons, Glenn L., 86, 94, 286, 294, 297,
    336n1
epilepsy, 138, 298
Esther Ross: Stillaguamish Champion (Ruby
    and Brown), lxvi

face and body painting, 63, 65, 115, 246

Fairburn, Mr., 80
Fairburn, Mrs., 231
fans, 183, 187, 188, 189, 235
Fast Wolf, Todd, 222, 295
feathers: in dance costumes, 138, 240, 323; in
    peyote meetings, 183, 185, 187, 188, 266; used
    by medicine men, 120
Feehan, John J., 139
Ferraca, Steve, 255
field nurses, xxvii, xxxvi, liii, 131
fire starters, 230
Fire Thunder, William, 76, 89, 90, 106, 125
Fitzgerald, William, 191–92
Flesh, 119, 121, 123
Flying Hawk, Joe, 176
food and nutrition: food supplies for
    boarding schools, 27; government rations
    to Indians, lii, 47, 61, 75; reservation food
    sources, 25; tuberculosis and, xxxviii–xxxix,
    lii, lviii; warrior food, 64; wild fruits and
    berries, 19
Fools Crow, Andrew, 118, 161, 166, 214, 238,
    239, 241
Fools Crow, Frank, 84
Fools Crow, Mrs., 165
Forshey, Elizabeth: Adult Education lectures
    by, 61, 67, 70; as agency social worker,
    37, 44, 57; assessment for reservation
    socioeconomic changes, 201; attending
    Yuwipi ceremonies, 118, 123; on bootleggers,
    171–72; dealing with complaints, 128; Edgar
    Red Cloud's relationship with, 238, 260–61,
    275–76; on Indians hiding food supplies,
    177–78; issuing relief money, 71, 82, 221, 284,
    285; observing Horse Dance, 60; observing
    peyote meetings, 180, 182; opinions of Mr.
    Sande, 68, 81; political views of, 68; on
    school advisor handling student funds,
    282–83; verifying eligibility for medical
    care, 168, 172–73
Fort Berthold, 92, 163
Fort Thompson, 232
Fort Yates, 27, 28, 31, 93, 136, 166, 283
From the Deep Woods to Civilization
    (Eastman), xxxi

Fuller, Harold, 212
funerals and burials, lvii, 23, 52

Gage, Crescentia, 173
gallbladder disease, 11, 16, 322
gangrenous bowel, 107
Gap, Eva, 193
Gap, George, 193
Garreau, Manson A., 261
Gassman, Harvey S.: assignment as Pine
    Ridge physician, 44, 90–91, 204, 254, 276;
    dog of, 217; end of tour at Pine Ridge, 252,
    293, 342n2; snowy emergency calls by, 140;
    tuberculosis cases handled by, 192
Gassman, Yetta, 44, 273
gastrectomy, 303–4, 305, 310, 312
gastritis, 295
gastroenteritis, 130
Geboe, Jim, 206–7
Gerbers, xviii
germ theory, 104, 130
Ghost Dance, 51, 138, 142
Ghost Dog, Kenneth, 301
Gildersleeve, Jo Ann, 212
Gildersleeve, Mrs., 285
Goings, Bill, 251
Goings, "Fish," 80
Goings, Keva, 278
Golden, Glyndine F., 209, 218, 228, 254, 255,
    273, 314
gourds: Indian dances using, 156; in peyote
    ceremonies, 183, 185, 187, 188, 189, 235; in
    Yuwipi meetings, 110, 114, 121, 123, 267, 268,
    269, 270
Grace, Mother, 305, 308
Gray Eagle, Clarence, 27, 28
The Great Sioux Uprising (1953), 132
Greene, Felix, 267, 272
Griot, Dr., 72
ground hogs, 37
Grueb, Mr., 277

Hagel, Mr., 304
Hagels grocery store, xviii
Half Moon peyote sect: competing with
    Cross Fire, 104, 193; healing ceremonies by,

161; members of, 196, 253; prayer meetings
    of, 179; using peace pipe, 108; water bird
    symbol of, 159, 160; water calls in, 176
*Half-Sun on the Columbia: A Biography of
    Chief Moses* (Ruby and Brown), lxvi
Hampton Indian School, xxxix
Hand, Marie, 200, 265, 269
Happy Hunting Ground, 115, 116
Harris, Mr., 155
Harris, Mrs., 155
Has No Horses, 196
Has No Water, George, 196
Hawk, Lewis, 254
headaches, 119
head injuries, 74, 161, 175–76, 198, 261
head lice, 293
Hearst, William Randolph, Jr., 178, 197, 323
Heinemann, Ruth K., 53, 238, 298
Hemingway, Mrs., 285
Hemingway Texaco, xviii, *112–1*
Henderson, Jeanne: birth and childhood,
    lxxii; marriage to Robert Ruby, lxvi
Henderson, Mrs., 223, 224
hepatitis, 275
Herbert, Rudolph C., 260
Herd Camp, 254, 258
Herman, Jake: on government rations, 47;
    powwow held by, 84; relationship with
    Dr. Ruby, 202, 237, 280, 323; stories told
    by, 50–52; in Sun Dance festivities, 243; as
    translator, 322; on tribal council, 49, 73, 89,
    92, 106, 162, 163, 172, 201
hernia, 38, 280
Hickock, Wild Bill, 206
High White Man, Angelique, 178
Hobby, Oveta Culp, 68, 71, 337n3
Hockenberry, Mr., 244
Holden, Sara E.: back ailment of, 155; dealing
    with patients, 85; as director of nursing at
    Pine Ridge Hospital, 30–31, 44, 69, 79, 80,
    81, 93, 205; on disruptive staff, 87, 95; on
    Mr. Sande, 36; ordering supplies, 107, 208,
    215; replacement for, 315; retirement of, 208,
    211, 213; sanitation lecture trips, 101, 102; on
    staffing the hospital, 56, 57, 87, 95

Holmes, Graham, 100, 298

Holmes, Orrin, 150–51, 206, 207, 293, 296, 339n3

Holy Rosary Mission, xviii, xlix, 19, 93, 233, 305, 308, 322, 325. *See also* Red Cloud Indian School

Hoop Dance, 155

Horn Cloud, Joe, 7, 278

Horn Cloud, John, 5

Horn Cloud, Mrs., 283

Horse, Douglas, 107–8, 126, 195

Horse Dance, 60

horses: accidents and injuries related to, 27; Dr. Ruby riding, 197–98; hairs in ceremonial items, 188; injuries to, 205, 217; as measurement of wealth, 229; Morgan Gold, 305; open grazing, 195; owned by Indians, 12, 26, 172; for physicians, xlv; Red Correl, 305; saddle blankets, 244; school herds of, 205, 217; stealing, 132; as transportation, xv, 27, 112–7, 146; wagon teams of, xv, 112–7, 233; as wedding gifts, 64

Hudgins, Herbert A., 252, 298, 305, 310, 311

Hudspeth, Mrs., 279

Hump, Rebecca, 253

Hunt, G. H., 164

Hunter, Lawrence, 179

hypertension, 24

hyperthyroidism, 252

Idaho: McCall, xii, *lxxi*; River of No Return, xi; White Bird Canyon, xi, xii

"Indian giver," 302, 307

Indian Health Service: African American physicians and nurses, 324; formation of, xxix; revolving door of medical personnel, xlvii–xlviii

"Indian Love Call," 154, 158, 212

Indian New Deal, xv

infectious hepatitis, 275

influenza, xlviii

intramedullary nail, 71

intussusception, 144

Iron Boulder, Jack, 31

Iron Cloud, Agnes, 204, 241, 314, 320

Iron Cloud, George, 26, 207

Iron Cloud, James, 242

Iron Cloud, Philip, 168

Iron Crow, 238

Iron Nail, 221

Irving, Ben, 201, 202, 203, 241, 243, 245

Jackson, Joe, 315, 317

Jamruszka, Mr., 146, 303

Janis, Boob, 207, 254, 274, 280, 342n1

Janis, Leroy, 207

Janis, Miss, 237–38, 341–42n7

joblessness, lxx

Joe's Market, xviii

Johnson, Brent, 145, 150, 155, 157

Johnson, Craig, 145, 150, 155, 157

Johnson, Emery, lx

Johnson, Marion Ruby: as "Chowder," 10, 334n10; Dr. Ruby's letters to, xii–xvi; as "Graceful Woman," 157; in McCall, Idaho, xii, *lxxi*; visit to Pine Ridge, 145, 147

Johnson, Mrs. B. T., 16

Jones, Gordon, 307

Jones, Rosalie, as Public Health nurse in Wanblee, 204, 206, 209, 210, 215, 227

Journal of the American Medical Association, 312

Julesburg CO, 314

Keevan, Brother, 29

Kehna, Miss, 56

Kelly, William H., 276

Kessis, Michael: as Area Health administrator, 29, 30, 42, 84, 86, 250, 259, 261; locating missing items and funds, 41, 44, 128, 251, 252

Kicking Bear, 51

Kicking Bear, Nancy, 27, 28

Klinker, Dolores H., 303–4

Korean War, xvii, lxvi, 22, 25, 72, 116, 240, 242

Kurilecz, Michael, 84, 195, 196, 206, 211

Kyle SD, xix, *lxxiv*; availability of doctors, xxxvii, xlv, xlviii, xlix, 102; field nurses in, 31, 111–12, 117; schools, xxxvii, 33–34 lacerations, 55–56, 141, 169, 194, 195, 205, 256, 308

LaCompt, Dennis, 206–7

LaCourse, Eldon: as BIA administrative officer, 39, 56, 89, 90, 91, 96, 164, 216, 226; fiscal concerns of, 128, 165, 208; leaving position, 280, 283; staffing the hospital, 56, 79; on supply issues, 107, 237

LaDeaux, Waup, 80

La Flesche, Susan, xxvi

Lakota language, 137

Lam, Dr., 36

Lame Deer MT, 176, 240, 245, 246, 293

LaPointe, Angelique, 27, 28

LaPointe, James, 280

Lautzenheiser, Mr., 67

LaVizzio, Dr., 259

Leading Eagle Jr., 241

LeCompt, Dennis, 307–8

LeGrande, Pierre, 223, 251, 308

leg ulcer, 179

Lehner, Joseph, 255–56, 290, 297, 302

Leupp, Francis E., xliv

Levine Tube, 310–11

lightning, 50

lipoma, 307

Little Bear, Charlie, 43

Little Bear, Dixon, 5

Little Bighorn, Battle of, 221, 222

Little Goose, Henry, 40

Little Spotted Horse, Sarah, 27, 28

Little Thunder, Marvin, 40

Little Wound, 65

Lone Dog, John, 259

Looks Twice, Sara, 133, 244

Lund, John, 214

MacDonald, Elizabeth, 225

MacGregor, James: *The Wounded Knee Massacre*, 141

marriage, past tribal practices, 63

Martin, Roy, 253, 295

Mast, Joe, 81, 92–93, 118, 288, 301, 318, 323

Mast, Lorie, 301

Mast, Vicky, 301

Mathews, Miss, 76, 79

Mathews, Mrs., 95, 96, 97, 226

Mature, Victor, 214

McCall, Jack, 206

McDowell, Duane, 303

McGill, Margaret: as acting director of nursing at Pine Ridge Hospital, 17, 196, 213; professional and personal behaviors, 85, 87, 95, 250–51, 254, 315; purchase of school horses, 305; request for transfer, 106–7, 209

McGillycuddy, Agent: A Biography of Dr. Valentine T. McGillycuddy (McGillycuddy), 135

McGillycuddy, Julia B.: *McGillycuddy, Agent*, 135

McGillycuddy, V. T., xxx, 135, 167, 209, 339–40n3

McKay, James Douglas, 68, 337n4

McKinley, William, 157

McLaughlin, James, xxxvii

Means, John, 220, 221, 222

measles, lviii, 1

Medicine, Antoine, 206

medicine men, xlii–xliii; becoming a healer, 218–19; government views of, xxiii; healing practices of, 43, 44, 110–11, 113, 119, 120, 121, 122; inherited roles of, 43; licensing of, 219; Yuwipi practices of, 42–44, 48, 59, 60, 73

Meier, Joseph, 21

meningitis, 94

mental problems, 298, 314

Meriam Report, liii

Merrill's Marauders, 173, 340n6

Merrival, Ethel: on barking dogs, 277–78, 279; cattle herd of, 81; as champion of Indians, 29; complaints against medical staff, 78–79, 80, 84, 85, 86, 87, 97; criticisms by, 72, 73, 93; education issues, 254; employment maneuvering by, 76; meeting with Ben Reifel, 165; on patient transportation, 30, 95; relationship with tribal council, 73, 83, 106; requesting commodities, 316; singing "Indian Love Call," 154, 158

Mickelson, Lawrence T., 112–6; arranging clinics for students, 273; discovering

Mickelson, Lawrence T. (*continued*)
duplicate employees, 274; Fort Yates
position, 136; friendship with Dr. and Mrs.
Ruby, 44, 157–58, 254, 255; as godparent
to Edna Ruby, 288; keeping up student
attendance, 25, 93; managing teacher issues,
150, 286; as school principal, 22, 140, 173,
205; working with Mr. Pyles, 151, 152
Mickelson, Lillian, *112–6*; friendship
with Dr. and Mrs. Ruby, 27, 44, 157–58,
257–58; as godparent to Edna Ruby, 288;
on reservation violence, 136; on school
attendance, 25, 243
Miles, Nelson A., 49
Miles, Sidney, 287
Miller, Dave, 212, 213
Mills, Bud, 106
Mills, Sydney, 319
Minnesota: Leech Lake Reservation, xlii;
White Earth, lx
Miss Indian America, 107
mitral valve murmurs, 24
moccasins, 25, 118, 244
Montana: Blackfeet Agency, xxxv; Red
Lodge, 2
Montezuma, Carlos, xxvi
Morgan, Thomas J.: as Commissioner
of Indian Affairs, xxii, xxiii–xxiv, xxix,
330nn18–27; on duties of reservation
doctors, xxvi, xxvii; Indian health care
initiatives, xix, xxii–xxvii, xxix; on neglect
of Indian medical care, xxvi, xxvii
Morrell, Warren, 241
Moss, General, 49
Mosseau, Louis, 43–44, 168
Mundt, Karl E., 20, 225, 297, 303, 335n17,
341n3

National Congress of American Indians,
249
Native American Church: aboriginal and
Christian features of, 58, 228n1, 336n2;
altar arrangement of, *184*, 233, *233*; drums
in ceremonies of, 186, *187*; members of,
182; national charter, 182; peyote practices

of, 58, 73, 106, 125, 176, 182–91, 212, 233–37,
336n2, 338n1
Navajo Indians, xxiii
Nebraska: Alliance, 297–98; Chadron, xviii,
10, 12; Crawford, 46, 47, 215; Gordon, xviii,
131, 196, 332n72; Hastings State Hospital,
298; Omaha, 293; Rushville, xviii, 145,
280; Scottsbluff, 216, 219, 289; Valentine,
228; White Clay, xv, lxxiv, 15, 258. *See also*
Chadron NE
Nelson, Bob, 296
Nelson, Cleveland, 80
Nelson, Emma, 56–57, 297
Nelson, Florence, 296
Nelson, John, 241
Nelson, Moot, 106, 165
Newkirk, Morris, 262
Nez Perce Indian War, xi
Nichols, Eva, 128, 319
Nierenhauser, Mrs., 238
No More, Morris, 196
Noralf, Mr., 192
North Dakota: Devils Lake, 165; Fort Yates,
27, 28, 31, 93, 136, 166, 283; Hettinger, 2;
San Haven, 199, 224, 313; Standing Rock
Reservation, 27, 28, 31, 62, 251
Northwest Museum of Arts and Cultures
(Spokane WA), lxix
nurses: patient assault of, 29–30; reservation
field nurse programs, xxvii, xxxvi, liii, 131.
See also specific reservation hospitals

Obert, Reverend, 244
obstetric cases and deliveries, xlix, 11, 12, 124,
129–30, 142–44, 277, 321
O'Clock, George, 135, 136
Oehmcke, Dick, 258
Oehmcke, Mick, 258
of Whose Horses They Are Afraid, Young
Man, 209
Oglala Presbyterian Church, 244
The Oglala Sioux: Warriors in Transition
(Ruby), lxvi, 306
Oglala Sioux Indians: beliefs about the
dead, 50; braids, xix, xx, 18, 28–29, 40, 51,

119; chiefs and tribal councils, 26; dancers, 126, 133, 178, 197; full-blooded and mixed blooded, xxxix, 94; grandmother spirit, 50; history of health care, xxi–xxii; Horse Dance, 60; "Indian time" of, 130–31; living off the reservation, 61; marriage and divorce, 40; military service of, 22, 25, 170, 173, 178–79, 240, 293, 295, 304, 308, 335n4; as seasonal laborers, 131, 148–49, 288–89, 303; spiritual world of, 43; Sun Dance of, xx, 46–47, 146, 209, 220, 235, 237, 239, 240–42, 245, 246, 292, 320, 323; warrior traditions of, 46, 64–65

Oglala Sioux Tribal Health Administration, 324, 325

Oglala Wi, Edna Ruby as, 218

Old Age Assistance (OAA), 285

Olinger, Josephine: on Indian expectations of field nurses, 111; as Kyle field nurse, 31, 166, 169, 199, 222, 307; professional and personal behaviors, 261, 286–87; quarrel with boss farmer, 147

Olinger, Mr., 148

One Feather, Jackson, 256

One Feather, Joe, 104, 219

open reduction with plate, 38

Orchot, Reverend, 276, 288

Oregon, Chemawa Indian School, xxviii, xliii, xliv

otitis media, 192

Our Lady of Lourdes Hospital, 94, 151, 194

out-of-wedlock sexual activity, lxx

owls, 63, 114, 115, 188

Pahin Santi, 71

Palmier, Buster, 217

Palmier, Taylor, 216

Parks, Mrs., 228

Parks, Stephen A.: on efficiency of agency health care, 232; as Rosebud Reservation physician, 227, 228, 229, 230, 231, 256, 259, 273

Paulson, Dr., 148

Pawluk, Valerie, 196, 209, 218, 314, 321

peace pipe: carving of, 148; as exchange gifts, 64; in Half Moon ceremonies, 159; in Sun Dances, 240; in Yuwipi ceremonies, 60, 111, 114, 115, 120, 122, 267, 268, 269, 270

Pease, Laurella, 178

Pease, Miss, 196

Pede, J. S., xxxv

pediatrics, 18

Peg Leg, 305

Pejuta Tepee, xviii, 112–1

Penney, Chas. G., xxix–xxx, xli

Penny, 217

peptic ulcers, 16, 23

peritonitis, 23

Peyjuta, 160

peyote: Cross Fire sect, 108, 159, 160, 171, 176, 180, 190, 193, 205, 239, 253; Half Moon sect, 159, 160, 161, 169, 176, 179, 193, 196, 205, 253; in healing practices, 104, 106, 107–8; ritual use of, 37, 52, 58, 99, 112, 124–25, 217

pheasant, 188

Pike, Charlie, 82

Pine Ridge, 61, 107, 147

Pine Ridge Hospital, 112–2; blood supplies, 25–26, 143–44; clinic days, 13, 18; as community and healing place, xiii; complaints against staff or care, 78, 83–84, 85, 88, 97, 128; field hospitals, xxxiv, xxxvi; funding and appropriations, xiii; new hospital building, xlvi, liv; OB cases and deliveries, 11, 12, 124, 129–30, 277, 321; Oglala beliefs and, xxxvi; pediatric care, 18; phone system of, 95; relatives camping with patients, xxxv; site and layout of, xxxiv–xxxv, liv, 17–18; staffing of, 17, 32, 35, 45, 56–57, 79, 209, 213, 218, 223, 238; supplying, 18, 107, 208, 215; transportation and gas for, xlv, 31–32, 41–42, 45; water supply, xxxiv–xxxv

Pine Ridge Indian Reservation, lxxi, lxxiii, lxxiv; alcoholism, xv, 12, 25, 134, 135, 168, 274, 275, 325; Badlands bordering, xxi, 22, 38, 51, 52, 157, 172; BIA office, xix; "Big Issue" events, xxxii–xxxiii; Blindman Table, 22; Cedar Creek, 51; celebrations and dances, 22, 25, 159; chief and tribal council, 65;

Pine Ridge Indian Reservation (*continued*)
child mortality, lvii; churches, 3, 26;
communities in, *lxxiv*; Cooley Table,
22; crime, xv, 50–51; cultural and social
repression, xx; dancers, 126, 178, 197;
dances, 239–42, 244; Denby Dam, 19;
districts of, 15; economic conditions,
lii–liii; eligibility for health services, 87;
employment on, 78, 82; enrollment and
eligibility of, 140; family size, liii; federal
influences, xix–xx; geographic location,
xviii, xix; goods and services, xviii; Holy
Rosary Mission, xlviii, 33, 93, 233, 305,
308, 322, 325; hunger and malnutrition,
lii–liii; hunting on, 52, 55; Indian justice,
26; infant mortality, lii, lvii; influenza
epidemic, xlviii–xlix; lands as home
and traditions, xx–xxi; life expectancy,
lx–lxi; living conditions, xix, xli, liii, lviii,
27–28, 51, *112–7*, 134, 295–96; maternal
deaths, lxi; Oglala Boarding School, xxxiv,
xxxvii; phone service, 8, 39, 51, 75, 143,
245; Porcupine Butte, 51; promiscuity and
prostitution, 24–25, 320; Red Cloud Agency
moved to, xxix; Red Shirt Table, 22, 57, 65,
66, 139, 142, 157, 213, 215, 222, 249, 295, 310;
Rehabilitation Program, 52, 152; relocation
program, 54; renting grazing lands, 81; safe
water, xxx, xl, xli, l; sanitation, xxx, xl, xli,
l; Slim Buttes, *lxxiv*, 128, 146, 171, 172, 174,
175, 303; snowstorms and blizzards, 139–40,
142, 145, 146; socioeconomic conditions,
xiv, 78, 82; transportation, xv, 27, *112–7*,
146; unprobated estates on, 248; villages,
xix; violence and shootings on, 49, 91–92,
136, 170, 215; Wakpamni district, 15, 80, 104,
109; White Clay Creek, xxix, l, 195, 233, 272;
White Clay Dam, 19; White Horse Creek,
51; women's auxiliary, liii; word of mouth
communication, 22–23; Wounded Knee
Butte, 51; Wounded Knee Creek, 51. *See also*
Pine Ridge Hospital
pipes, 230
Pitner, Will J., 228
Plenty Wolf: conducting Yuwipi meetings,

60, 113, 114, 115, 116, 264, 265, 267, 268,
272, 273; as medicine man, 198, 269, 270;
suitcase of ceremonial items, 266; tattoos
of, 271
Plenty Wolf, George, 200
Plenty Wounds, 161
pneumonia, lviii, 219
Pons, Lily, xvii
Poor Bear, Bob, 116, 117
Poor Thunder, Charlie, 239
Poor Thunder, George, 119, 126–27, 161,
196–97, 212, 219, 240, 242, 245
porcupine quills, 62, 267
postpartum psychosis, 284
Potato Creek Joe, 206
Pourier, Bat, 51
Pourier, Mr., 143
Powers, Mr., 200, 279
powwows, 37, 84–85, 90
Pratt, Miss, 17
Public Health Service: Commissioned Corps
of, xxviii, 71; transfer of Indian health care
to, lix–lx, 68, 124
Public Law 67–85, xxviii
Pueblo Indians, 241, 244
Pyles, Albert T.: administrative abilities of,
53, 93, 151–52, 192, 194, 215, 263, 287, 318,
319; control of housing, 216; as head of
Education, 31, 57, 67; on Relocation policy,
277; reservation education program of, 174

Quinn, Mr., 192, 197, 198
Quint, Harley: as Pine Ridge Hospital eye
doctor, 71, 154, 167, 251, 276, 313, 315, 316–17;
skiing to work, 139
Quiver, 192

Rabbit Dance, 155
Randall, Charlie, 105, 145
Rapid City SD, xviii, *lxxiii*; Crippled
Children's Clinic, 195; hospitals, 30;
Indian populations in, 133; Indian School,
liv; School of Mines, 225. *See also* Sioux
Sanitarium
Rapid City Journal, 241

rattles, 230

Red Bear, 209

Red Bear, Joe, 220

Red Bear, Mrs., 220, 341n1

Red Cherries, Adolph, 245, 246

Red Cloud: band of, 124; descendants of, xiv, 46, 65, 156; on Indians working, 135; trading the Black Hills, 49, 55

Red Cloud, Dick, 233

Red Cloud, Edgar: attending tribal council sessions, 88, 191; bailing people out of jail, 171, 200; as Catholic, 113; friendship with Dr. Ruby, 69, 80, 117, 180, 317; fundraising by, 245, 275; as great-grandson of Red Cloud, 58–59; as interpreter, 190; in the movies, 207–8, 213, 238; opinion of Ben Reifel, 109, 172, 256; relationship with Mrs. Forshey, 302; as seasonal worker, 312; stories told by, 74–75, 156, 322–23; Sun Dance participation, 239; white guest of, 239, 244, 255, 290, 294, 302; on Yuwipi practices, 73, 118–19, 179

Red Cloud, James: Catholic and Yuwipi practices, 204; as dancer, 84; distributing commodities, 316; hospitalization of, 198, 199–200, 203; as old chief, 155, 156, 157, 158, 297, 322; opinion of Ben Reifel, 168, 256, 340n4; sweathouse of, 264, 265; Yuwipi ceremony at home of, 264–68, 268, 269–73

Red Cloud, Mary Ann, 155, 178, 200, 208, 272, 317, 323

Red Cloud, Reno: as dancer, 155, 245, 255, 260, 261, 290, 294, 302; in the movies, 208, 222; as son of Edgar Red Cloud, 200, 323

Red Cloud, Vincent, 130, 171, 200, 233, 239, 271, 293, 294, 323

Red Cloud Indian School, 325

red measles, l

Red Owl, Cordelia, 107

Reed, Bob, 194

Reifel, Benjamin: on benefits of reservation, 247–48; complaints about poor student behaviors, 256–57, 258–59; daily news sheets by, 94, 109, 130, 136, 141, 162, 255, 313; on discrimination, 112; expectations of behaviors on reservation, 97–98; on getting kids to schools, 288, 289, 290; handling complaints by, 146–47; Indian feelings and attitudes toward, 220, 222, 243, 248, 249, 286; inspecting jails by, 225–26, 227, 253–54; job performance ratings by, 205; liquor policies of, 158, 171; plans for socioeconomic changes, 129–30, 149, 163–64, 174; policy on barking dogs, 275, 276, 278–79, 286; recommendations for Bimson Report, 124; as superintendent of Pine Ridge, 82, 84, 92, 93, 94, 96, 100–101, 102–3, 117, 118, 128, 129–30, 337–38n1

Reifel, Loyce, 212, 228

Reifel, Alice (Mrs. Benjamin), 100, 105, 118, 127, 208

Reinhardt, Siegfried, 7, 334n7

Resineck, Miss, 86, 95

rheumatic fever, 24

Richard, Brady, 155, 156

Richards, John, 199, 215, 216

Rising Sun, 184, 187, 189

Roberts, Mr., 259, 298, 299

Roberts, W. O., 14, 165

Robeson, Paul, xvii

Rocking Bear, 52

rodeos: injuries related to, 12, 261, 285–86, 296, 307; jobs in, 198; pregnancies related to, 24; rowdy crowds with, 25, 229, 231

Rolfe, Weldon, 215, 280

"rosaries," 59, 113, 120–21, 122, 123, 265, 267

Rosebud Indian Reservation: Burning Breast Lake, 228; communities, lxxiv; Heffer Lake, 229; Rosebud Hospital, 152; St. Francis Mission, lxxiv, 136, 137, 154, 228; Soldier Creek, 229, 231; violence on, 136, 207; White Lake, 231

Rosseau, Louis, 135

Rowland, Eugene, 22, 25, 72, 116–17, 155, 242, 335n4

Ruby, Edna Phyllis, 112–4, 112–5, 112–6; baptism of, 292; birth of, lxvii, 207; Dr. Ruby's observations of, 216, 263, 287, 291, 305–6; as Oglala Wi, 218

Ruby, Jeanne, *112–3, 112–5*; accompanying husband on lecture trips, 101; baby Edna, 207, 211, 218, 223–24; finding fresh fruits and vegetables, 19; house water problems, 35, 38–39, 41, 70; laundry and cleaning challenges, 5, 6; setting home in Pine Ridge, 4–6, 11–12, 16; teaching at reservation schools, xi, xii, xiv, 24; tea for Mrs. Reifel, 126

Ruby, Robert, *112–3, 112–4, 112–6, 112–8*; as American College of Surgeons fellow, 222, 303, 313, 316, 341n2; assignment to Pine Ridge Indian Hospital, xi, xii; on assimilation policies, 14–15; birth and childhood of, xvi, lxv, *lxxi*; commission with U.S. Public Health Service, xvii, 1; on daily reservation life, lxi–lxii; education of, xvii, lxv; on government attitudes and practices, lxi, 1, 16; *Esther Ross*, lxvi; *Half-Sun on the Columbia*, lxvi; hosting dance and powwow at home, 155–56; interests in Indian histories, xiv, 16; job performance ratings of, 205; journalism experience, xvi–xvii, 329n6; living quarters at Pine Ridge, 4–6, *112–3*; marriage to Jeanne Henderson, lxvi; medical and surgical training of, xvii, lxv, lxvi; as medical director at Pine Ridge Hospital, xii, xxi, 10, 20, 34; Moses Lake practice of, lxiii, lxvi, *lxxii*; observations of Indian behaviors, lxiii, 89–91, 94, 135–36, 223, 290–91, 292–93, 296, 301, 302, 307–9, 342–43; *The Oglala Sioux: Warriors in Transition*, lxvi, 306; one week duty at Rosebud, 226, 227; peyote meeting observations of, 180–84, *184*, 185–87, *187*, 188–91, 233, *233*, 234–37; Pine Ridge letters to sister Marion, xii–xiii, lxix, 324–25; playing in pep band, 80; public relations trips, 65–77; return visit to Pine Ridge Hospital, *112–4*; school physicals by, 23–24, 33–34, 276, 277, 291; service in U.S. Army Air Corps, xvii, lxv, lxvi; Sun Dance observations by, 220–21; on unnecessary surgery, 36; views on Withdrawal policy, 36,

37; Yuwipi ceremony observations, 118–23, 127, 264–68, *268*, 269–73

Running Bear, Dick, 182, 183, 184, 185–86, 187, 189, 190, 193

Running Bear, Mrs., 185

Running Bear, Oscar, 101

Running Hawk, Dorothy, 253

Running Hawk, Joe, 169, 189, 244, 253

Rural Electric Administration (rea), 66

Russell, Oliver, 228, 229, 231

Ryder, Manning C., 80, 173, 318, 320

sage: in peyote meetings, 190–91, 235; in Sun Dance, 240, 245; in Yuwipi ceremonies, 111, 114, 120, 121, 266, 267, 269, 271

St. Elizabeth's Hospital, 253

St. Francis Mission, *lxxiv*, 136, 137, 154, 228

St. Joseph's Hospital, 293

Salaway's barbershop, xviii

Salvation Army, 128

Sande, O. R.: in Area Education Office, 243, 257; dispensing money, 23; on economic depression, 78, 82; staffing the hospital, 79; as superintendent of Pine Ridge, 9, 10, 20, 26, 56, 57, 67, 68; transfer of, 81, 85–86; using hospital car, 32, 39, 42; views on Withdrawal policy, 36, 37

Sandoz, Mari: *Crazy Horse*, 197

Santee Sioux, xxxi, 125

Sauser, Emmaline, 94, 254, 256, 257, 262, 283

scabies, lviii

scalping, past tribal practices, 64

scarlet fever, 118

Schindlebower, Moses, 101, 102, 287, 314

Schlinger, Brother, 19

schools and education: bia schools, xx; church schools, xx; classes for handicapped, 194; complaints about poor student behaviors, 256–57, 258–59; Day School Number 4, 218, 295; Day School Number 5, liv, 28, 243, 257; Day School Number 6, 295; disease and absenteeism, lvi; Grass Creek Day School, liv; herds of horses, 205, 217, 254; historic repression of Native life ways, xx; Holy Rosary Mission,

29, 137, 140, 148, 233, 305, 308, 322; Indian folklore taught, 125; Lone Man Day School, liv; medical care of Indian children, xxv; off-reservation boarding schools, xxvii, xxviii, xxxix; Oglala Boarding School, xxxiv, xxxvii; Oglala Community School, 23–24, 27, 55, 80; operating expenses, 161; reservation boarding schools, xxii, 33; school physicals, 23–24, 33, 276, 277, 291; seasonal work by students, 33–34, 288–89, 303; state funding per pupil, 67, 336n1; student athletics, 27; supplies for boarding schools, 27, 73; teachers as unofficial nurses, lv–lvii

Scott, Dick, 223, 228

Scott, Ella, 223, 224

scrofula, xl–xli

Searles, Mamie, 88

shamans, xxx

Shaw, James R., lx

Shaw, Mr., 139, 142, 295

Shelby, Dr., 30

Sheppard, Stanley L., 45, 95–96

Sherman, Mr., 214

Shield, Grace, 116

Shield, Hazel, 119, 269, 271, 272, 312

shootings, 49, 91–92, 136, 170, 215

Simms, Mary E., 250–51, 259, 322

Sioux Sanitarium: deaths, 172; opening of, liv; patients signing out against medical advice, 53, 141, 175, 193, 224, 305, 313–14; spirits reporting on patients, 270; staffing of, 86, 197, 209, 231, 238, 250; transporting patients to, 253, 302

Sioux Uprising, 118

Sitting Bull, 27, 28, 31, 40, 214

Sitting Hawk, Joe, 323

Sitting Hawk, Levi, 176, 181, 182, 190, 196, 217, 219

Sitting Holy, Russell, 253

skull fracture, 161

skunks, 313

Small, Daniel, 232

smallpox, xxi

Smith, Gerald K., 68

Smith, Lynn, 136

Smoke, Lena, 253

smoking, 325

snakes, 43

Snyder Act, xxviii

Soil and Moisture Conservation, 36

South Dakota, lxxiii; Allen, xix, liii, lxxiv, 57, 76; Badlands, xxi, 22, 38, 52, 157, 172, 221, 224; Black Hills, li, 20–21, 49, 54–55, 105, 140, 150, 206, 296–97; Chamberlain, 232; Cheyenne Creek, 49; Crazy Horse monument, 150–51; Custer, 47, 150; Custer State Park, 212, 213; Deadwood, 206; Denby, 180; Department of Crippled Children, 300, 301; Department of Health, 39, 40; Hill City, 150; Hot Springs, xviii, 91, 135, 136, 194; Kadoka, 224; Lakeview, lxxiv; Manderson, xlviii, liii, lxxiv, 51, 57, 70; Martin, lxxiv, 2, 67; Medicine Root, 15; Mission, lxxiv; Mobridge, 27, 28; Mount Rushmore, 20–21, 125, 150; Oglala, liii, lxxiv, 28; Parmalee, lxxiv; Passion Play, 21; Pierre, lxxiii; Pine Ridge, 69, 112–1; Porcupine, xix, liii, lxxiv, 15, 33, 57, 71–72, 74, 101–4; Sisseton, 210; Smithwick, 309; Spearfish, 21, 206; tourism, 105, 125; Vetal, lxxiv; Veterans Administration Hospitals in, 91, 102, 136, 173, 179, 303; Wounded Knee, xxxi, lxxiv, 15, 22, 25, 77; Yankton State Hospital, 298, 299; Yellow Bear, xix. See also Aberdeen; Pine Ridge Indian Reservation; Rapid City; Rosebud Indian Reservation

Southerton, Don, xliii

Speaking of Indians (Deloria), 229

Spider, Melvin, 277

Spider, Serena, 277

spiders, 50

spinal fluid leak, 256

spine, ruptured disc, 142

spleen, ruptured, 315

Spotted Tail, 51, 232

sprains, 198–99

"squaw coolers," 220, 341n1

stabbings, 55–56

staffs, ceremonial, 188, 235

Standing Bear, xiv, 51

Standing Bear, Henry, 47–48, 141, 151, 207, 241

Standing Rock Reservation, 27, 28, 31, 62, 251

Standing Soldier, Andrew, 62, 123–24, 127–28, 138, 141, 212

Stands, Homer, 224

Stands, Samuel, 26

Stands Up, Peter, 269–70, 272

Steed, Jess, 161

Stevenson, Robert Louis, 101

Stiff Tail, 169

Stoldt, Butch, 155, 278, 279, 303

Stomley, Vera, 310, 311

strangulated hernia, 280

stroke, 43, 47, 219

substance abuse, lxx

Sun Dance: Dr. Ruby's observations of, 240–42, 245, 323; participants of, 235, 240–42, 245, 293; as personal vow, 220, 246; public practice of, xx, 209, 237; sacred pole of, 239; sweat baths and, 245; traditional, 46–47

Swallow, Charles, 205

sweat baths, 54, 113–15, 240, 241, 264, 265, 272, 339n5

sweet grass, 130, 266, 267

Swift Bird, George, 177–78, 255

Swift Bird, Joe, 127, 133–34, 169, 182, 207, 308

Swift Bird, Mr., 67

Talcott, Margaret, 87, 88, 173

talipes equinavarus, 300, 301

tattoos, 13, 271

Teton Sioux, 125

Theise, Mrs., 304

Theisz, Miss, 213

Thompson, J. Ashley, xxx–xxxi

thyroid disease, 38

thyroid surgery, 254, 261

Time, 27

toads, 237

tobacco: in peyote meetings, 183, *184*, 185, 188, 189, 234, 236; in Yuwipi ceremonies, 43, 59, 113, 120, 265, 267

Tomahawk (1951), 214

tomahawks, 138

tonsils and adenoids, liii, 312, 332–33n78

Tracey, John, 213, 214

trachoma, liii, lv, lvi, 332–33n78

travois, 62

Trennert, Robert A., xxiii

tuberculosis: compliance with treatment, 39–40, 53, 133, 141, 174–75, 192, 193, 199, 224–25, 305, 314; forms of, xxxviii, xl–xli, 22; nutrition and, xxxviii–xxxix, lii, lviii; open-air treatment for, xliii, xlvi; as primary cause of Oglala deaths, xxxvii–xxxviii, xl–xli, lviii; sanatoriums, l, lviii, 40; school infirmaries treating, xxviii; scrofula, xl–xli; smoking and, xxxviii; virulence of, xxxviii, xl–xli

Turkey, Oliver, 231

Turtle Mountain Reservation, 312

Two Bulls, Matthew, 214–15

Two Bulls, Moses, 77, 89, 106, 129, 154, 158, 259

Two Bulls, Stern, 66

Two Dogs, Mrs., 279

Two Tails, 188

Tylee, Harry, 245

typhoid, xl

Umatilla Indians, 164, 339n1

Under Baggage, Charles, 26

Under Baggage, Nancy, 224

Under Baggage, William, 213

United States: Agricultural Extension agencies, 26; assimilation of Indians, xv, xxii; Commissioner of Indian Affairs, xxii, xxiii; Department of Health, Education, and Welfare, xxix, 71, 94, 124, 199, 215, 225, 247, 255; Department of the Interior, xxviii, 1, 26, 68; Doctor-Dentist Draft Law, xvii; Federal Bureau of Investigation (FBI), 135, 136; Great Depression, liv; Health and Human Services, xxix; Indian health care system, xxi–xxii, xxv; Indian New Deal, xv, xxviii–xxix; Indians as citizens, 34; Public Law 67–85, xxviii; Public Law 568 (HR 303), 215; Sanitary Commission, xlii; Snyder Act, xxviii; Termination and Withdrawal policies, xv, 31, 34, 36–37, 83, 193; Wheeler-

Howard Act, 65, 106. *See also* Bureau of Indian Affairs (BIA); Indian Health Service; Public Health Service. *See also specific reservation*
United States Army, Criminal Investigation Command (CID), 196
Universal Studios, 215
Unsigned, Linda, 275
uterus, ruptured, 143–44

vaccinations, liii
vein ligation, 32
venereal disease, 284–85, 303, 320
vision and glasses, 44–45, 53, 71, 162, 168, 252, 263

Walker, James R.: appearance of undermining medicine men, xlii–xliii; measures against TB, xlii–xliv; as reservation physician, xl–xlv
Walker, Mr., 96
Walker, Stanley, 20, 128
Walking, Felix, 29, 40, 148, 159, 160, 169, 176, 273
Walter, Joseph: assessing calls for ambulances, 167; health lectures and speeches, 155; living quarters in Pine Ridge, 4, 6, 7, 96, 216, 238; making snowy house calls, 142; maternity and gynecology cases handled by, 101, 124, 261; observing a Sun Dance, 220; one week duty at Rosebud, 227; as Pine Ridge Hospital physician, 2, 30, 67, 304; temporary duty in Cheyenne, 263, 276, 291
Walter, Mrs., 101
Wanblee SD: Public Health nurse in, 147–48, 205, 209, 210, 215, 227; reservation community of, xix, lxxiv, 57, 67
Wanek, Dr., 196
Wankan Tanka, 185, 189, 121
Wanna, Miss, 88
Warwick, Robert, 214, 340n3
Washington: Chelan, lxxii; Mabton, lxxi, lxxii, 8; Puyallup Reservation, xlii; Yakama Indian Reservation, xvi

Wasicu, 123, 132, 244
wasna, 176, 257
water bird, 159–60
Wayne, Miss Walborg: as acting Area medical director, 29, 89, 192, 195, 305, 310; finding lost hospital items, 30; handling Congressional inquiries, 90; monitoring nursing issues, 42, 84, 87, 197, 250; placing Public Health nurses, 204, 208–9, 210; staffing reservation hospitals, 196, 211, 218, 252
Weasel Bear, 267, 268, 269, 270
Wells, interpreter, 49
West, Mrs., 26
West, W. E., 82, 196, 250
Weston, C. B., 232
Weston, Reverend, 101
Wheeler-Howard Act, 65, 106
Whirlwind Horse, Mrs., 277
whistles, 183, 189, 235, 240, 245
White, Julie, 117
White Bull, Mr., 104
White Clay NE, xv, lxxiv, 15, 258
White Coyote, *112–7*
White Indian Soldier, 52
White Man, 245
white owls, 63
White Whirlwind, 113, 114, 115, 116
White Whirlwind, Leroy, 323
White Wolf, 233, 235
White Wolf, Calvin, 245, 246
whooping cough, l
Wilkinson, Charles, xix, xx, xxi; *Blood Struggles*, xix
Wilson, Frank, 89, 92, 106
Wilson, Jim, 106
Wilson, Mrs., 96
Winnebago Indians, 234, 236
Wisconsin, Green Bay Agency, xxxv
witch doctor, 106
Woman Dress family, 242
Woodworth-Ney, Laura, lv, lvi
Wounded, Narcisse, 267, 268, 269, 271, 272
Wounded, Willie, 161, 197, 218–19, 224, 267, 272

Wounded Knee, Battle of, xxxi, 25, 33, 124, 127, 141–42, 145, 212, 221, 222

The Wounded Knee Massacre (MacGregor), 141

Wyoming: Cheyenne River Agency, 7, 87; Red Cloud Agency, xxix

Yankton Sioux, 125

Yellow Boy, Charlie, 112–5; with Buffalo Bill Cody Show, 60, 118; complaining to Ben Reifel, 256; as drummer, 242; healing meeting for, 317; hospitalization of, 133; medicine for, 242, 301; naming Dr. Ruby's daughter and sister, 157, 218; stories told by, 167–68; as visitor at Ruby home, 155; Yuwipi meeting at home of, 119–20

Yellow Boy, Mrs., 119

Yellow Boy, Silas, 118, 119, 120, 121, 123, 196, 197

Yellowstone National Park, 2, 73

Yohe, Dr., 299

Young, Sid, 278, 307, 308

Young Bull Bear, Mrs. Dan, 161

Yuwipi: ceremonies of, 60, 110–11, 264–68, 268, 269–73; contacting spirits of deceased, 48; licensed medicine men for, 73; members of, 197; purifying with sweet grass, 130; "rosaries" used in, 59, 113, 120–21, 122, 123, 270; singing in, 121, 122; summoning medicine men for, 42–43; sweat baths and, 58–59; traditional practices of, 126

Zephier, Alvin, 57, 61, 202, 203

Ziolkowski, Korczak, 151, 339n4

Zumwalt, A. John, 259

Zumwalt, Dr., 195

9 780803 226258